Early Detection and Intervention in Psychosis

Key Issues in Mental Health

Vol. 181

Series Editors

Anita Riecher-Rössler Basel
Norman Sartorius Geneva

Early Detection and Intervention in Psychosis

State of the Art and Future Perspectives

Volume Editors

Anita Riecher-Rössler Basel
Patrick D. McGorry Parkville, Vic.

16 figures, 10 in color, and 11 tables, 2016

KARGER Basel · Freiburg · Paris · London · New York · Chennai · New Delhi · Bangkok · Beijing · Shanghai · Tokyo · Kuala Lumpur · Singapore · Sydney

Key Issues in Mental Health
Formerly published as 'Bibliotheca Psychiatrica' (founded 1917)

Prof. Anita Riecher-Rössler
Center for Gender Research and Early Detection
University of Basel Psychiatric Clinics
CH–4051 Basel (Switzerland)

Prof. Patrick D. McGorry
Orygen, the National Centre for Excellence in
Youth Mental Health, University of Melbourne
Parkville, VIC 3052 (Australia)

Library of Congress Cataloging-in-Publication Data

Names: Riecher-Rössler, Anita, editor. | McGorry, Patrick D., editor.
Title: Early detection and intervention in psychosis : state of the art and
    future perspectives / volume editors, Anita Riecher-Rössler, Patrick D.
    McGorry.
Other titles: Key issues in mental health ; v. 181. 1662-4874
Description: Basel ; New York : Karger, 2016. | Series: Key issues in mental
    health, ISSN 1662-4874 ; vol. 181 | Includes bibliographical references
    and indexes.
Identifiers: LCCN 2015039541| ISBN 9783318056204 (hard cover : alk. paper) |
    ISBN 9783318056211 (electronic version : alk. paper)
Subjects: | MESH: Psychotic Disorders--diagnosis. | Early Diagnosis. | Early
    Medical Intervention.
Classification: LCC RC473.D54 | NLM WM 200 | DDC 616.89/075--dc23 LC record available at
http://lccn.loc.gov/2015039541

Bibliographic Indices. This publication is listed in bibliographic services, including Current Contents® and MEDLINE/Pubmed.

Disclaimer. The statements, opinions and data contained in this publication are solely those of the individual authors and contributors and not of the publisher and the editor(s). The appearance of advertisements in the book is not a warranty, endorsement, or approval of the products or services advertised or of their effectiveness, quality or safety. The publisher and the editor(s) disclaim responsibility for any injury to persons or property resulting from any ideas, methods, instructions or products referred to in the content or advertisements.

Drug Dosage. The authors and the publisher have exerted every effort to ensure that drug selection and dosage set forth in this text are in accord with current recommendations and practice at the time of publication. However, in view of ongoing research, changes in government regulations, and the constant flow of information relating to drug therapy and drug reactions, the reader is urged to check the package insert for each drug for any change in indications and dosage and for added warnings and precautions. This is particularly important when the recommended agent is a new and/or infrequently employed drug.

© Copyright 2016 by S. Karger AG, P.O. Box, CH–4009 Basel (Switzerland)
www.karger.com
Printed in Germany on acid-free and non-aging paper (ISO 9706) by Kraft Druck GmbH, Ettlingen
ISSN 1662–4874
eISSN 1662–4882
ISBN 978–3–318–05620–4
e-ISBN 978–3–318–05621–1

Contents

Foreword

The Near Future

The care and study of persons with psychotic illness has a rich history. The acquisition of knowledge has accelerated, and application with life-altering potential for patients is now established in expert centers and ready for broader application in health care systems. Material in this book details the relevant advances in knowledge and understanding and enables the reader to view the near future with optimism. Presented in this Foreword is a brief outline of how the field has arrived at this point. Knowledge developed in the context of schizophrenia is critical, but so is the extension across disorders associated with psychosis or psychotic-like experiences. The reader will gain an appreciation of rapidly changing concepts in mental illness research and the implications for clinical application.

Kraepelin defined two fundamental psychotic disorders, dementia praecox and manic-depressive illness, providing a profound conceptual framework still influential in current classification, research, and clinical care. But the combination of 'weakening the well-springs of volition' with dissociative thought and a poor prognosis set the stage for 100 years of pessimism regarding clinical course. Bleuler's view of dissociative pathology as fundamental and primary in all cases reinforced the disease entity concept even while the 'group of disorders' seemed to suggest a syndrome. Decades later, Schneider's symptoms of first rank suggested that true schizophrenia was identified with special forms of reality distortion. This emphasis did not deny the importance of what we now term negative symptoms and disorganized thought and behavior, nor did it change presumptions regarding poor prognosis. These concepts, combined with limited effectiveness of treatment and concern about stigma, resulted in emphasis on schizophrenia as a brain disease where antipsychotic medication for symptom control and relapse prevention was the central issue, and expectations were of a chronic course for most patients.

A very different picture emerges from careful consideration of the actual data available for over a half century. First, schizophrenia has never been validated as a disease entity. The diagnostic class is a heterogeneous clinical syndrome. With various pathophysiologies, substantial individual variation is expected. This was shown to be the case with onset, manifestations, and course data in long-term studies including Manfred Bleuler's 40-year follow-up of his father's patients. More recent studies have shown that not all patients have a poor developmental history and many do not have a chronic course. Despite psychotic symptoms being unifying at the level of diagnostic criteria, the nature of the psychotic experience and associated features have also varied between cases. In short, there is a profound heterogeneity that is not addressed in public or clinical concepts of schizophrenia, nor is it addressed in treatment guidelines or therapeutic discovery.

If the above snapshot generally captures our history (and, of course, there are many exceptions), it is about to change. This change is driven by a combination of new concepts and accumulated knowledge of early morbid/prodromal pathologies in the schizophrenia spectrum.

The following concepts are relevant to the care of persons with a psychotic illness: clinical syndromes are not adequately informative about individual patients, clinical targets for treatment go well beyond psychotic symptoms, recovery as a personal process and recovery as a goal of medical treatment, stress reduction, emphasis on the individual's resilience and support network, and reduction in adverse factors such as substance abuse. These and other issues related to understanding the individual patient provide a basis of personalized and integrated therapeutics. These concepts are not new, but what has changed the landscape is a body of work focused on detecting clinical high risk in persons before full psychosis. It is the personalized application of these therapeutic concepts at the earliest point in a psychosis and moving clinical intervention to a prepsychosis phase of illness that will enable young people vulnerable to psychosis to gain a better future.

Much is known about early morbid features such as impaired cognition, declining social engagement, negative symptoms, aggressive and inappropriate behaviors, deteriorating role performance, and the experience of psychotic-like phenomena. These manifestations of psychopathology were traditionally viewed as prognostic factors or the developmental pathway to schizophrenia. The paradigm shift involves viewing this early phase as defining the need for clinical care with the goal of secondary prevention of psychosis. Throughout medicine, early detection and intervention is time honored as an approach to reducing morbidity/mortality. Clinical scientists such as this book's editors and its contributors have produced an astounding growth in knowledge over the past quarter century that includes identifying at-risk individuals, organizing model programs for clinical care, validating the clinical high-risk construct with the full range of methods used to study established illness including electrophysiology, neuroimaging of structure, function and biochemistry, phenotypic information, associated negative symptoms, impaired cognition, and more. In addition to reliable and valid methods for identifying cases of clinical high risk, the initial random assignment controlled clinical trials support efficacy for symptom reduction, secondary prevention of full psychosis, and perhaps improved function. This is accomplished with minimum-risk therapeutics reserving risk/

benefit decisions for antipsychotic medications to a stage where full psychosis is emerging.

Specialized clinical care programs are growing internationally at a rapid rate. Model programs creating friendly clinical environments for young people and staging treatment according to what is wrong and where in the pathway to psychosis the individual fits provides a common-sense approach, but one that is challenging in traditional clinical care systems.

I think our field can make the future for persons who may be on a path to psychotic illness substantially better. To date we have no therapeutic approach that cures the pathology once established. We know that early intervention in the first psychotic episode is better for the person and for society. There are proven advantages to reducing the duration of untreated psychosis. Identifying and providing care for clinical high-risk individuals may benefit each person with the psychopathology already present and, for those who are on the path to full psychosis, may delay or prevent a first episode. If psychosis emerges, institution of treatment specific for psychosis will be immediate rather than the usual delay of months or years.

We do not yet know if intervention in the prepsychotic phase will alter the long-term pathophysiology. If so, this will be an unparalleled accomplishment. But if not, clinical intervention may enable the person to be successful with life milestones that are essential to future well-being such as successful education, being employed, having a love relationship, and supportive social network.

The field does not yet have the knowledge base to launch large-scale public health initiatives at primary prevention. But the knowledge base reviewed in this book provides the basis for an aggressive shift in the timing and nature of clinical care for persons who merit clinical attention and may be vulnerable to a psychotic disorder.

William T. Carpenter, Baltimore, Md.

Preface and Introduction

"I was extremely scared when the symptoms occurred for the first time. From one moment to the next, everything changed massively. That was extremely bizarre and scary at the time – this change in perception. At that time, the fear was predominant. What can I do about it? Why did this happen now and as suddenly? I consulted my family doctor a couple of times hoping to be referred to psychiatric services. But from what I felt, he thought that I just did not feel like going to work and wanted a sick note. He then put me on sick leave for a couple of days each time. After moving, I saw an advertisement of a psychiatric emergency service in the tram. I called and got an appointment for the next day. From there I got referred to the early intervention service very quickly – and finally, I felt that I was being taken seriously for the first time. I was really seeking help before. There was something seriously wrong with me and I had not been taken seriously. I felt desperate.

Prior to my first appointment at the early detection clinic, I was insecure. What is next? What will happen to me there? But to not do anything would not have been the solution either, and my symptoms were very severe at the time. That's why I said to myself: 'I need to seek help now! I do not want to continue like this!' You go to the hospital too when you break an arm or a leg, and in my case something else was broken. After my first appointment at the early detection clinic, I felt seen for the first time and at last taken seriously, which I was very glad about.

When I was informed that I had a risk of developing psychosis and received information about the possible outcomes and about psychosis and schizophrenia in general, I could finally evaluate myself again. Up to the time I received this information, there had always been a certain insecurity that felt like an empty space in which I didn't know where I stood. I knew a lot from my education as a health care worker, but I had not been able to integrate the information properly. To know what was happening to me was a great relief. It took a lot of the fear away. Afterwards, my energy increased, I took back control over my life, I cleaned up my apartment and dedicated myself to my hobbies again. I thought that since I had completed my education and performed well so far despite my symptoms, I would not let myself down now! I knew chronically ill patients with schizophrenia from work and I could see the difference between them and myself, standing with both feet on the ground – despite the insecurity and everything that I had been through! Some insecurity stayed – I knew that I could possibly slide down into schizophrenia. But then I thought that the probability was not that high, and that, if the symptoms stayed as they were I could live with them quite fine. Step by step, with successive appointments at the early detection clinic, I found explanations and answers for the changes I perceived. Then, I slowly managed to cope with them. From the initial exhausting additional burden of the symptoms on top of my everyday stress, they became with time something that I perceived as less and less scary and in the end as interesting, even. I perceived the support I received from the early detection center as friendly, enjoyable and obliging – exactly what I had so often needed. While I was dealing with what had happened to me, someone was standing behind me the whole time. Someone neutral, who I could call if something happened. That support in the background helped me a lot in my search for answers. I am a lot better now compared to how I was half

a year ago when I first came to the early detection clinic. I still suffer from certain problems, but I can cope quite well. After long days, I get tired faster than before, but I can live with that. I was really glad for the support I got and would like to express a great thank you for it!"
Patient of the FePsy Early Detection Clinic, Basel, Switzerland

Psychiatry during the last decades has achieved enormous progress. One of the major steps certainly was the overdue recognition of the concept of early detection and intervention as in other medical disciplines.

Interest first arose in the field of schizophrenia research. In these disorders, it had been described for some decades that they do not arise all of a sudden but, in most cases, very slowly with early subthreshold features. Kraepelin and Bleuler both described this pattern of onset, but the first to focus on it specifically was Harry Stack Sullivan [1] in 1927. Later, German authors recognized the so-called 'Vorposten' (outpost syndromes) and prodromal symptoms as well as a new concept of basic symptoms [2, 3]. Influenced by these early descriptive clinical studies, Häfner et al. [4] developed a semistructured interview to assess the prodromal phase of schizophrenia, the IRAOS. In 1986, they started a first representative study in a population of 232 first-admitted psychosis patients in and around Mannheim, Germany, and found that in 73% of all patients the disorder had begun with a prodromal phase which lasted on average for 5 years [5, 6]. An emerging research focus on first-episode patients through the 1980s (Crow, Kane, Lieberman) helped to show that treatment delay was substantial even for clear-cut first-episode psychosis [7, 8].

Clinical services based on early intervention principles began to develop in the 1990s, beginning with the EPPIC program in 1992, which not only aimed to reduce the duration of untreated psychosis, but also to engage and treat prodromal patients and to ensure that all early psychosis patients had the best chance of recovery in the early 'critical' period after diagnosis. In 1994, McGorry, Yung and colleagues [9, 10] established the PACE Clinic as part of EPPIC, the first clinical and research program for potentially prodromal individuals in Australia. They began to investigate the predictive validity of prospectively defined risk criteria, developing the ultra-high-risk (UHR) criteria and the first psychometric instrument [11]. Similar services and instruments were later developed in the United States, e.g. by Miller et al. [12] and in Switzerland by Riecher-Rössler and colleagues [13–15].

In Germany, Klosterkötter et al. [16] have especially pursued the predictive power of basic symptoms as very early risk indicators. Other major contributions to the field have come from the United Kingdom and Scandinavia, and similar clinical services for early detection and intervention have been established worldwide, often accompanied by research projects. So far, it has been shown quite clearly that (1) the disease, even in these very early stages, can – if untreated – have very severe consequences for the patient, (2) early detection of the disease, even in its prodromal phase, is possible, and (3) early treatment not only ameliorates presenting symptoms, but also improves illness course and psychosocial outcome [for reviews, see 17–24].

However, despite significant advances in the field, early detection of psychosis still faces some problems and obstacles. Thus, the accuracy of identifying those at risk for psychosis could certainly be improved. Existing risk-prediction approaches have achieved only modest predictive accuracy with 3-year transition rates of 30–43% of those originally identified as being 'at risk' [19]. These have even been falling in recent times. This means that many 'false positives' are identified who will in fact not develop frank psychosis. It was argued by critics that these individuals are not only exposed to the unnecessary stress of being confronted with such a diagnosis and the potential stigma associated with it, but potentially also to unnecessary treatment [18].

On the other hand, we now know that even the patients without later transition to psychosis often suffer from severe symptoms and functional impairment, are seeking help and treatment, and have a longer-term need for care [25–27]. It was suggested that the stigma associated with being identified as having a risk for psychosis was more related to the behavior associated with the illness rather than the diagnosis. Educating patients and clinicians and providing care in stigma-free settings might actually reduce stigma and unnecessary treatment [25]. In any case, it would be of utmost importance to improve the accuracy of the risk assessment. This should involve a 'staging' of the emerging disease and profiling of the patients, which would allow interventions tailored to the respective stage and personalized for the individual patient.

At the same time, there is a clear need for better evidence regarding therapeutic approaches in the different stages, which has prompted several questions. How shall we treat patients with suspected early prodromal symptoms and low risk, and how should we treat those with subthreshold psychotic symptoms and high risk? How should we treat patients with predominantly negative symptoms or cognitive deficits? An initial wave of intervention trials have indicated that certain psychological, pharmacological and other intervention strategies may be of value in terms of symptom reduction and delay or prevention of transition to frank psychosis. However, clear guidelines for clinicians as to which treatment to offer to which patient with which symptoms and impairments and in which sequence have not yet been established. This volume will give the reader a state-of-the-art overview on the current knowledge, developments, questions and discussions in the area of early detection and intervention for psychosis. It will also provide perspectives on how to improve early detection as well as early intervention.

In this context, the reader will learn how to recognize the very first signs of emerging psychosis. The significance and correlates of the high-risk state in adolescence and early adulthood will be outlined. Some debates and controversies will be captured, such as whether the 'high risk for a psychosis state' is really a valid entity, a question which stirred huge controversy when DSM-5 was being finalized [18]. Furthermore, the question of whether being informed about the risk for psychosis in fact is a negative, stigmatizing experience for patients – or rather a helpful one – will be considered.

Several authors will discuss in different chapters the possibilities to improve the accuracy of early detection by using different domains in addition to the clinical assessments such as neurocognition, fine motor functioning and neurophysiology. Also, structural and functional MRI, including the use of new methods such as pattern recognition methods or the analysis of connectivity abnormalities will be discussed regarding their values for improving the prediction of psychosis. Finally, different methods for early intervention will be presented – psychological methods as well as other nonpharmacological interventions including potentially neuroprotective substances for early intervention in the at-risk mental state, as well as pharmacological, psychosocial and other interventions in first-episode psychosis.

This volume will hopefully stimulate clinicians as well as researchers to further develop the field, which, in our opinion, is one of the most promising areas of current psychiatry. If performed correctly and wisely, early detection and intervention should extend to a transdiagnostic focus and could prevent enormous suffering in patients and their families.

This early intervention focus and spreading the concept of staging and stepwise intervention across the current diagnostic silos may well help to modernize psychiatry to become a 21st-century medical discipline with a truly preventative approach, and in the process further reduce the stigma that still holds the field back. Last but not least, intensive research in this relatively new field of emerging illness will hopefully contribute to a better understanding of the pathogenetic mechanisms leading to psychosis.

Anita Riecher-Rössler, Basel, Switzerland
Patrick D. McGorry, Parkville, Vic., Australia

References

1 Sullivan HS: Affective experience in early schizophrenia. Am J Psychiatry 1927;83:467–483.

2 Mayer-Gross W: Die Klinik der Schizophrenie; in Bunke O (ed): Handbuch der Geisteskrankheiten. Berlin, Germany, Springer, 1932, IX.

3 Huber G, Gross G: The concept of basic symptoms in schizophrenic and schizoaffective psychoses. Recenti Prog Med 1989;80:646–652.

4 Häfner H, Riecher-Rössler A, Hambrecht M, Maurer K, Meissner S, Schmidtke A, Fätkenheuer B, Löffler W, van der Heiden W: IRAOS: an instrument for the assessment of the onset and early course of schizophrenia. Schizophr Res 1992;6: 209–223.

5 Häfner H, Maurer K, Löffler W, an der Heiden W, Munk-Jørgensen P, Hambrecht M, Riecher-Rössler A: The ABC Schizophrenia Study: a preliminary overview of the results. Soc Psychiatry Psychiatr Epidemiol 1998;33:380–386.

6 Häfner H, Maurer K, Löffler W, Riecher-Rössler A: The influence of age and sex on the onset and early course of schizophrenia. Br J Psychiatry 1993;162: 80–86.

7 Wyatt RJ: Early intervention with neuroleptics may decrease the long-term morbidity of schizophrenia. Schizophr Res 1991;5:201–202.

8 Loebel AD, Alvir JMJ, Mayerhoff DI, Geisler SH, Szymanski SR: Duration of psychosis and outcome in first-episode schizophrenia. Am J Psychiatry 1992;149:1183–1188.

9 Yung AR, McGorry PD, McFarlane CA, Jackson HJ, Patton GC, Rakkar A: Monitoring and care of young people at incipient risk of psychosis. Schizophr Bull 1996;22:283–303.

10 McGorry PD, Edwards J, Mihalopoulos C, Harrigan SM, Jackson HJ: EPPIC: an evolving system of early detection and optimal management. Schizophr Bull 1996;22:305–326.

11 Yung AR, McGorry PD: The prodromal phase of first-episode psychosis: past and current conceptualizations. Schizophr Bull 1996;22:353–370.

12 Miller TJ, McGlashan TH, Woods SW, Stein K, Driesen N, Corcoran CM, Hoffman R, Davidson L: Symptom assessment in schizophrenic prodromal states. Psychiatr Q 1999;70:273–287.

13 Riecher-Rössler A: Die beginnende Schizophrenie als 'Knick in der Lebenslinie' [Emerging Schizophrenia as 'kink in the lifeline']; in Schneider H (ed): Lieben und Arbeiten – Der junge Erwachsene und der Ernst des Lebens. Schriftenreihe des Psychotherapie-Seminars Freudenstadt. Heidelberg, Mattes, 1999, pp 23–40.

14 Riecher-Rössler A, Gschwandtner U, Aston J, Borgwardt S, Drewe M, Fuhr P, Pflüger M, Radü W, Schindler C, Stieglitz RD: The Basel early-detection-of-psychosis (FEPSY)-study – design and preliminary results. Acta Psychiatr Scand 2007;115: 114–125.

15 Riecher-Rössler A, Aston J, Ventura J, Merlo M, Borgwardt S, Gschwandtner U, Stieglitz RD: Das Basel Screening Instrument für Psychosen (BSIP): Entwicklung, Aufbau, Reliabilität und Validität. [The Basel Screening Instrument for Psychosis (BSIP): Development, Structure, Reliability and Validity]. Fortschritte der Neurologie und Psychiatrie 2008;76:207–216.

16 Klosterkötter J, Hellmich M, Steinmeyer EM, Schultze-Lutter F: Diagnosing schizophrenia in the initial prodromal phase. Arch Gen Psychiatry 2001; 58:158–164.

17 Riecher-Rössler A, Gschwandtner U, Borgwardt S, Aston J, Pflüger M, Rössler W: Early detection and treatment of schizophrenia: how early? Acta Psychiatr Scand Suppl, 2006, pp 73–80.

18 Tsuang MT, Van Os J, Tandon R, Barch DM, Bustillo J, Gaebel W, Gur RE, Heckers S, Malaspina D, Owen MJ, Schultz S, Carpenter W: Attenuated psychosis syndrome in DSM-5. Schizophr Res 2013; 150:31–35.

19 Fusar-Poli P, Borgwardt S, Bechdolf A, Addington J, Riecher-Rössler A, Schultze-Lutter F, Keshavan M, Wood S, Ruhrmann S, Seidman LJ, Valmaggia L, Cannon T, Velthorst E, De Haan L, Cornblatt B, Bonoldi I, Birchwood M, McGlashan T, Carpenter W, McGorry P, Klosterkötter J, McGuire P, Yung A: The psychosis high-risk state: a comprehensive state-of-the-art review. JAMA Psychiatry 2013;70: 107–120.

20 McGorry PD, Nelson B, Amminger GP, Bechdolf A, Francey SM, Berger G, Riecher-Rössler A, Klosterkötter J, Ruhrmann S, Schultze-Lutter F, Nordentoft M, Hickie I, McGuire P, Berk M, Chen EY, Keshavan MS, Yung AR: Intervention in individuals at ultra-high risk for psychosis: a review and future directions. J Clin Psychiatry 2009;70:1206–1212.

21 van der Gaag M, Smit F, Bechdolf A, French P, Linszen DH, Yung AR, McGorry P, Cuijpers P: Preventing a first episode of psychosis: meta-analysis of randomized controlled prevention trials of 12 months and longer-term follow-ups. Schizophr Res 2013;149:56–62.

22 Schultze-Lutter F, Michel C, Schmidt SJ, Schimmelmann BG, Maric NP, Salokangas RK, Riecher-Rössler A, van der Gaag M, Nordentoft M, Raballo A, Meneghelli A, Marshall M, Morrison A, Ruhrmann S, Klosterkötter J: EPA guidance on the early detection of clinical high risk states of psychoses. Eur Psychiatry 2015;30:405–416.

23 Schmidt SJ, Schultze-Lutter F, Schimmelmann BG, Maric NP, Salokangas RKR, Riecher-Rössler A, van der Gaag M, Meneghelli A, Nordentoft M, Marshall M, Morrison A, Raballo A, Klosterkötter J, Ruhrmann S: EPA guidance on the early intervention in clinical high risk states of psychoses. Eur Psychiatry 2015;30:388–404.

24 McGorry PD, Killackey E, Yung A: Early intervention in psychosis: concepts, evidence and future directions. World Psychiatry 2008;7:148–156.

25 Addington J, Cornblatt BA, Cadenhead KS, Cannon TD, McGlashan TH, Perkins DO, Seidman LJ, Tsuang MT, Walker EF, Woods SW, Heinssen R: At clinical high risk for psychosis: outcome for nonconverters. Am J Psychiatry 2011;168:800–805.

26 Riecher-Rössler A, Pflueger MO, Aston J, Borgwardt SJ, Brewer WJ, Gschwandtner U, Stieglitz RD: Efficacy of using cognitive status in predicting psychosis: a 7-year follow-up. Biol Psychiatry 2009; 66:1023–1030.

27 Lin A, Wood SJ, Nelson B, Beavan A, McGorry P, Yung AR: Outcomes of non-transitioned cases in a sample at ultra-high risk for psychosis. Am J Psychiatry 2015;172:249–258.

Riecher-Rössler A, McGorry PD (eds): Early Detection and Intervention in Psychosis: State of the Art and Future Perspectives. Key Issues Ment Health. Basel, Karger, 2016, vol 181, pp 1–14 (DOI: 10.1159/000440910)

Early Detection of Psychosis – State of the Art and Future Perspectives

Joachim Klosterkötter

Department of Psychiatry and Psychotherapy, University of Cologne, Cologne, Germany

Abstract

The worldwide established early detection and prevention centers for psychosis follow the modern approach of predictive, preventive and personalized medicine. If primary prevention is to succeed, the individual risk of the disease has to be estimated correctly and the psychosis onset has to be predicted accurately. Accordingly, this chapter provides an overview on the recent prediction analyses in clinical high risk for psychosis research. The previously identified high-risk criteria achieved considerable predictive power, which can further be enhanced by their combined use as well as other strategies of risk enrichment and risk stratification. Clinical prediction already allows risk-adapted prevention measures and is currently being enhanced even further by additional biological brain diagnostics.   © 2016 S. Karger AG, Basel

With the replacement of the traditional clinical paradigm by the modern molecular one, medicine has set off into new directions. 'Prediction', 'prevention' and 'personalization' are the programmatic keywords of this new approach. Like other medical disciplines, psychiatry has broadened its focus from diagnosis and treatment to the detection and estimation of the risk of disease development, the prediction of its onset, and strategies to avoid its manifestation [1].

Severe mental disorders such as psychoses and especially schizophrenia are suitable candidates for the application of this program. The lifetime prevalence of psychoses is estimated to be between 0.2 and 3.5%, and their annual incidence between 0.01 and 0.035%, with growing numbers reported in Europe where, within 12 months, approximately 3.7 million adults (0.8%) were affected in 2005 and as many as 5 million (1.2%) in 2011. Although treatment has greatly advanced over the last decades, a significant number of patients continue to take an unfavorable chronic course. Following psychotic episodes, negative symptoms are commonly present and are associated with cognitive impairments and psychosocial disabilities. This is the main reason why this relatively infrequent disorder is responsible for the sixth largest share of disability-adjusted life years (DALYs) in adults in Europe (i.e. 637,693 DALYs), and the third largest (16.8 million DALYs) of all main brain disorders worldwide. Thus, at EUR 93.9 billion for total direct health care, direct non-medical and indirect costs of brain disorders in Europe in 2010 attributed to psychoses, only the cost for mood disorders and dementia were higher. In addition, the burden caused by stigma and discrimination is also among the highest in psychosis [2].

First-episode psychosis (FEP) research has shown that the outbreak of the disease is preceded in about 70% to nearly 100% of cases by an initial prodrome, which lasts for an average of 5–6 years. Even in highly developed health care systems, an average of 1 year thereafter elapses from the first manifestation of psychotic positive symptoms to the initiation of adequate treatment. The period over which the FEP remains untreated (duration of untreated psychosis) correlates with delayed and incomplete remission of the symptoms; necessity of more protracted treatment and greater risk of relapse; lower compliance, greater burden on the family and a higher level of 'expressed emotion'; increased risk of depression and suicide; greater impact on the individual's employment or education; increased drug abuse and delinquent behavior, and markedly increased costs of treatment [3].

This not only provides strong arguments in favor of treating the FEP as early as possible, but has also led to a systematic effort to decrease the incidence of psychosis through primary prevention (fig. 1).

Early Detection of Risk

In principle, primary prevention can be offered universally to the general unselected population, selectively to healthy individuals with a known risk factor of the disease, or by indication to persons already suffering from first complaints and impairments and who are actively seeking advice and help. The universal and the selective approach cannot be implemented effectively – at least to date – due to the low incidence of psychosis in the general population and lack of sufficient etiological knowledge and of risk factors of sufficiently large effect [4].

Psychosis is increasingly considered as a complex brain development disorder with polygenetic heredity. Its pathogenesis seems to be greatly influenced by interactions between different genes and between genes and environment. Associations to variants of the genes for dysbindin and neuregulin-1, the genetic locus G72, and the DAOA (D-amino acid oxidase activator) gene, for example, have been repeatedly confirmed. As with other complex diseases, research is focusing now on characterizing the polygenetic factors and clarifying their variable phenotypic

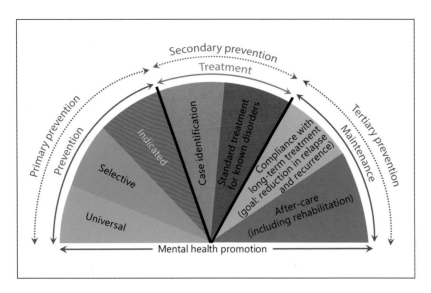

Fig. 1. Prevention of mental disorders according to Mrazek and Haggerty [4].

expression. Research methods range from molecular genetics via proteome research to cell biology, neurophysiology, brain structural and functional imaging, and neuropsychology. With all these methods, several indicators for an increased risk of psychosis have been identified. However, the currently recognized neurobiological risk factors are not sufficiently predictive to allow the development and application of 'selective' prevention measures targeting asymptomatic persons at risk. There are also established environmental risk factors for psychosis, such as exposure to viral agents in the second trimester of pregnancy, birth complications, childhood trauma, migration, the quality of the rearing environment, environment, socioeconomic disadvantage, urban birth, living in urban areas and using illicit drugs, particularly cannabis [5]. However, with odds ratios of around 2, each of these factors increases lifetime risk for psychosis only slightly, and causality can be difficult to determine. Thus, the currently known genetic and environmental risk factors, either alone or taken together, cannot be used for prediction and prevention (fig. 2).

Only longitudinal research including big cohorts followed up for many years, or better decennia, can eventually inform us about whether or when a certain constellation of risk factors might fuel progression into psychosis. Furthermore, this kind of research might help us in drawing conclusions about the adequacy and the most reasonable time point for either universal or selective preventive actions. It remains to be seen whether the currently promoted intensive elucidation of gene-environment interaction might shed a different light on this matter [6].

Today, it appears that comprising the initial prodromal phase into the risk assessment when studying psychosis has been especially helpful. Here, the initial impulse

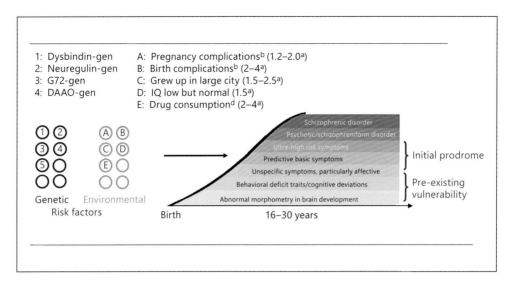

Fig. 2. Indicators for increased risk of schizophrenia. [a] Relative lifetime risk in the presence of a risk factor in percent (general population: 0.5–1.0%). [b] Infections or malnutrition of the mother during pregnancy (possible effect: neuronal migration disorder in the 2nd trimenon). [c] Especially birth weight, lack of oxygen. [d] Especially cannabis. [e] Average duration of 5 years.

came from centers that were specifically founded to focus on early recognition and prevention, as for example in Melbourne, Australia, the first center worldwide, and in Cologne, Germany, the first center in Europe. Many more centers at various sites have followed this example and now offer support and advice to individuals showing first complaints. In the course of this movement, it has been possible to extract risk symptoms with a high predictive power, which are able to narrow down the expected time frame for a psychotic breakout. These risk symptoms, in contrast to the risk factors characterizing the asymptomatic state of psychosis development, go hand in hand with distress, psychosocial impairment and reduced quality of life, which already make them candidates for treatment. This, however, allows the easy and methodologically solid monitoring of success of corresponding preventive actions. In turn, these preventive actions can then be more easily implemented into patient care in the form of indicated interventions. In addition, indicated preventive actions might be able to shorten the otherwise rather long scientific way to selective or eventually even universal preventive actions. At the same time, the approach offers the possibility to investigate the assumed risk mechanisms, indicated by genetic-epigenetic, neurobiological and environment-focused research, during the time frame preceding a psychotic breakout [1, 3].

However, only a minor part of the phenomena usually referred to as initial prodromal symptoms is of predictive value at all, and not even a well-suited sample progresses 100% to an FEP. Therefore, the traditional definition of a prodromal state has accordingly been replaced by the concept of a psychosis high-risk state (HRS) [7].

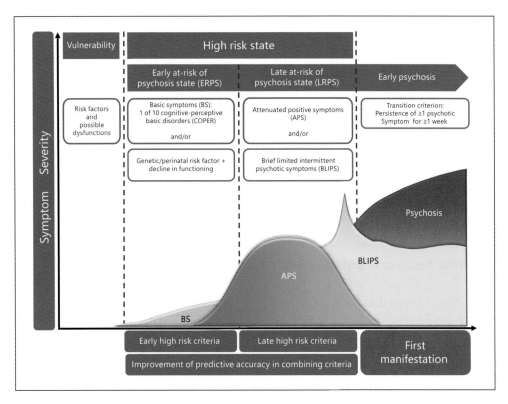

Fig. 3. Prediction of psychosis in an HRS (modified according to Fusar-Poli et al. [7]).

Psychosis High-Risk State

Two lines of scientific development have led to the characterization of a psychosis HRS, which lies between premorbid vulnerability and a full psychotic outbreak. The first emanated from the German Basic Symptom (BS) Research, which probably generated the most comprehensive and detailed description of alterations in psychological functioning during this time frame. These alterations are not only self-perceived but also described as a personal deficit by the affected individuals.

The second is of more pragmatic origin and initially aimed at making the DSM-III criteria for prodromal symptomatology and schizotypal disorders useful for early detection and intervention [8]. The differentiation between the resulting definitions of attenuated positive symptoms (APS) or brief limited intermittent psychotic symptoms (BLIPS) and delusional states, hallucinations or formal thought disorder is only gradual and quantitative. On the other hand, BS are explicitly distinguishable from positive psychotic symptoms on a qualitative and phenomenological base (fig. 3).

Support for the notion that BS reflect an earlier and more remote state of psychosis development, while APS and BLIPS characterize a more advanced state, came from subtle reconstructions of the initial time point and sequence of their occurrence [9]. Therefore, the current version of the HRS concept, emerging from these two lines of research, differentiates between an early at-risk of psychosis state (ERPS) and a late at-risk of psychosis state (LRPS). Here, the ERPS follows the long phase of premorbid vulnerability, which is presumably of prenatal origin, while the LRPS characterizes a state passing on to a first psychotic episode. Of course, the genetic, epigenetic, neurobiological and environmental risk factors, and early dysfunctions of the premorbid phase, which have been extracted in a multitude of both older and recent investigations, can also be classified as predictors. However, whether and in how far these predictors do justice to this appraisal in individuals at risk who are symptom-free cannot be evaluated at this time point due to the methodological reasons mentioned before [1].

Predictive Accuracy of Early High-Risk Symptoms

In contrast to this, the risk symptoms of the HRS and among them also the early BS can be included in systematic predictive analyses. The first predictive large-scale investigation of the Cologne Early Recognition (CER) project [10], which included 385 individuals with or without BS and no prior history of psychosis, was able to document a surprisingly high transition rate into first psychotic episodes. 160 of these individuals could be followed up over the whole study time frame of 10 years. 20% of them had developed a schizophrenic first manifestation after 12 months, and another 17 and 13% after 24 and 36 months, respectively. After approximately 4.5 years, 70% of the individuals in this vulnerable group had developed a schizophrenic dysfunction.

Transition rates as high as these and the presence of a control group consisting of help-seeking individuals with various complaints but without definite BS enabled a detailed predictive analysis on a syndrome and symptom level for the first time.

The actual predictive symptomatology was cognitively coined and characterized by 10 types of thought, language and perceptive disorders. They were observable in more than a quarter of the help-seeking individuals and had a positive predictive power of ≥70% and a minor false-positive predictive rate of ≤7.5%.

The results of further methodological analyses, as well as content analyses, comprising systematic examinations in another prospective predictive investigation on 146 persons at risk over a time frame of 24 months gave way to the formulation of the generally accepted high-risk criteria for ERPS of today (table 1).

Depending on the purpose of psychosis prediction, it is possible to choose between the more sensitive predictive accuracy of a cognitive-perceptive approach of risk criteria (COPER) and the more specific predictive one of a pure cognitive approach (COGDIS). Both have almost identical transition rates after 24 months (COPER 32.9%, COGDIS 33.1%).

Well-established instruments such as the Bonn Basic Symptom Scale (BSABS) and the Schizophrenia Proneness Instrument, available as both an adult version

Table 1. BS-based definitions of an at-risk mental state of psychosis and their predictive accuracy in the CER study

Criterion	Predictive accuracy[a]
COPER	
At least any 1 of the following 10 BS with an SPI-A/SPI-CY score of ≥3	sensitivity = 0.87
within the last 3 months *and* first occurrence ≥12 months ago:	specificity = 0.54
Thought interference	positive predictive value = 0.65
Thought perseveration	negative predictive value = 0.82
Thought pressure	positive likelihood ratio = 1.89
Thought blockages	negative likelihood ratio = 0.24
Disturbance of receptive speech	odds ratio = 7.86
Decreased ability to discriminate between ideas and	false positives = 23.1%
perception, fantasy and true memories	false negatives = 6.3%
Unstable ideas of reference	
Derealization	
Visual perception disturbances (excl. blurred vision and	
hypersensitivity to light)	
Acoustic perception disturbances (excl. hypersensitivity to	
sounds/noises)	
COGDIS	
At least any 2 of the following 9 BS with a SPI-A/SPI-CY score of	sensitivity = 0.67
≥3 within the last 3 months:	specificity = 0.83
Inability to divide attention	positive predictive value = 0.79
Thought interference	negative predictive value = 0.72
Thought pressure	positive likelihood ratio = 3.94
Thought blockages	negative likelihood ratio = 0.40
Disturbance of receptive speech	odds ratio = 9.91
Disturbance of expressive speech	false positives = 8.8%
Unstable ideas of reference	false negatives = 16.3%
Disturbances of abstract thinking	
Captivation of attention by details of the visual field	

[a] For BSABS rating of presence, irrespective of recency and frequency.

(SPI-A) and a child and youth version (SPI-CY), have been translated into various languages and are available worldwide for the assessment of these criteria [11].

Predictive Accuracy of Late High-Risk Symptoms

According to the concept of HRS, LRPS are supposedly at hand when symptoms have reached the level of APS or BLIPS. The Melbourne Early Prediction Centre has consciously chosen very precise definitions for these two symptom constellations, which are only gradually distinguishable from full psychosis [8]. It was their aim to develop

Table 2. The UHR criteria according to SIPS

UHR criterion APS
At least any 1 of the following 5 symptoms with a SIPS score of 3–5
Unusual thought content/delusional ideas (P1)
Suspiciousness/persecutory ideas (P2)
Grandiosity (P3)
Perceptual abnormalities/hallucinations (P4)
Disorganized communication (P5)
First occurrence or worsening within past 12 months
At least weekly occurrence within past month
UHR criterion BLIPS
At least any 1 of the above 5 symptoms (P1–P5) with a SIPS score of 6
Psychotic level of intensity, i.e. a score of 6 was reached within past 3 months
At least present for several minutes per day at a frequency of at least once per month
UHR 'trait-state' criterion
At least any 1 of the following risk criteria
1st-degree biological relative with a history of psychotic disorder
Schizotypal personality disorder in the patient[a]
At least a 30% drop in GAF score over the last month as compared to 12 months ago

GAF = Global Assessment of Functioning scale. SIPS = Structured Interview of Prodromal Syndromes.
[a] In the German Research Network on Schizophrenia, this criterion was replaced with 'obstetric complications' in July 2000.

ultra-high-risk (UHR) criteria that are able to predict an impending psychotic outbreak 12 months in advance during the mean 5-year period where HRS symptoms occurred. Therefore, these criteria should be able to assess the effectiveness of indicated preventive measures in a short time (table 2).

The utilization of UHR criteria has widely, but not always in an identical manner, been accepted by most centers worldwide. Initially, there was still another category of risk symptoms next to APS and BLIPS that included familial risk factors and assured the closeness to psychosis by referring to already existing functional deficits. However, this category has taken a back seat and has merged into the category of ERPS or is amended by birth complications in some centers.

Considering the data gathered over the past 10 years, transition rates of individuals at risk with either APS and/or BLIPS criteria vary tremendously between studies. In line with the initial expectations, early studies documented transition rates over 40% in 12 months, while later studies sometimes indicated rates of 20% or less (fig. 4). However, the better publicly established a center was, the more their offers and preventive measures were perceived by the public, which eventually led to smaller transition rates.

This observation suggests that the included at-risk individuals were more likely to be in an earlier phase of the UHR state in the more recent investigations as

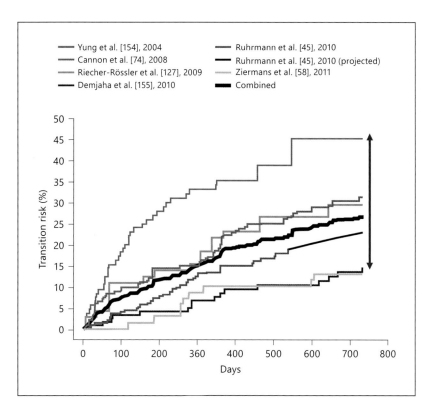

Fig. 4. Meta-analysis of transition risks in studies reporting Kaplan-Meier estimates of psychosis: transition over time in an HRS (n = 984 individuals; adapted according to Fusar-Poli et al. [7]).

compared to the older ones. Hence, they should have been followed up for periods longer than 12 months in order to obtain a more accurate transition rate. In fact, investigations with longer follow-up phases do indicate comparably high transition rates after 12 months once APS and BLIPS have been displayed. Two large-scale studies, which investigated the predictive power of UHR criteria, should be highlighted within this context. Like the CER study, they both included a sufficiently big control group not displaying these high-risk criteria [12]. One of these investigations focused on 6 and 24 months of follow-up Melbourne data from both UHR-positive and UHR-negative patients coming from either an early prediction or a specialized center. Here, the predictive power of the UHR criteria was excellent and partly comparable to the CER study's longitudinal data. The other investigation was the large-scale North American Prodrome Longitudinal Study (NAPLS). The content of this investigation consisted of pooled data gathered from studies conducted at eight independent centers, with an observation phase of 30 months each. Again, the presence of a sufficiently big UHR-negative control group allowed a methodologically solid evaluation of both sensitivity and specificity of the UHR criteria [13].

Next to the original Melbourne Comprehensive Assessment of At-Risk Mental States (CAARMS) [14], the Basel FePsy Study [15] uses similar criteria, but has developed a shorter instrument for assessing them, the Basel Screening Instrument for Psychosis (BSIP) [16]. A workgroup at Yale University has meanwhile also developed a series of widely accepted interviews, scales and criteria (SIPS, SOPS, COPS) for the assessment of criteria [17].

Moreover, a similar program was developed in New York [18] and, based on proper criteria and assessment tools and the Mannheim Interview for the Retrospective Assessment of the Onset and Course of Schizophrenia and Other Psychoses, has meanwhile been complemented by the Early Recognition Inventory (ERIraos), which allows the assessment of both BS and UHR criteria at the same time [19].

Improvement of Predictive Accuracy by Combining Criteria

That a shared application of clinical high-risk criteria might be reasonable was shown in the European Prediction of Psychosis Study (EPOS) for the first time [20]. In terms of significance, this project was comparable to the NAPLS project. The study sample consisted of adolescents and young adults from six European centers, all displaying either UHR criteria or the BS-confounded COGDIS, or both. A predictive analysis of UHR symptoms and COGDIS, after an 18-month follow-up period, generated values that were to be expected based on the previous state of knowledge.

Interestingly, a somewhat higher positive predictive power could be achieved by combining different types of criteria. A combination of criteria led to improved sensitivity regarding the ability to detect individuals with an imminent risk for a first psychotic episode. The advantage of combining criteria has just recently been impressively attested. In a 48-month follow-up examination of 246 individuals at risk, the combined approach led to explicitly higher transition rates and significantly improved sensitivity, and a likewise reduced percentage of false-positive predictions [21].

Until now, the best information on predictive accuracy of both high-risk criteria approaches was provided in a meta-analysis comprising the years 1996 to January 2011. Among these 27 studies, comprising a total of 2,502 individuals at risk, there were – besides EPOS – only two investigations on smaller samples that were based on both criteria approaches. The mean risk for a transition to psychosis in the otherwise BS- or UHR-based studies was 18, 22, 29 or 36% after 6, 12, 24 or 36 months, respectively [22]. As soon as studies with a simultaneous use of criteria and longer observation periods are available, future meta-analyses will surely yield even higher transition rates. In the meantime, further analysis has already been performed for *European Psychiatry*, which will be published shortly in a guidance paper of the European Psychiatric Association [2].

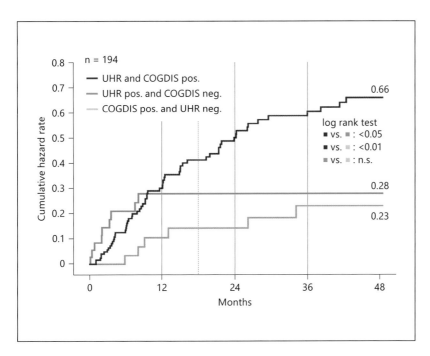

Fig. 5. Kaplan-Meier analysis: baseline risk conditions. Orange line: 'only COGDIS' (n = 30); green line: 'only UHR' (n = 37); red line: 'COGDIS + UHR' (n = 127); small vertical lines: censored cases (adapted according to Schultze-Lutter [21]).

The percentage of individuals at risk of transitioning into psychosis in the predictive analyses mentioned above, which were the first of this kind since EPOS [20], has meanwhile, after 4 years, reached 66%. This is a dimension that has so far, by applying a separate criteria approach, only been documented by the longitudinal CER study, which had transition rates of 70% after 4.5 years (fig. 5).

Next to better risk enrichment, due to the application of a combined criteria approach, and the development of a plausible clinical prediction model with excellent predictive power, EPOS has also opened many other doors. In order to prepare means for individualized risk estimations and corresponding preventive actions, an individual prognostic score has been calculated for each included person at risk based on clinical and demographic variables. These risk scores could be stratified by means of data modeling in four classes with a 0.67–1.62 increased risk of disease compared to the relative risk of the general population.

Neurobiological and environmental risk factors can also be included into these stratified models, like this four-stage prognostic index, in order to yield even more exact and refined individualized prognoses. A first example is a stratified predictive model for psychosis, which is, next to clinical variables, also based on the outcomes of conventional neurocognitive test procedures. Due to its feasibility, it is already well embedded inthe work of early prediction centers [23].

Improving Predictive Accuracy by Biomarkers

Recent meta-analytic works on HRS indicate that transition rates into a first psychotic episode approximately equal those for Alzheimer's dementia once mild cognitive impairment has been detected. Here, imaging procedures and cerebrospinal fluid analyses offer a possibility for predicting dementia with almost absolute certainty, especially if memory dysfunctions are subjectively perceived as being highly burdensome [24]. It is exactly this improvement of clinical risk estimation by additional diagnostic procedures that is being aspired to by early detection and prevention centers for psychosis. Accordingly, the clinical high-risk research has long been occupied with identifying biomarkers with their own predictive power. So far, principally useful deviations have been found on all relevant levels in individuals showing ERPS and LRPS symptoms. Among these are meta-analytically confirmed neuropsychological impairments, as well as a reduced speed of cognitive processing [7], alterations of EEG power spectrums [25], deviances from action-related potentials, such as the P300 [26] or especially mismatch negativity [27]; structural changes in terms of density in orbitofrontal, hippocampal, cerebral and adjacent regions [28]; results from model classifications of brain-structural magnetic resonance tomographies receiving so much attention lately [29], and other neurobiological-genetic findings.

The development of predictive models, comprising several levels of investigation [30] along with the just-mentioned potential biomarkers, for risk-stratification continues on [23, 25].

Singular studies could already verify that the combination of UHR as well as BScriteria with neuropsychological, neurophysiological and structural parameters can achieve a clinical predictive power that is comparable to that of mild cognitive impairment if complemented by additional diagnostics [23, 24, 29]. Several international but independent and well-designed studies could verify that EEG deviation, particularly mismatch negativity, is a biomarker with its own predictive power and is well suited as an additional diagnostic parameter in HRS [27].

The accumulated knowledge regarding possibilities of risk enrichment and stratification has gradually reached a level that allows consensus decisions on the application of additional diagnostic parameters in HRS. The model classification of neurobiological data aided by machine learning algorithms might further enrich and improve this possibility substantially. Hence, the upcoming application of these procedures on structural magnetic resonance tomography data from PREVENT, the biggest German investigation on indicated prevention [31], which is almost complete, as well as the just-initiated large-scale systematic examination of the suitability of imaging models for improving prediction should be evaluated before complementing the clinical high-risk criteria for psychoses with obligatory additional diagnostics [1].

References

1 Klosterkötter J, Schultze-Lutter F, Bechdolf A, et al: Prediction and prevention of schizophrenia: what has been achieved and where to go next? World Psychiatry 2011;10:165–174.

2 Schultze-Lutter F, Michel C, Schmidt SJ, Schimmelmann BG, Maric NP, Salokangas RRK, Riecher-Rössler A, van der Gaag M, Nordentoft M, Raballo A, Meneghelli A, Marshall M, Morrison A, Ruhrmann S, Klosterkötter J: EPA guidance on the early detection of clinical high risk states of psychoses. Eur Psychiatry 2015;30:405–416.

3 Klosterkötter J: Prevention of psychotic disorders. Nervenarzt 2013;84:1299, 1302–1309.

4 Mrazek PJ, Haggerty HJ: Reducing Risks for Mental Disorders: Frontiers for Preventive Research. Washington, Academy Press, 1994.

5 van Os J, Kenis G, Rutten BP: The environment and schizophrenia. Nature 2010;468:203–212.

6 The European Network of Schizophrenia Networks for the Study of Gene-Environment Interactions (EU-GEI): Schizophrenia aetiology: do gene-environment interactions hold the key? Schizophr Res 2008;102:21–26.

7 Fusar-Poli P, Borgwardt S, Bechdolf A, et al: The psychosis high-risk state: a comprehensive state-of-the-art review. JAMA Psychiatry 2013;70:107–120.

8 Yung AR, Phillips LJ, McGorry PD, et al: Prediction of psychosis. Br J Psychiatry 1998;172(suppl 33):14–20.

9 Schultze-Lutter F, Ruhrmann S, Berning J, Maier W, Klosterkötter J: Basic symptoms and ultrahigh risk criteria: symptom development in the initial prodromal state. Schizophr Bull 2010;36:182–191.

10 Klosterkötter J, Hellmich M, Steinmeyer EM, Schultze-Lutter F: Diagnosing schizophrenia in the initial prodromal phase. Arch Gen Psychiatry 2001;58:158–164.

11 Schultze-Lutter F, Klosterkötter J, Picker H, Steinmeyer E, Ruhrmann S: Predicting first-episode psychosis by basic symptom criteria. Clin Neuropsychiatry 2007;4:11–22.

12 Ruhrmann S, Schultze-Lutter F, Klosterkötter J: Probably at-risk, but certainly ill – advocating the introduction of a psychosis spectrum disorder in DSM-V. Schizophr Res 2010;120:23–37.

13 Cannon TD, Cadenhead K, Cornblatt B, et al: Prediction of psychosis in youth at high clinical risk: a multisite longitudinal study in North America. Arch Gen Psychiatry 2008;65:28–37.

14 Yung AR, Yuen HP, McGorry PD, et al: Mapping the onset of psychosis: the comprehensive assessment of at-risk mental states. Aust NZ J Psychiatry 2005;39:964–971.

15 Riecher-Rössler A, Geschwandtner U, Aston J, et al: The Basel early detection-of-psychosis (FEPSY)-study – design and preliminary results. Acta Psychiatr Scand 2007;115:114–125.

16 Riecher-Rössler A, Aston J, Ventura J, Merlo M, Borgwardt S, Gschwandtner U, Stieglitz RD: Das Basel Screening Instrument für Psychosen (BSIP): Entwicklung, Aufbau, Reliabilität und Validität. Fortschr Neurol Psychiatr 2008;76:207–216.

17 McGlashan T, Walsh B, Woods S: The Psychosis-Risk Syndrome. Handbook for Diagnosis and Follow-Up. New York, Oxford University Press, 2010.

18 Cornblatt B: The New York High-Risk Project to the Hillside Recognition and Prevention (RAP) Program. Am J Med Genet 2002;114:956–966.

19 Häfner H, Bechdolf A, Klosterkötter J, et al: Psychosen – Früherkennung und Frühintervention. Stuttgart, Schattauer, 2012.

20 Ruhrmann S, Schultze-Lutter F, Salokangas RK, et al: Prediction of psychosis in adolescents and young adults at high risk: results from the prospective European Prediction of Psychosis Study (EPOS). Arch Gen Psychiatry 2010;67:241–251.

21 Schultze-Lutter F, Klosterkötter J, Ruhrmann S: Improving the clinical prediction of psychosis by combining ultra-high risk criteria and cognitive basic symptoms. Schizophr Res 2014;154:100–106.

22 Fusar-Poli P, Bonoldi I, Yung AR, Borgwardt S, Kempton MJ, Valmaggia L, Barale F, Caverzasi E, McGuire P: Predicting psychosis: meta-analysis of transition outcomes in individuals at high clinical risk. Arch Gen Psychiatry 2012;69:220–229.

23 Michel C, Ruhrmann S, Schimmelmann BG, Klosterkötter J, Schultze-Lutter F: A stratified model for psychosis prediction in clinical practice. Schizophr Bull 2014;40:1533–1542.

24 Jessen F, Wiese B, Bachmann C, Eifflaender-Gorfer S, Haller F, Kölsch H, Luck T, Mösch E, van den Bussche H, Wagner M, Wollny A, Zimmermann T, Pentzek M, Riedel-Heller SG, Romberg HP, Weyerer S, Kaduszkiewicz H, Maier W, Bickel H; German Study on Aging, Cognition and Dementia in Primary Care Patients Study Group: AD dementia risk in late MCI, in early MCI, and in subjective memory impairment. Alzheimers Dement 2014;10:76–83.

25 van Tricht MJ, Ruhrmann S, Arns M, Müller R, Bodatsch M, Velthorst E, Koelman JH, Bour LJ, Zurek K, Schultze-Lutter F, Klosterkötter J, Linszen DH, de Haan L, Brockhaus-Dumke A, Nieman DH: Can quantitative EEG measures predict clinical outcome in subjects at clinical high risk for psychosis? A prospective multicenter study. Schizophr Res 2014;153:42–47.

26 Nieman DH, Ruhrmann S, Dragt S, Soen F, van Tricht MJ, Koelman JH, Bour LJ, Velthorst E, Becker HE, Weiser M, Linszen DH, de Haan L: Psychosis prediction: stratification of risk estimation with information-processing and premorbid functioning variables. Schizophr Bull 2014;40:1482–1490.

27 Bodatsch M, Ruhrmann S, Wagner M, et al: Prediction of psychosis by mismatch negativity. Biol Psychiatry 2011;69:959–966.

28 Pantelis C, Velakoulis D, McGorry PD, et al: Neuroanatomical abnormalities before and after onset of psychosis: a cross-sectional and longitudinal MRI comparison. Lancet 2003;361:281–288.

29 Koutsouleris N, Borgwardt S, Meisenzahl EM, Bottlender R, Möller HJ, Riecher-Rössler A: Disease prediction in the at-risk mental state for psychosis using neuroanatomical biomarkers: results from the FePsy study. Schizophr Bull 2012;38:1234–1246.

30 Riecher-Rössler A, Aston J, Borgwardt S, Bugra H, Fuhr P, Gschwandtner U, Koutsouleris N, Pflueger M, Tamagni C, Radü EW, Rapp C, Smieskova R, Studerus E, Walter A, Zimmermann R: Prediction of psychosis by stepwise multilevel assessment – the Basel FePsy (Early Recognition of Psychosis)-Project (in German). Fortschr Neurol Psychiatr 2013;81: 265–275.

31 Bechdolf A, Müller H, Stützer H, et al: Rationale and baseline characteristics of PREVENT: a second-generation intervention trial in subjects at-risk (prodromal) of developing first-episode psychosis evaluating cognitive behavior therapy, aripiprazole, and placebo for the prevention of psychosis. Schizophr Bull 2011;37(suppl 2):S111–S121.

Prof. Dr. Joachim Klosterkötter
Department of Psychiatry and Psychotherapy, University of Cologne
Kerpener Strasse 62
DE–50924 Cologne (Germany)
E-Mail joachim.klosterkoetter@uk-koeln.de

Riecher-Rössler A, McGorry PD (eds): Early Detection and Intervention in Psychosis: State of the Art and Future Perspectives. Key Issues Ment Health. Basel, Karger, 2016, vol 181, pp 15–28 (DOI: 10.1159/000440911)

Early Intervention in Emerging Psychosis: State of the Art and Future Perspectives

Patrick D. McGorry · Sherilyn Goldstone

Orygen, The National Centre for Excellence in Youth Mental Health, University of Melbourne, Parkville, Vic., Australia

Abstract

Today's outlook for a young person experiencing the onset of a psychotic illness can – and should – be very different from that of just three decades ago. Over this time, basic research into the epidemiology and neurobiology of the psychotic illnesses has allowed the development of improved medical treatments, while innovative clinical research has led to the development of better services that are specifically designed around the unique needs of this particularly vulnerable group. This has led to a shift in focus from the historical, and largely palliative, approach to the care of those living with psychosis, to an emphasis on early intervention with evidence-based care that is appropriate to the stage of illness, and delivered within an optimistic, recovery-oriented framework. Here, we outline current thinking on early intervention and the service reforms that have led to these advances in the management of the psychotic illnesses, which the available evidence indicates offer the best chance for these young people to achieve a full functional recovery and live meaningful, connected, and satisfying lives.   © 2016 S. Karger AG, Basel

'The best hope now for the prevention of schizophrenia lies with indicated preventive interventions targeted at individuals manifesting precursor signs and symptoms who have not yet met full criteria for diagnosis. The identification of individuals at this early stage, coupled with the introduction of pharmacological and psychosocial interventions, may prevent the development of the full-blown disorder' [1].

Over the last three decades our historic view of schizophrenia as a catastrophic illness, with progressive and inevitable decline the usual outcome, has changed significantly. This shift in thinking began with a series of long-term outcome studies from the 1980s that showed that up to two thirds of those with schizophrenia achieve significant recovery [2–4]. Since then, a combination of better pharmaceutical treatments and a greater understanding of the epidemiology and neurobiology of psychosis has led to the development of more appropriate treatments and better services for those experiencing a psychotic illness, as well as a shift in our approach to managing these potentially devastating illnesses [5]. Now, the focus of treatment is no longer exclusively on managing symptoms, but largely on promoting the best possible recovery to enable those who experience psychosis to live meaningful and contributing lives within their communities.

It is the timing of onset of the psychotic disorders that is a major reason for their destructive potential. Epidemiological studies have shown that the vast majority of those with a psychotic illness experience its onset during their late teens to early twenties [6, 7], a time in life when most young people are finishing their education and beginning their working lives, developing intimate relationships, and moving from their families of origin to establish themselves as independent adults. Disrupting a young person's life during this crucial transition inevitably affects their social, educational, and vocational development, which if left unrecognised and unremedied, has the potential to cause significant and ongoing secondary disability [8].

Seminal studies from the 1980s have highlighted the special clinical needs of young people experiencing a first episode of psychosis [9–11]. Since then a growing body of evidence has shown that the course of the psychotic disorders is not fixed, with deterioration being the norm and a poor prognosis inevitable, but instead is fluid and potentially malleable [12–21]. Examination of the risk factors that influence outcome has revealed that many of these may be reversible, and that attention to these factors as part of treatment has the potential to limit or repair the damage. This has driven an explosion of interest in early intervention and phase-specific, recovery-focused treatment for early psychosis. Indeed, the current paradigm shift towards preventive, or at least pre-emptive, psychiatry has largely been driven by the last two decades of research in early psychosis [22].

Defining the Sub-Threshold Stage of Psychotic Illness and Its Consequences

Clinical criteria based on a combination of trait and state markers able to identify help-seeking young people who may be at ultra-high risk of psychosis were first developed and validated in a series of studies beginning in the 1990s [23]. These criteria are divided into three groups on the basis of the young person's presenting symptoms: attenuated psychotic symptoms; brief, self-limiting intermittent psychotic symptoms, and genetic risk of schizophrenia (a first-degree relative with schizophrenia/schizoaffective disorder) with a recent significant decrease in functioning. While early studies showed that up to 40% of the young people who met the ultra-high-risk criteria made a transition to psychosis within the following year [24], more recent data have revealed that the 12-month transition rate has fallen to around 22% in recent cohorts, yet over a 3-year period it remains at around 36% [25, 26]. By comparison, in a meta-analysis of six prospective studies of the non-help-seeking general population, Kaymaz et al. [27] calculated the 12-month rate of transition to psychotic illness in those reporting psychotic-like experiences as 0.56%, compared to 0.16% in those who did not report such symptoms, thereby providing a useful baseline against which to compare the rate of transition in those considered to be at ultra-high risk.

The Psychosis Prodrome or a Pluripotential Risk Syndrome?

Although the ultra-high-risk criteria show good relative specificity for transition to psychosis, the majority of young people who fulfil these criteria do not develop a full-threshold psychotic disorder, and a significant proportion (up to approximately 50%) experience remission of their psychotic symptoms within a year of seeking help [28, 29]. However, most of these young people continue to report clinically relevant symptoms, primarily a blend of anxiety and depression, as well as difficulties in social and occupational functioning, highlighting their need for ongoing care [26]. Furthermore, long-term follow-up has shown that transition to psychosis can occur up to 10 years following the initial diagnosis, clearly indicating that these young people may remain vulnerable for long periods of time [26], and again emphasising the need for careful monitoring and clinical care.

What then is the relationship between sub-threshold psychotic phenomena and psychotic illness? While sub-threshold psychotic phenomena are universally present prior to the onset of schizophrenia, epidemiological studies have shown that transient sub-threshold psychotic experiences are common in healthy young people from the general population [30–32], although only a minority of these cases evolve into a diagnosable mental illness each year, whether this be psychotic or otherwise. Moreover, a significant proportion (approximately 27%) of young people with depressive or anxiety disorders also report psychotic-like experiences [31, 33], with the presence of psychotic symptoms being associated with a poorer course of illness [31, 33]. Furthermore, the vast majority of young people who fulfil the ultra-high-risk criteria also have at least one diagnosable Axis I disorder [34]. There may also be other pathways to psychosis onset, not solely via the ultra-high-risk route [35, 36]. Thus, there is considerable overlap between the psychopathological dimensions represented in the ultra-high-risk state, and it has become increasingly evident that the concept of 'ultra-high risk' might usefully be broadened to one of a 'pluripotential risk state', rather than being considered specific to psychosis alone [37]. Psychotic phenomena could be perhaps more usefully considered an indication of severity of illness rather than a specific indicator of imminent risk of a full-threshold psychotic illness [38–40]. This has obvious implications for the treatment approach for these young people. Here, the presence of psychotic phenomena per se should not be the primary determinant of treatment selection (i.e. prescription of antipsychotic medication). Instead, first-line treatment should favour supportive psychosocial interventions, in line with the clinical staging model [41], with careful ongoing monitoring of the young person's mental state. Persistence and worsening of psychotic symptoms and impairment despite use of evidence-based non-drug therapies could then prove a reasonable guide and justification for moving to antipsychotic medications, especially if these reach full threshold.

Interventions in the Sub-Threshold Stage

The early intervention strategies that have been trialled to date range from the psychologically based, including psychoeducation, supportive psychotherapy, cognitive behavioural therapy (CBT), and family work, to the biologically based, including symptomatic treatment for depression, anxiety, and any sub-threshold psychotic symptoms, through to experimental biological neuroprotective approaches. The global aim of treatment in this phase is to provide comprehensive clinical care designed to reduce distressing symptoms and improve functioning, and if possible, to prevent these symptoms from worsening and developing into fully fledged and sustained psychosis. If a first episode of psychosis does occur, the aims of treatment are to minimise the duration of untreated psychosis, to attain and maintain remission of psychotic symptoms, and to promote maximum recovery without residual disability [41].

Ten intervention studies have now been conducted with ultra-high-risk young people worldwide, investigating the use of medications (low-dose antipsychotics and/or antidepressants), psychosocial treatments, or both, to prevent the onset of psychosis. A recent meta-analysis of these trials has shown that each of these treatments are effective, with an overall number needed to treat of 9 (95% CI: 6–15) and an overall risk reduction at 12 months of 54% [42]. However, risk-benefit concerns related to the use of antipsychotic medication, even at low doses, means that psychosocial interventions, including supportive therapy and CBT, and other benign interventions, such as treatment with omega-3 fatty acids [43], are currently recommended as the first-line therapy in this patient group [41]. Drug therapies should only be considered if distressing symptoms *and* impairment persist or worsen. Antipsychotic medication may have a place in the treatment of those who fail to respond to initial intervention with psychosocial therapies; symptom severity alone, as the definition of 'transition to psychosis', may not be a perfect guide for the need for antipsychotic medication. Other factors, such as symptom type and pattern, and other clinical phenomena, including patient choice, comorbid substance use, triggers and stressors, genetic and other biomarkers, etc., will also determine the optimal treatment for a given patient. When antipsychotics are prescribed, the best candidates are those with a more favourable metabolic and neurological safety profile such as aripiprazole [44]. The results of these intervention trials are promising, but there is a need to carefully study other strategies such as cognitive remediation and benign biotherapies targeting candidate neurobiological mechanisms such as inflammation and oxidative stress. Determination of the optimal sequence of interventions and definition of therapeutically relevant subgroups via sophisticated clinical trial designs is necessary to build a solid evidence base to inform future therapeutic strategies for this particularly vulnerable patient group.

Interventions for First-Episode Psychosis: Pharmacological and Psychosocial

The management of first-episode psychosis (FEP) requires great sensitivity and clinical skill and is optimally delivered in specialised services that stream younger patients and families separately from older people at later stages of illness. Low-dose antipsychotic medications and a range of intensive psychological and social interventions are essential to maximise recovery and minimise secondary morbidity. These clinical interventions have been heavily researched in recent years and incorporated into detailed clinical practice guidelines [45, 46], and so detailed exposition of the management of FEP will not be provided here, though it is vital that this phase of illness is optimally managed in order that speedy and sustained recovery is more likely.

Recovery and the Critical Period

Most young people who experience their first episode of psychosis achieve symptomatic remission [47]. However, they remain at high risk for relapse, with a recent meta-analysis of 29 longitudinal follow-up studies showing a pooled prevalence relapse rate of 54% (40–63%) by 3 years [48]. Furthermore, discontinuation of treatment is associated with relapse rates of at least 80% within 5 years with treatment in mainstream services [e.g. 49–51].

Current expert consensus treatment guidelines for early psychosis recommend that following remission, maintenance antipsychotic medication is prescribed for at least 12 months before discontinuation is attempted [52]. This has become accepted practice due to the risks of disease progression, further disruption to psychosocial functioning, and the development of treatment resistance [53, 54]. However, there is a growing debate about the balance between the risks and benefits of maintenance medication and its optimum duration in order to maximise recovery and prevent relapse. The argument for long-term standard-dose maintenance antipsychotic medication as a uniform approach for all FEP cases has been challenged by two key recent findings. First, a recent 7-year follow-up study of first-episode patients who had achieved remission in their first year of treatment has shown that long-term recovery was not jeopardised, but rather improved, when their total exposure to antipsychotic medication was controlled via a dose reduction/discontinuation strategy [55]. This study involved randomising 128 patients who had achieved remission to either a dose reduction/discontinuation strategy or maintenance treatment for 18 months. At 18 months, the relapse rate in the dose reduction/discontinuation group was more than double that in the maintenance treatment group (43 vs. 21%), with functional outcomes similar in both groups [56]. However, at the 7-year follow-up, the outcomes had changed dramatically: the relapse rates in both groups were not significantly different, with the excess in the dose reduction/discontinuation group being confined to the first 3 years, while those in the dose reduction/discontinuation group had achieved twice the level of functional recovery than those in the maintenance therapy group (40.4 vs. 17.6%). Second, there is new correlational evidence for an association between level of exposure to antipsychotic medication over time and reductions in brain volume in early psychosis [57, 58], possibly adding to the established list of physical health, tolerability, and acceptability problems (see below).

Relapse prevention has long been the main goal of treatment. This is not surprising, given that relapses are risky, distressing, and can set back recovery in all domains. The high rate of medication non-adherence/discontinuation in young people with early psychosis is one of the strongest risk factors for relapses in young people with early psychosis [48]. However, modest exacerbations of symptoms, which are more common in the first 3–5 years after diagnosis, may be a price worth paying in the subset of early remitters at least for better longer-term functional recovery [59], particularly as young people tend to give more weight to the recovery of their social functioning, as opposed to symptom recovery alone [60, 61]. Furthermore, there is good evidence to suggest that a significant percentage of young people who experience a first psychotic episode can achieve full functional recovery, even in the presence of residual positive symptoms [19].

The emphasis on relapse prevention should therefore be balanced with a focus on functional recovery and the cost of long-term continuous antipsychotic treatment, which evidence suggests may contribute to the longer-term suppression of functioning. A promising balanced strategy includes a dose minimisation strategy, combined with intensive and recovery-focused psychosocial treatments with vigilant monitoring for early signs of relapse [51]. However, whether some FEP patients can be safely treated with minimal maintenance antipsychotic medication within a narrow 'window' (not too much, but not too little either in most patients), especially when a more intensive psychosocial safety net is provided, remains an open question that needs to be addressed in further large-scale studies. One of the drivers of our unquestioning universal use of medication is our current lack of evidence-based intensive psychosocial interventions that can be regularly used in routine clinical care; further exploration of this area is a key issue for future research.

Successful relapse prevention [62, 63] and vocational [64] programs have been developed that focus on functional recovery rather than symptomatic recovery alone, and programs like these could be offered in the context of medication discontinuation with careful monitoring for signs of relapse. Our EPISODE II study was the first randomised controlled trial comparing CBT for relapse prevention plus recommended FEP treatment with recommended treatment alone [63]. A significant treatment effect on relapse rates was shown at the 7-month follow-up in young people who had reached remission on positive symptoms. We also showed that this effect was sustained at 12 months, and beyond this relapse rates were kept to historically very low levels [63]. Importantly, and in accordance with the dose reduction/withdrawal trial discussed above, adherence to maintenance antipsychotic medication in our randomised controlled trial appears to have constrained psychosocial functioning, suggesting that a strong focus on medication maintenance may interfere with long-term recovery [62].

Despite wanting to work, more than 40% of young people with early psychosis are unemployed. Employment is an important pathway to other areas of functioning, and increases the opportunities for social and economic participation. Supported employment, and in particular individual placement and support, is currently the most effective model for promoting vocational recovery. The key elements of this model are that it focuses on the competitive job market; it is open to anyone with a mental illness who wants to look for work, irrespective of their mental state; job searching begins immediately, with potential jobs being chosen on the basis of the young person's preferences; the program is integrated within the mental health service's treatment team, and support is available for as long as it is needed and continues after employment is obtained, depending on the individual's needs [65]. We have successfully trialled this program in young people with early psychosis and found that those who received 6 months of individual placement and support for vocational recovery plus their recommended usual treatment had significantly better outcomes on the level of employment (85 vs. 28% in the control group), hours worked per week, jobs acquired, and longevity of employment compared to those who received their usual treatment alone [64]. This model can also be applied to educational settings as well, as a study from the United Kingdom has shown [66].

Intensive psychosocial interventions to promote, support, and maintain a meaningful recovery are particularly important for young people with early psychosis, as this age group is uniquely vulnerable to ongoing secondary disability. Ideally, these interventions should be maintained at an appropriate level of intensity for each individual for the critical period of the first 5 years after diagnosis [67], when the risk of ongoing and entrenched secondary disability is highest. Strategies targeted at maximising functional recovery, such as the relapse prevention and vocational interventions outlined here, may complement and enhance each other, and when combined with an appropriate approach to medication, can significantly improve the outcome for many young people. Our group is now studying the translation of many of these psychosocial interventions to online formats which may allow more effective maintenance of recovery after discharge from specialised early psychosis settings [68, 69].

Identifying and Responding to Early Treatment Resistance
Despite the availability of a wide range of medications and psychosocial care as described above, a percentage of patients (up to 20%) will fail to achieve remission and recovery from their first episode of psychosis [70]. They need to be proactively

screened for and identified, and intensive CBT and clozapine should be offered from around the 6-month point following entry to care [71]. We have described how this safety net strategy operates within a first-episode program [45, 70].

Physical Health in Those with a Psychotic Illness
Young people who are taking antipsychotic medication are at increased risk of weight gain and metabolic abnormalities, which may appear in the first few weeks of treatment and can lead to metabolic syndrome (insulin resistance, abdominal obesity, dyslipidaemia, hyperglycaemia, and hypertension) [44, 72, 73]. There are a range of reasons for this, such as genetic predisposition, poor nutrition, lack of exercise, smoking, and substance abuse, as well as the side effects of antipsychotic medication [72, 73]. Moreover, there is strong evidence to suggest that people with psychotic illnesses receive inferior quality physical health care to those with chronic physical illnesses [74]. Apart from these effects on physical health, the weight gain associated with antipsychotic treatment can affect a young person's self-esteem, increase self-stigma, and increase the chances of them discontinuing their medication, increasing the risk of relapse. Together, these factors mean that it is crucial to take measures to prevent and treat weight gain, preferably prior to it becoming an issue. A pre-emptive approach is crucial to addressing the physical health needs of these young people and preventing the antipsychotic-induced metabolic disturbances that contribute so strongly to poor physical health before this becomes entrenched and a self-perpetuating cycle.

Monitoring of weight, waist circumference, and blood glucose and lipid levels is essential from the time that antipsychotics are initiated, with weight gain being assessed every week, or at least once every 2 weeks, for the first 8 weeks of treatment; then all parameters should be assessed every 3 months for the first year of treatment [74]. Switching antipsychotic medication may be necessary for those who experience rapid and significant weight gain [75]. Interventions promoting a healthy lifestyle and behavioural change are particularly important for young people and are generally well accepted [74, 76, 77], and medication, such as metformin, may also be considered.

Novel Service Approaches to Maximise Recovery

Specialised mental health services for young people are warranted on several grounds. Young people with emerging illness usually present with complex and evolving patterns of morbidity and fluctuating symptoms, which often means that they do not fit the entry criteria applied in adult services, and even if they are accepted, they often find these services inappropriate and alienating. The complexity and relative non-specificity of their symptom profiles means that different treatment approaches are required than those for full-threshold illness, with the emphasis being on offering care that is appropriate to the very early stages of illness, is pre-emptive in nature, and with a strong preventive and recovery-oriented focus [78, 79]. This requires a different culture of care to that of the child and adolescent mental health care system, centred as it is on young children in their family environment, or the adult system, which is primarily designed for adults with more established illness. Young people's unique individual and group identity and their help-seeking needs and behaviours must be central to any care model, which must recognise that developmentally and culturally appropriate approaches are essential for the management of emerging illness in young people. Furthermore, these unique clinical and cultural needs means that youth mental health services must blur the distinctions between the tiers of primary and specialist care in order to allow a flexible and appropriate response for each young person (and their family), depending on their own unique needs [79].

All available evidence shows that youth-specific services should be provided in an accessible, community-based, non-judgmental, and non-stigmatising setting, where young people feel comfortable, have a say in how their care is provided, and can feel a sense of trust [79, 80]. For young people experiencing the early stages of a psychotic illness, these services must offer three core functions: (1) early detection, (2) acute care during and immediately following a crisis, and (3) recovery-focused continuing care, featuring multimodal interventions to enable a young person to maintain or regain their social, academic, and career trajectory during the critical first 2–5 years following the onset of illness [81]. The key features of an appropriate service are:

- Easy access to care, ensured by simple referral pathways, close links with local providers, and the 'youth-friendliness' of the service and its structure
- A holistic and integrated biopsychosocial approach to clinical intervention, which takes into account the developmental stage of the young person, as well as the stage of their illness; the focus of treatment is not only on the amelioration of distressing symptoms and achieving symptomatic remission, but also strongly emphasises psychosocial interventions designed to assist the young person to maintain or regain their normal educational, vocational, and social developmental trajectory to enable a full functional recovery
- A high level of partnerships with local service providers to ensure effective and timely pathways into and out of the service, as well as supporting service delivery during the critical period of care [82]

Long-term follow-up studies from Australia [16], Canada [18], Norway [15], Denmark [12], and Hong Kong [21] have shown significantly better clinical and functional outcomes for young people treated within a specialised early psychosis service compared to those who were treated in standard mental health services. Furthermore, these services are more cost-effective than traditional services [e.g. 83, 84]. More importantly, they are highly valued by clients and their families [85]. It is the culture of hope and optimism, combined with intensive evidence-based biopsychosocial care featuring collaboration with the young person and their family, plus the nature of the environment in which it is provided, that is crucial to their success.

Conclusion

The outlook for a young person experiencing a first episode of psychosis today should be very different to that of two decades ago. The research effort dedicated towards a better understanding of the psychoses and improved clinical care for patients with psychotic disorders has not only largely driven the shift to our current recovery-focused models of care, but has also contributed to the transformation of psychiatry towards a more preventive therapeutic focus. Early, stage-appropriate, evidence-based care, delivered within an optimistic, recovery-oriented framework offers the best chance for a young person to achieve functional recovery and live a meaningful, connected, and satisfying life. While this level of recovery is well within reach, even given our existing knowledge, all too often our current health care systems do not provide the appropriate care to support it. This is an unfortunate consequence of a combination of factors, primarily the chronic underinvestment in mental health care and the absence of political will for change, both by our policy-makers and those within the health care system itself. Because of the silence still produced by shame and stigma, the community has not yet found its voice fully as in other health domains. Perhaps economists will prove to be effective allies in the future [86]. This failure of public policy certainly needs to be urgently addressed if we are to achieve better outcomes for our young people and a stronger, healthier, and more productive society.

While the ultimate aim in psychiatry, as in all clinical endeavour, is a truly personalised, predictive, and pre-emptive medicine, we are still a long way from reaching this goal. The last two decades have seen major advances in our understanding of the neurobiology of the major mental illnesses, but as yet we still lack the necessary biomarkers able to clearly define the pathological processes underlying mental illness, an individual's risk of illness, or their likely response to treatment, making personalised medicine largely aspirational at this stage. To reach this goal we need a much better understanding of both the basic neurobiology underlying serious mental illness, as well as the complexity of the interactions between the biological, psychological, and social factors that contribute to the development of mental illness. However, this should not be a barrier to achieving better outcomes for our patients in the short term. Here, there is much to be learnt from other areas of medicine, such as oncology, where the great improvements seen in recovery and outcomes have largely resulted not from dramatic breakthroughs or novel treatments, but from the much earlier and more timely deployment of existing treatments, which are then delivered in a more sustained and comprehensive fashion for as long as evidence indicates they are needed. We are still some way away in psychiatry from such a scenario; however, we are within reach and if this were pursued seriously, we would rapidly transform outcomes and see so many more young people being enabled to live fulfilling and productive lives. We could then focus, as in cancer, on prevention and the search for safer, personalised, and more effective cures and treatments.

References

1 Mrazek PJ, Haggerty RJ: Reducing the risks for mental disorders: frontiers for preventive intervention research. Washington DC, National Academy Press, 1994, p 15.

2 Ciompi L: The natural history of schizophrenia in the long term. Br J Psychiatry 1980;136:413–420.

3 Huber G, Gross G, Schüttler R, Linz M: Longitudinal studies of schizophrenic patients. Schizophr Bull 1980;6:592–605.

4 Harding CM, Brooks GW, Ashikaga T, Strauss JS, Breier A: The Vermont longitudinal study of persons with severe mental illness, II: long-term outcome of subjects who retrospectively met DSM-III criteria for schizophrenia. Am J Psychiatry 1987;144:727–735.

5 McGorry PD, Killackey E, Yung A: Early intervention in psychosis: concepts, evidence and future directions. World Psychiatry 2008;7:148–156.

6 Kessler RC, Berglund P, Demler O, Jin R, Merikangas KR, Walters EE: Lifetime prevalence and age-of-onset distributions of DSM-IV disorders in the National Comorbidity Survey Replication. Arch Gen Psychiatry 2005;62:593–602.

7 McGorry PD, Purcell R, Goldstone S, Amminger GP: Age of onset and timing of treatment for mental and substance use disorders: implications for preventive intervention strategies and models of care. Curr Opin Psychiatry 2011;24:301–306.

8 McGorry P: Transition to adulthood: the critical period for pre-emptive, disease-modifying care for schizophrenia and related disorders. Schizophr Bull 2011;37:524–530.

9 Crow TJ, MacMillan JF, Johnson AL, Johnstone EC: A randomised controlled trial of prophylactic neuroleptic treatment. Br J Psychiatry 1986;148:120–127.

10 Kane JM, Rifkin A, Quitkin F, Nayak D, Ramos-Lorenzi J: Fluphenazine vs placebo in patients with remitted, acute first-episode schizophrenia. Arch Gen Psychiatry 1982;39:70–73.

11 Lieberman JA, Alvir JM, Woerner M, Degreef G, Bilder RM, Ashtari M, et al: Prospective study of psychobiology in first-episode schizophrenia at Hillside Hospital. Schizophr Bull 1992;18:351–371.

12 Bertelsen M, Jeppesen P, Petersen L, Thorup A, Ohlenschlaeger J, le Quach P, et al: Five-year follow-up of a randomised multicenter trial of intensive early intervention vs standard treatment for patients with a first episode of psychotic illness: the OPUS trial. Arch Gen Psychiatry 2008;65:762–771.

13 Crumlish N, Whitty P, Clarke M, Browne S, Kamali M, Gervin M, et al: Beyond the critical period: longitudinal study of 8-year outcome in first-episode non-affective psychosis. Br J Psychiatry 2009;194:18–24.

14 Menezes NM, Malla AM, Norman RM, Archie S, Roy P, Zipursky RB: A multi-site Canadian perspective: examining the functional outcome from first-episode psychosis. Acta Psychiatr Scand 2009;120:138–146.

15 Hegelstad WT, Larsen TK, Auestad B, Evensen J, Haahr U, Joa I, et al: Long-term follow-up of the TIPS early detection in psychosis study: effects on 10-year outcome. Am J Psychiatry 2012;169:374–380.

16 Henry LP, Amminger GP, Harris MG, Yuen HP, Harrigan SM, Prosser AL, et al: The EPPIC follow-up study of first-episode psychosis: longer-term clinical and functional outcome 7 years after index admission. J Clin Psychiatry 2010;71:716–728.

17 Larsen TK, Melle I, Auestad B, Haahr U, Joa I, Johannessen JO, et al: Early detection of psychosis: positive effects on 5-year outcome. Psychol Med 2011;41:1461–1469.

18 Norman RM, Manchanda R, Malla AK, Windell D, Harricharan R, Northcott S: Symptom and functional outcomes for a 5 year early intervention program for psychoses. Schizophr Res 2011;129:111–115.

19 Alvarez-Jimenez M, Gleeson JF, Henry LP, Harrigan SM, Harris MG, Killackey E, et al: Road to full recovery: longitudinal relationship between symptomatic remission and psychosocial recovery in first-episode psychosis over 7.5 years. Psychol Med 2012;42:595–606.

20 Morgan C, Lappin J, Heslin M, Donohoe K, Lomas B, Reininghaus U, et al: Reappraising the long-term course and outcome of psychotic disorders: the AESOP-10 study. Psychol Med 2014;44:2713–2726.

21 Chan SK, So HC, Hui CL, Chang WC, Lee EH, Chung DW, et al: 10-year outcome study of an early intervention program for psychosis compared with standard care service. Psychol Med 2015;45:1181–1193.

22 Insel TR: The arrival of pre-emptive psychiatry. Early Interv Psychiatry 2007;1:5–6.

23 Fusar-Poli P, Borgwardt S, Bechdolf A, Addington J, Riecher-Rossler A, Schultze-Lutter F, et al: the psychosis high-risk state: a comprehensive state-of-the-art review. JAMA Psychiatry 2013;70:107–120.

24 Yung AR, McGorry PD: The initial prodrome in psychosis: descriptive and qualitative aspects. Aust NZ J Psychiatry 1996;30:587–599.

25 Fusar-Poli P, Bonoldi I, Yung AR, Borgwardt S, Kempton MJ, Barale F, et al: Predicting psychosis: a meta-analysis of evidence. Arch Gen Psychiatry 2012;69:220–229.

26 Nelson B, Yuen HP, Wood SJ, Lin A, Spiliotacopoulos D, Bruxner A, et al: Long-term follow-up of a group at ultra high risk ('prodromal') for psychosis: the PACE 400 study. JAMA Psychiatry 2013;70:793–802.

27 Kaymaz N, Drukker M, Lieb R, Wittchen HU, Werbeloff N, Weiser M, et al: Do subthreshold psychotic experiences predict clinical outcomes in unselected non-help-seeking population-based samples? A systematic review and meta-analysis, enriched with new results. Psychol Med 2012;42:2239–2253.

28 Addington J, Cornblatt BA, Cadenhead KS, Cannon TD, McGlashan TH, Perkins DO, et al: At clinical high risk for psychosis: outcome for nonconverters. Am J Psychiatry 2011;168:800–805.

29 Simon AE, Borgwardt S, Riecher-Rossler A, Velthorst E, de Haan L, Fusar-Poli P: Moving beyond transition outcomes: meta-analysis of remission rates in individuals at high clinical risk for psychosis. Psychiatry Res 2013;209:266–272.

30 van Os J, Linscott RJ: Introduction: the extended psychosis phenotype –relationship with schizophrenia and with ultrahigh risk status for psychosis. Schizophr Bull 2012;38:227–230.

31 van Rossum I, Dominguez MD, Lieb R, Wittchen HU, van Os J: Affective dysregulation and reality distortion: a 10-year prospective study of their association and clinical relevance. Schizophr Bull 2011;37:561–571.

32 Varghese D, Scott J, Welham J, Bor W, Najman J, O'Callaghan M, et al: Psychotic-like experiences in major depression and anxiety disorders: a population-based survey in young adults. Schizophr Bull 2011;37:389–393.

33 Wigman JT, Lin A, Vollebergh WA, van Os J, Raaijmakers QA, Nelson B, et al: Subclinical psychosis and depression: co-occurring phenomena that do not predict each other over time. Schizophr Res 2011;130:277–281.

34 Fusar-Poli P, Yung AR, McGorry P, van Os J: Lessons learned from the psychosis high-risk state: towards a general staging model of prodromal intervention. Psychol Med 2014;44:17–24.

35 Schultze-Lutter F: Subjective symptoms of schizophrenia in research and the clinic: the basic symptom concept. Schizophr Bull 2009;35:5–8.

36 Schultze-Lutter F, Ruhrmann S, Berning J, Maier W, Klosterkotter J: Basic symptoms and ultrahigh risk criteria: symptom development in the initial prodromal state. Schizophr Bull 2010;36:182–191.

37 McGorry PD: Risk syndromes, clinical staging and DSM V: new diagnostic infrastructure for early intervention in psychiatry. Schizophr Res 2010;120:49–53.

38 Stochl J, Khandaker GM, Lewis G, Perez J, Goodyer IM, Zammit S, et al: Mood, anxiety and psychotic phenomena measure a common psychopathological factor. Psychol Med 2015;45:1483–1493.

39 Foulds GA, Bedford A: Hierarchy of classes of personal illness. Psychol Med 1975;5:181–192.

40 Kelleher I, Keeley H, Corcoran P, Lynch F, Fitzpatrick C, Devlin N, et al: Clinicopathological significance of psychotic experiences in non-psychotic young people: evidence from four population-based studies. Br J Psychiatry 2012;201:26–32.

41 McGorry PD, Nelson B, Goldstone S: Providing care to young people with emerging risk of psychosis: balancing potential risks and benefits. Clin Pract 2012;9:669–682.

42 Van Der Gaag M, Smit F, Bechdolf A, French P, Linszen D, Yung AR, et al: Preventing a first episode of psychosis: meta-analysis of randomised controlled prevention trials of 12 month and medium-term follow-ups. Schizophr Res 2013;149:56–62.

43 Amminger GP, Schafer MR, Papageorgiou K, Klier CM, Cotton SM, Harrigan SM, et al: Long-chain omega-3 fatty acids for indicated prevention of psychotic disorders: a randomised, placebo-controlled trial. Arch Gen Psychiatry 2010;67:146–154.

44 Kahn RS, Fleischhacker WW, Boter H, Davidson M, Vergouwe Y, Keet IP, et al: Effectiveness of antipsychotic drugs in first-episode schizophrenia and schizophreniform disorder: an open randomised clinical trial. Lancet 2008;371:1085–1097.

45 Early Psychosis Writing Group: Australian Clinical Guidelines for Early Psychosis, ed 2. Melbourne, Orygen Youth Health Research Centre, 2010.

46 IRIS: IRIS Early Intervention in Psychosis Guidelines, Revised 2012. 2012 www.iris-initiative.org.uk/.

47 Emsley R, Rabinowitz J, Medori R: Remission in early psychosis: rates, predictors, and clinical and functional outcome correlates. Schizophr Res 2007;89:129–139.

48 Alvarez-Jimenez M, Priede A, Hetrick SE, Bendall S, Killackey E, Parker AG, et al: Risk factors for relapse following treatment for first episode psychosis: a systematic review and meta-analysis of longitudinal studies. Schizophr Res 2012;139:116–128.

49 Chen EY, Hui CL, Lam MM, Chiu CP, Law CW, Chung DW, et al: Maintenance treatment with quetiapine versus discontinuation after one year of treatment in patients with remitted first episode psychosis: randomised controlled trial. BMJ 2010;341:c4024.

50 Emsley R, Nuamah I, Hough D, Gopal S: Treatment response after relapse in a placebo-controlled maintenance trial in schizophrenia. Schizophr Res 2012;138:29–34.

51 Gitlin M, Nuechterlein K, Subotnik K, Ventura J, Mintz J, Fogelson D, et al: Clinical outcome following neuroleptic discontinuation in patients with remitted recent-onset schizophrenia. Am J Psychiatry 2001;158:1835–1842.

52 Takeuchi H, Suzuki T, Uchida H, Watanabe K, Mimura M: Antipsychotic treatment for schizophrenia in the maintenance phase: a systematic review of the guidelines and algorithms. Schizophr Res 2012;134:219–225.

53 Emsley R, Chiliza B, Asmal L, Harvey BH: The nature of relapse in schizophrenia. BMC Psychiatry 2013;13:50.

54 Zipursky RB, Menezes NM, Streiner DL: Risk of symptom recurrence with medication discontinuation in first-episode psychosis: a systematic review. Schizophr Res 2014;152:408–414.

55 Wunderink L, Nieboer RM, Wiersma D, Sytema S, Nienhuis FJ: Recovery in remitted first episode psychosis at 7 years of follow-up of an early dose-reduction/discontinuation or maintenance strategy. JAMA Psychiatry 2013;70:913–920.

56 Wunderink L, Nienhuis FJ, Sytema S, Slooff CJ, Knegtering R, Wiersma D: Guided discontinuation versus maintenance treatment in remitted first-episode psychosis: relapse rates and functional outcome. J Clin Psychiatry 2007;68:654–661.

57 Andreasen NC, Liu D, Ziebell S, Vora A, Ho BC: Relapse duration, treatment intensity, and brain tissue loss in schizophrenia: a prospective longitudinal MRI study. Am J Psychiatry 2013;170:609–615.

58 Andreasen NC, Nopoulos P, Magnotta V, Pierson R, Ziebell S, Ho BC: Progressive brain change in schizophrenia: a prospective longitudinal study of first-episode schizophrenia. Biol Psychiatry 2011;70:672–679.

59 McGorry P, Alvarez-Jimenez M, Killackey E: Antipsychotic medication during the critical period following remission from first-episode psychosis: less is more. JAMA Psychiatry 2013;70:898–900.

60 Iyer SN, Loohuis H, Pawliuk N, Joober R, Malla AK: Concerns reported by family members of individuals with first-episode psychosis. Early Interv Psychiatry 2011;5:163–167.

61 Ramsay CE, Broussard B, Goulding SM, Cristofaro S, Hall D, Kaslow NJ, et al: Life and treatment goals of individuals hospitalised for first-episode nonaffective psychosis. Psychiatry Res 2011;189:344–348.

62 Gleeson JF, Cotton SM, Alvarez-Jimenez M, Wade D, Gee D, Crisp K, et al: A randomised controlled trial of relapse prevention therapy for first-episode psychosis patients: outcome at 30-month follow-up. Schizophr Bull 2013;39:436–448.

63 Gleeson JF, Cotton SM, Alvarez-Jimenez M, Wade D, Gee D, Crisp K, et al: A randomised controlled trial of relapse prevention therapy for first-episode psychosis patients. J Clin Psychiatry 2009;70:477–486.

64 Killackey E, Jackson HJ, McGorry PD: Vocational intervention in first-episode psychosis: individual placement and support v. treatment as usual. Br J Psychiatry 2008;193:114–120.

65 Bond GR: Supported employment: evidence for an evidence-based practice. Psychiatr Rehab J 2004;27:345–359.

66 Rinaldi M, Perkins R, McNeil K, Hickman N, Singh SP: The Individual Placement and Support approach to vocational rehabilitation for young people with first episode psychosis in the UK. J Ment Health 2010;19:483–491.

67 Birchwood M, Todd P, Jackson C: Early intervention in psychosis. The critical period hypothesis. Br J Psychiatry 1998;172:53–59.

68 Alvarez-Jimenez M, Bendall S, Lederman R, Wadley G, Chinnery G, Vargas S, et al: On the HORYZON: moderated online social therapy for long-term recovery in first episode psychosis. Schizophr Res 2013;2013:143–149.

69 Gleeson JF, Alvarez-Jimenez M, Lederman R: Moderated online social therapy for recovery from early psychosis. Psychiatr Serv 2012;63:719.

70 Edwards J, Cocks J, Burnett P, Maud D, Wong L, Yuen HP, et al: Randomised controlled trial of clozapine and CBT for first-episode psychosis with enduring positive symptoms: a pilot study. Schizophr Res Treatment 2011;2011:394896.

71 Agid O, Remington G, Kapur S, Arenovich T, Zipursky RB: Early use of clozapine for poorly responding first-episode psychosis. J Clin Psychopharmacol 2007;27:369–373.

72 Alvarez-Jimenez M, Gonzalez-Blanch C, Crespo-Facorro B, Hetrick S, Rodriguez-Sanchez JM, Perez-Iglesias R, et al: Antipsychotic-induced weight gain in chronic and first-episode psychotic disorders: a systematic critical reappraisal. CNS Drugs 2008;22:547–562.

73 Foley DL, Morley KI: Systematic review of early cardiometabolic outcomes of the first treated episode of psychosis. Arch Gen Psychiatry 2011;68:609–616.

74 Eapen V, Shiers D, Curtis J: Bridging the gap from evidence to policy and practice: reducing the progression to metabolic syndrome for children and adolescents on antipsychotic medication. Aust NZ J Psychiatry 2013;47:435–442.

75 Correll CU, Penzner JB, Parikh UH, Mughal T, Javed T, Carbon M, et al: Recognising and monitoring adverse events of second-generation antipsychotics in children and adolescents. Child Adolesc Psychiatr Clin North America 2006;15:177–206.

76 Alvarez-Jimenez M, Hetrick SE, Gonzalez-Blanch C, Gleeson JF, McGorry PD: Non-pharmacological management of antipsychotic-induced weight gain: systematic review and meta-analysis of randomised controlled trials. Br J Psychiatry 2008;193:101–107.

77 Alvarez-Jimenez M, Martinez-Garcia O, Perez-Iglesias R, Ramirez ML, Vazquez-Barquero JL, Crespo-Facorro B: Prevention of antipsychotic-induced weight gain with early behavioural intervention in first-episode psychosis: 2-year results of a randomised controlled trial. Schizophr Res 2010;116:16–19.

78 McGorry PD: The specialist youth mental health model: strengthening the weakest link in the public mental health system. Med J Aust 2007;187:S53–S56.

79 McGorry P, Bates T, Birchwood M: Designing youth mental health services for the 21st century: examples from Australia, Ireland and the UK. Br J Psychiatry 2013;54:s30–s35.

80 McGorry PD, Tanti C, Stokes R, Hickie IB, Carnell K, Littlefield LK, et al: headspace: Australia's National Youth Mental Health Foundation – where young minds come first. Med J Aust 2007;187:S68–S70.

81 Edwards J, McGorry P: Implementing Early Intervention in Psychosis: A Guide to Establishing Early Psychosis Services. London, Martin Dunitz, 2002.

82 Hughes F, Stavely H, Simpson R, Goldstone S, Pennell K, McGorry P: At the heart of an early psychosis centre: the core components of the 2014 Early Psychosis Prevention and Intervention Centre model for Australian communities. Australas Psychiatry 2014;22:228–234.

83 McCrone P, Craig TK, Power P, Garety PA: Cost-effectiveness of an early intervention service for people with psychosis. Br J Psychiatry 2010;196:377–382.

84 Mihalopoulos C, Harris M, Henry L, Harrigan S, McGorry P: Is early intervention in psychosis cost-effective over the long term? Schizophr Bull 2009;35:909–918.

85 Garety PA, Craig TK, Dunn G, Fornells-Ambrojo M, Colbert S, Rahaman N, et al: Specialised care for early psychosis: symptoms, social functioning and patient satisfaction: randomised controlled trial. Br J Psychiatry 2006;188:37–45.

86 Bloom DE, Cafiero ET, Jane-Llopis E, Abrahams-Gessel S, Bloom LR, Fathima S, et al: The global economic burden of non-communicable disease. Geneva, World Economic Forum, 2011.

Prof. Patrick D. McGorry
Orygen, The National Centre of Excellence in Youth Mental Health
University of Melbourne, 35 Poplar Road
Parkville, VIC 3052 (Australia)
E-Mail pmcgorry@unimelb.edu.au

Riecher-Rössler A, McGorry PD (eds): Early Detection and Intervention in Psychosis: State of the Art and Future Perspectives. Key Issues Ment Health. Basel, Karger, 2016, vol 181, pp 29–41 (DOI: 10.1159/000440912)

First Signs of Emerging Psychosis

Frauke Schultze-Lutter

University Hospital of Child and Adolescent Psychiatry and Psychotherapy, University of Bern, Bern, Switzerland

Abstract

The majority of first-episode psychoses are preceded by a prodromal phase that is several years on average, frequently leads to some decline in psychosocial functioning and offers the opportunity for early detection within the framework of an indicated prevention. To this, two approaches are currently mainly followed. The ultra-high-risk (UHR) criteria were explicitly developed to predict first-episode psychosis within 12 months, and indeed the majority of conversions in clinical UHR samples seem to occur within the first 12 months of initial assessment. Their main criterion, the attenuated psychotic symptoms criterion, captures symptoms that resemble positive symptoms of psychosis (i.e. delusions, hallucinations and formal thought disorders) with the exception that some level of insight is still maintained, and these frequently compromise functioning already. In contrast, the basic symptom criteria try to catch patients at increased risk of psychoses at the earliest possible time, i.e. ideally when only the first subtle disturbances in information processing have developed that are experienced with full insight and do not yet overload the person's coping abilities, and thus have not yet resulted in any functional decline. First results from prospective studies not only support this view, but indicate that the combination of both approaches might be a more favorable way to increase sensitivity and detect risk earlier, as well as to establish a change-sensitive risk stratification approach.
© 2016 S. Karger AG, Basel

The idea to detect psychosis early, desirably even before the onset of the first frank psychotic episode, goes far back. As early as 1932, the German psychiatrist Wilhelm Mayer-Gross (1889–1961), an important member of the 'Heidelberg school' of psychopathology until his emigration to the UK in 1933, wondered 'why hitherto one has so infrequently made use of the impressive experience that is represented by the first irruption of a thought disorder, a decrease in activity, an aberration in sympathy and other emotions into the healthy personality' [1, p. 296; translation by the author] of persons with emerging psychosis. His detailed and illustrated description of the subtle first symptoms of an insidious onset was one of the first comprehensive descriptions of prodromal symptoms of first-episode psychosis and a main source of inspiration for the subsequent works of Gerd Huber (1921–2012), i.e. for the development of the concept of basic symptoms [2–4].

The Concept of Basic Symptoms

Starting in the 1960s, Gerd Huber gradually developed the concept of basic symptoms from two different lines of his work [2]: from the detailed psychopathological reconstruction of the development of first-episode schizophrenia and its subsequent course in the Bonn Schizophrenia Study [5], and from his pioneer pneumoencephalographic study showing enlarged third ventricles in schizophrenic patients [6, 7]. In presumption of two main aspects of the basic symptom concept, Mayer-Gross [1] had already conceptually distinguished between first uncharacteristic (e.g. lack of motivation and obsessive-compulsive phenomena) and first characteristic signs of developing schizophrenia (e.g. subtle disturbances in thinking, salience, affect and interpersonal relatedness). Moreover, he considered these early symptoms not as part of the premorbid personality that – equal to basic symptoms – would be present 'already pre-*psychotically* but precisely not pre-*morbidly*' [2, p.134; translated by the author; italics as in original]. Against this background, Huber [2, 8] later introduced the term 'substrate-close basic symptoms' to delineate his conviction that these early and often initially occurring subjective symptoms would form the basis for the development of psychotic 'end phenomena' and be the most immediate reportable self-experience of the somatic processes underlying the illness, i.e. disturbances in cortical information processing. Therefore, Huber regarded basic symptoms as '*micro-productive* positive symptoms in statu nascendi' [2, p.135; translated by the author; italics as in original] that had a closer association to neurobiological aberrations than positive psychotic and also negative symptoms [2, 8] (fig. 1). This assumption was recently supported by a functional magnetic resonance imaging study [9] that provided evidence for a cortical link between basic symptoms but not positive, negative or general symptoms and social cognition in first-episode schizophrenia. Aberrant functional interactions of the right ventral premotor cortex and bilateral posterior insula with the posterior cingulate cortex positively correlated with the total score of basic symptoms assessed with the Schizophrenia Proneness Instrument, Adult version (SPI-A) [10], but not with the any of the subscale totals of the Positive and Negative Syndrome Scale (PANSS) [11]. The authors suggested that this dysfunction might be closely related to basic symptoms and might help to disentangle the cortical basis of how self-experienced disturbances, i.e. basic symptoms, may effect social functioning [9].

Basic symptoms usually do not develop continuously and linearly into psychotic symptoms, but rather fluctuate in their appearance and severity, i.e. alternate between uncharacteristic 'stage 1' and more characteristic 'stage 2' basic symptoms as well as diagnostically subthreshold 'stage 3' symptoms [2, 12]. They might as well spontaneously remit completely, thus not strictly being part of a prodrome but rather of an 'outpost syndrome' (fig. 1). These symptom fluctuations are in response to endogenous factors as well as to situational factors such as daily stressors or even minimal affective arousal [2, 12]. Insufficient coping, including the development of inadequate explanatory models, then eventually leads to the development of stage 3 'end phenomena', i.e. attenuated

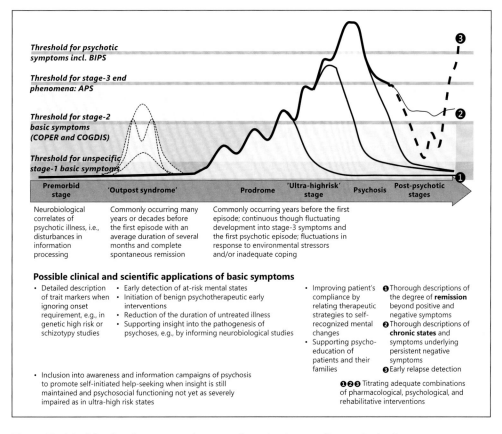

Fig. 1. Model of the development and course of psychosis according to the basic symptom concept and possible applications of basic symptoms in different illness stages [13, 14].

and frank psychotic symptoms. Basic symptoms and initiation of inadequate or lack of coping strategies for these also trigger negative symptoms such as withdrawal in response to a self-perceived decreased stress tolerance or desire for social contacts or even as a reaction to cognitive disturbances possibly impairing communication skills [2, 12].

Basic symptoms can be assessed by trained clinicians in a thorough clinical interview in all stages of psychotic disorders, and can thus serve multiple clinical and scientific purposes (fig. 1) [13]. However, their perception and assessment might be severely impaired by the loss of insight and of reality testing that commonly characterizes the acute psychotic episode [3, 4, 10, 14].

General Characteristics of Basic Symptoms

An obligate characteristic of basic symptoms is their subjectivity, i.e. their experience and report as disturbances or aberrations from 'normal' fluctuations in mental state known from the premorbid phase by patients themselves [10, 12–15]. Experienced with full insight, basic symptoms are thereby immediately recognized as dysfunctions in mental processes and not projected into the environment. As a result, basic symptoms either might be qualitatively new (in terms of a state marker) or might significantly increase in frequency while decreasing in their association to situational triggers at the same time (in terms of a trait-state marker). Consequently, phenomena that have clearly been present throughout life in the same severity or frequency (in terms of a trait marker) would not be considered basic symptoms by definition [3, 10, 13, 14], although they can be scored as a trait characteristic in both the SPI-A and the Schizophrenia Proneness Instrument, Child and Youth version (SPI-CY) [14].

Despite their conception as a direct expression of the underlying neurobiological dysfunction, a diagnosed neurological or another somatic disorder that might account for the disturbance is an exclusion criterion of basic symptoms. Further, phenomena that result from psychotropic substance use or that are a side effect of (psycho-)pharmacological medication are not considered basic symptoms [10, 14]. When these exclusion criteria were deliberately ignored, basic symptoms were reported to a degree similar to that of psychotic patients and clinical high-risk patients with later development of psychosis by patients with organic mental disorder [16] and patients with substance misuse, in particular of ketamine and cannabis [17], respectively.

Basic Symptoms in the Early Detection of First-Episode Psychosis

In the first long-term prospective early detection study, the Cologne Early Recognition (CER) study [18, 19], the predictive utility of basic symptoms was explored in 160 patients over an average 9.6-year follow-up (with a minimum follow-up of 5 years), and two basic symptom criteria were generated (tables 1, 2): the 'cognitive-perceptive basic symptoms' (COPER) criterion [18] and the 'cognitive disturbances' (COGDIS) criterion [19]. Within this sample, nearly 50% (n = 79) had converted to psychosis; the COPER criterion was associated with a conversion rate of 65%, while the COGDIS criterion was associated with one of 79% (fig. 2). COPER had a higher sensitivity and would have missed to detect only 13% of converters at baseline, while COGDIS would have missed 33% [20]. However, with no intermediate assessments, it remained unclear if these false-negative cases would have been detectable as risk cases at a later point in time before the development of psychosis. Further, due to the lack of subthreshold psychotic symptom assessment, it also remained unclear whether these cases had already developed some psychotic-like, yet not frank psychotic symptoms, in which only some insight was still remained [in terms of the later developing ultra-high-risk (UHR) criteria] and thus had already been compromised in their report of basic symptoms. For example, 'unstable ideas of reference' that are part of COPER and COGDIS (tables 1, 2) are defined as subjective, subclinical experiences of self-reference that are almost immediately rectified on further consideration without hav-

Table 1. Basic symptom criterion COPER according to the SPI-A [10] and SPI-CY [14]

COPER

Symptom criterion: presence of at least 1 of the following 10 basic symptoms:
    Thought interference (C2/D.9)[1]
    Thought perseveration (O1/D.14)
    Thought pressure (D3/D.10)
    Thought blockages (C3/D.15)
    Disturbance of receptive speech (C4/D.11)
    Disturbance in discriminating ideas and perception, phantasy and true memory contents (O2/B.1)
    Unstable ideas of reference (D4/B.2)
    Derealization (O8/B.7)
    Visual perception disturbances, excl. hypersensitivity to light and blurred vision (D5, F2-3, O4/B.3, O.1)
    Acoustic perception disturbances, excl. hypersensitivity to sound (F5, O5/B.4.2, B.5)

Onset criterion: the basic symptom has first been noted at least 12 months ago

Frequency criterion: for any period of time within the past 3 months, the basic symptom has occurred at a frequency of at least once per week (this corresponds to a severity rating on the SPI of at least 3)

[1] First item numbers are according to the SPI-A, second ones according to the SPI-CY.

Table 2. Basic symptom criterion COGDIS according to the SPI-A [10] and SPI-CY [14]

COGDIS

Symptom criterion: presence of at least 2 of the following 9 basic symptoms:
    Thought interference (C2/D.9)[1]
    Thought pressure (D3/D.10)
    Thought blockages (C3/D.15)
    Disturbance of receptive speech (C4/D.11)
    Disturbance of expressive speech (C5/D.12)
    Disturbance in abstract thinking (O3/D.7)
    Unstable ideas of reference (D4/B.2)
    Inability to divide attention (B1/D.8)
    Captivation of attention by details of the visual field (O7/O.2)

Frequency criterion: for any period of time within the past 3 months, each basic symptom has occurred at a frequency of at least once per week (this corresponds to a severity rating on the SPI of at least 3)

[1] First item numbers are according to the SPI-A, second ones according to the SPI-CY.

ing a clear explanation for this feeling or looking for one outside one's own mental processes. Thus, the development of 'ideas of reference' in terms of UHR-relevant attenuated psychotic symptoms (APS; i.e. relating random events to oneself, and at least for some time, considering this a correct experience and weighing pros and cons) excludes simultaneous rating of this basic symptom – although both can alternate depending on the level of stress and overall mental state [14].

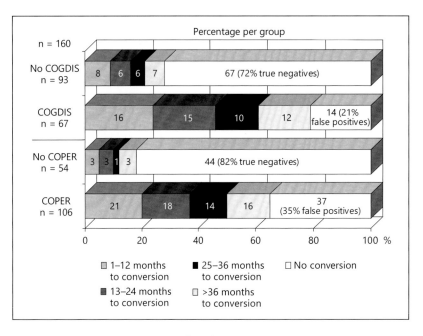

Fig. 2. Conversion rates and time of the basic symptom criteria COPER and COGDIS in the criteria generation sample (n = 160), irrespective of the potential presence of UHR criteria or of each other [18–20].

Other than the basic symptom approach that aims at the detection of emerging psychosis at the earliest possible time, i.e. desirably at the onset of the first sufficiently specific prodromal symptom, the UHR criteria [21] were developed with the explicit aim to predict conversion to psychosis within 1 year [22, 23] and were mainly modelled on subthreshold psychotic-like experiences as defined by Chapman and Chapman [24] and positive features of schizotypal personality disorder [25]. In light of the basic symptom concept, these symptoms [APS and brief intermittent psychotic symptoms (BIPS)] already represent stage-3 'end phenomena' that result from inadequate coping and search for an explanatory model (fig. 1). Thus, unsurprisingly, APS and BIPS are commonly associated with significant functional impairments [21, 26]. For the high long-term costs incurred by the functional impairments associated with psychotic disorders [27, 28], the prevention of persistent functional impairment has always been an important aim of preventive efforts and is increasingly moving into the focus of early intervention studies in psychosis-risk samples [29, 30].

The German Research Network Schizophrenia (GRNS) [31] followed this approach and established a related two-step intervention model: a cognitive-behavioral oriented psychotherapeutic intervention for the earlier risk stage characterized symptomatically by COPER, and a low-dose antipsychotic pharmacological intervention for the late risk stage characterized by APS and BIPS [32]. While development of a psychotic first episode was the main outcome measure in the late-stage project, in the early-stage project, any progression to a more severe, psychotic-like stage, i.e. to either frank psychosis or APS or BIPS, was the main outcome measure. In the early-stage supportive counselling control condition, 17% of COPER subjects not exhibiting APS or BIPS at baseline had converted to psychosis at the 2-year follow-up, with an additional 3% to a late-risk stage, i.e. had developed APS or BIPS [33]. Furthermore, the assumed sequence from unspecific symptoms (stage 1) to specific cognitive-perceptive basic symptoms (stage 2) and next via APS to BIPS and frank psychotic symptoms (stage 3) was broadly confirmed in a retrospective study of first-episode psychosis adult inpatients [34] conducted as part of the GRNS. This study also indicated a high sensitivity of COPER and APS for psychoses of more than 80% even in those not seeking help before the onset of the first psychotic episode. The authors discussed the results in support of the notion of COPER as at least a complementary approach to the UHR criteria, which may also allow for an earlier detection of psychosis [34].

Psychosis-Predictive Utility of Basic Symptom Criteria

A recent meta-analysis [22] conducted as part of the Guidance Project of the European Psychiatric Association (EPA) [35] supported the psychosis-predictive utility of both the basic symptom criteria, in particular COGDIS, and the UHR criteria, in particular APS and BIPS, and recommended these three criteria as sufficiently evidence-based alternative risk criteria in help-seeking patient samples. This meta-analysis of 42 samples including almost 5,000 patients (those lost to follow-up were conservatively regarded as nonconverters) revealed pooled conversion rates for COGDIS of 25.3% (95% CI: 22.5–28.1) at the 1-year follow-up, 28.4% (95% CI: 21.3–35.6) at the 2-year follow-up and 50.0% (95% CI: 39.7–60.4) at the 3-year follow-up, rising to 54.9% (95% CI: 41.8–68.1) at the 4-year follow-up and to 61.3% (95% CI: 43.9–78.9) beyond this time (fig. 3) [22]. For COPER, less studies were available (this being the main reason to not include it at present in risk criteria recommendations), and pooled conversion rates could only be calculated for 1- and 2-year follow-ups, where they were 14.4% (95% CI: 7.2–21.5) and 21.1% (95% CI: 10.7–31.5), respectively [22]. By comparison, based on a larger number of studies, in particular at the 1-, 2- and 3-year follow-ups, the UHR criteria irrespective of their assessment had pooled conversion rates of 15.0% (95% CI: 12.8–17.1) at the 1-year follow-up, 19.4% (95% CI: 17.6–21.1) at the 2-year follow-up and 29.1% (95% CI: 25.5–32.6) at the 3-year follow-up, but only rose to 37.0% (95% CI: 33.7–40.2) at follow-ups longer than 4 years [4] (fig. 3). Thereby, COGDIS and UHR samples – irrespective of the potential co-occurrence of criteria – did not significantly differ in 1- and 2-year conversion rates, but did in conversion rates at 3 years and beyond with significantly higher conversion rates in the COGDIS samples [22] (fig. 3). This indicates that basic symptoms or rather COGDIS are indeed able to detect the emerging psychotic disorder quite early, even years before its onset,

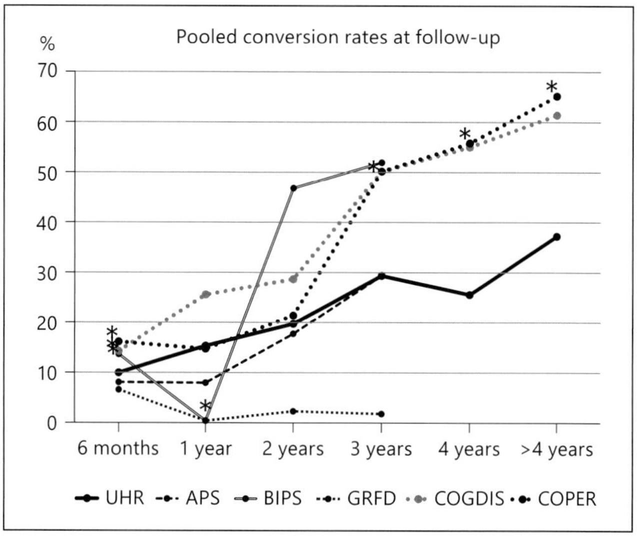

Fig. 3. Pooled conversion rates of risk criteria irrespective of each other at different follow-ups according to Schultze-Lutter et al. [22]. * Indicates not pooled but single-study conversion rates. GRFD = Genetic risk and functional decline criterion of the UHR criteria.

and do so at least as well as the UHR criteria. A trend towards higher conversion rates in studies including basic symptom criteria had also been described in an early meta-analysis [36] that further reported a higher rate of conversions to schizophrenia compared to other psychotic disorders in basic symptom studies compared to exclusive UHR studies.

Combining Basic Symptoms and Ultra-High-Risk Criteria

While many studies have employed either UHR or basic symptom criteria [22], studies that employed both approaches [37–40] consistently reported significantly higher conversion rates in patients simultaneously meeting UHR criteria, mainly APS, and basic symptom criteria, in all instances COGDIS, than in patients considered at increased risk for psychosis for one but not the other approach. For example, a study examining 4-year conversion rates in 246 patients presenting to an early detection service with and without an increased psychosis-risk according to COGDIS and/or symptomatic UHR criteria assessed with the Structured Interview for Prodromal Syndromes (SIPS) [41] reported a roughly 2.5-times higher conversion risk in patients with the combination of UHR and COGDIS at baseline compared to those with UHR or COGDIS alone [38]. Thereby, the hazard rates at 48 months were 0.66 for the combination that was met by a good 50% of patients, 0.28 for only UHR reported by 15% and 0.23 for the 12% of patients with only COGDIS. By contrast, the 21% of patients not reporting COGDIS or symptomatic UHR criteria only revealed a hazard rate of 0.14 at 4 years [38]. Interestingly, all conversions in the UHR-only group occurred within 8 months after baseline, while conversions in the COGDIS-only group

Schultze-Lutter

occurred within 6–34 months. The combination group exhibited a steady increase in the conversion rate throughout the 4 years that, however, leveled after 30 months [38]. From their results, and in line with other studies [37, 39, 40], the authors drew two main conclusions: (1) the alternative employment of symptomatic UHR criteria and COGDIS (APS/BIPS *or* COGDIS) in the detection of an increased risk for psychosis considerably increases sensitivity in persons truly at risk for psychosis by detecting those missed by employing only one approach, and (2) the combined employment of UHR criteria and COGDIS (APS/BIPS *and* COGDIS) clearly reduces the risk of false-positive predictions (i.e. considerably increases specificity). Furthermore, the consideration of both approaches might enable a risk stratification in terms of both overall risk for conversion and time to conversion [38] that might also inform the choice of intervention.

Basic Symptoms in Children and Adolescents

All but one early detection study using basic symptoms have been conducted so far in samples of mainly adult patients [42]. In this first early detection study on adolescents, 18% of those who had reported COGDIS had converted to psychosis at the 2-year follow-up [43]. Yet, it is so far unclear if the same criteria can be used in children and adolescents or if developmental aspects need to be considered in young age groups [42]. This is clearly the case for UHR criteria as the most recent meta-analysis [22] had already revealed a significant age effect in conversion rates. Compared to predominately adult samples of patients 18 years of age and older, and even compared to age-mixed samples with a majority of patients below age 18, samples including predominately or exclusively children and adolescents (mainly between 12 and 18 years of age) had significantly lower conversion rates across different follow-ups. Yet, for lack of data, it could not be explored whether these lower conversion rates were signaling a risk-diluting or a risk-delaying effect. A risk-delaying effect in children and adolescents might be related to the more insidious onset of early-onset compared to adult-onset psychosis [44]. A risk-diluting effect might be related to a lesser clinical significance of UHR criteria in adolescents that was indicated by the higher prevalence of perception-related phenomena in young age groups, particularly in those below the age of 16 years [45], in community studies [45, 46] and in a study of self-reported APS-like phenomena in an unselected clinical sample [47]. In either case, the same age-related pattern might be present in COPER samples as COPER also includes perception disturbances, but not in any case for COGDIS, which does not involve perception-related basic symptoms and thus might mainly be affected by a risk-delaying effect of young age.

The need to consider developmental peculiarities in the use of basic symptoms in children and adolescents has been indicated by various studies [4, 14, 42, 48]. These indications include the different dimensional structure of basic symptoms in children and adolescents compared to adults in different states of psychosis, i.e. from prodrome to multiepisode chronic schizophrenia [4]. The structural analyses implicated that adynamic features (disturbances in energy, motivation, interest, stress tolerance, mood and emotional responsiveness, as well as concentration, attention and memory problems) that were broadly unspecific for psychoses in adult samples play a central role in early-onset psychoses [4]. In support of this, the dimension 'adynamia' was clearly most pronounced in young risk patients compared to inpatients without indication of an increased risk for psychosis and controls from the community in a first pilot study [48] of the SPI-CY [13]. The SPI-CY was developed to account for the different dimensional structure in children and adolescents, and to accommodate the need to include third person/parent reports in the assessment of basic symptoms, in particular in children [14, 48]. So far, the SPI-CY is the only early detection instrument especially developed for children and adolescents [49]. In a first validation study of the SPI-CY on three groups of children and adolescents (8–18 years of age), the groups differed significantly on all four SPI-CY subscales [48]. Thereby, all subscales were most pronounced in patients considered at risk for psychosis for basic symptom and/or UHR criteria compared to both inpatient and community controls; in the latter group, subscales were least pronounced. The same pattern was also evident, at least on a descriptive level, for most items. Thus, the authors concluded that the SPI-CY might possess good concurrent validity and be a helpful tool for detecting and assessing basic symptoms in the psychosis spectrum in children and adolescents, by whom it was well received [48]. These results were in line with an earlier study of basic symptoms in patients with early-onset psychoses, inpatients with other disorders and controls of the community [50]. It also reported the highest number of basic symptoms in early-onset psychosis and by far the lowest in community controls [50]. Yet, these results require validation in larger samples of children and adolescents, and the psychosis-predictive ability of the SPI-CY subscales in different age groups will have to be explored in longitudinal studies.

Conclusion

Basic symptom criteria, in particular COGDIS, allow the identification of older adolescents and adults at high risk of developing psychosis in persons seeking help for mental problems already at a very early stage, and appear to be sufficiently sensitive, i.e. frequent prior to onset of the first psychotic episode in both adult-onset and early-onset psychosis. Further, COPER and COGDIS, and their included symptoms, also seem to be sufficiently rare in adolescents of the general population to be considered nonnormal, possibly psychopathological phenomena. With regard to the symptomatic UHR criteria, the combination of both approaches might be the most favorable way to increase sensitivity and earliness of risk detection, as well as to establish a change-sensitive risk stratification approach. However, the lower conversion rates, and possibly more frequent, less clinically significant perceptual phenomena – that are not included in COGDIS – in adolescent risk samples, call for caution with regard to communicating the possible risk for psychosis and the initiation of preventive treatment in minors [22, 30]. Therefore, there is a need for further studies of potential developmental peculiarities in the early detection of psychosis.

References

1 Mayer-Gross W: Die Schizophrenie. Die Klinik; in Bumke O (ed): Handbuch der Geisteskrankheiten. Berlin, Springer, 1932, pp 293–578.

2 Huber G: Prodrome der Schizophrenie. Fortschr Neurol Psychiatr 1995;63:131–137.

3 Schultze-Lutter F: Subjective symptoms of schizophrenia in research and the clinic: the basic symptom concept. Schizophr Bull 2009;35:5–8.

4 Schultze-Lutter F, Ruhrmann S, Fusar-Poli P, Bechdolf A, Schimmelmann B, Klosterkötter J: Basic symptoms and the prediction of first-episode psychosis. Curr Pharm Des 2012;18:351–357.

5 Huber G, Gross G, Schüttler R, Linz M: Longitudinal studies of schizophrenic patients. Schizophr Bull 1980;6:592–605.

6 Huber G: Klinische und neuroradiologische Untersuchungen an chronisch Schizophrenen. Nervenarzt 1961;32:7–15.

7 Huber G: Pneumoencephalographische und Psychopathologische Bilder bei Endogenen Psychosen. Berlin, Springer, 1957.

8 Huber G: Das Konzept substratnaher Basissymptome und seine Bedeutung für Theorie und Therapie schizophrener Erkrankungen. Nervenarzt 1983;54:23–32.

9 Ebisch SJ, Mantini D, Northoff G, Salone A, De Berardis D, Ferri F, Ferro FM, Di Giannantonio M, Romani GL, Gallese V: Altered brain long-range functional interactions underlying the link between aberrant self-experiences and self-other relationship in first-episode schizophrenia. Schizophr Bull 2014; 40:1072–1082.

10 Schultze-Lutter F, Addington J, Ruhrmann S, Klosterkötter J: Schizophrenia Proneness Instrument, Adult version (SPI-A). Rome, Giovanni Fioriti Editore, 2007.

11 Kay SR, Fiszbein A, Opler LA: The Positive and Negative Syndrome Scale (PANSS) for schizophrenia. Schizophr Bull 1987;13:261–276.

12 Gross G, Huber G: Das Basissymptomkonzept idiopathischer Psychosen. Zentralbl Neurol Psychiatr 1989;252:655–673.

13 Schultze-Lutter F, Schimmelmann BG: Early detection and treatment of psychosis: the Bern Child and Adolescent Psychiatric Perspective. Adv Psychiatry 2014, DOI: 10.1155/2014/365283.

14 Schultze-Lutter F, Marshall M, Koch E: Schizophrenia Proneness Instrument, Child and Youth version; extended English translation (SPI-CY EET). Rome, Giovanni Fioriti Editore, 2012.

15 Schultze-Lutter F, Ruhrmann S: Früherkennung und Frühbehandlung von Psychosen. Bremen, Uni-Med, 2008.

16 Klosterkötter J, Ebel H, Schultze-Lutter F, Steinmeyer EM: Diagnostic validity of basic symptoms. Eur Arch Psychiatry Clin Neurosci 1996;246:147–154.

17 Morgan CJ, Duffin S, Hunt S, Monaghan L, Mason O, Curran HV: Neurocognitive function and schizophrenia-proneness in individuals dependent on ketamine, on high potency cannabis ('skunk') or on cocaine. Pharmacopsychiatry 2012;45:269–274.

18 Klosterkötter J, Hellmich M, Steinmeyer EM, Schultze-Lutter F: Diagnosing schizophrenia in the initial prodromal phase. Arch Gen Psychiatry 2001;58: 158–164.

19 Schultze-Lutter F: Früherkennung der Schizophrenie anhand subjektiver Beschwerde-schilderungen: ein methoden-kritischer Vergleich der Vorhersageleistung nonparametrischer statistischer und alternativer Verfahren zur Generierung von Vorhersagemodellen (dissertation). Cologne, Universität zu Köln, 2001. http://kups.ub.uni-koeln.de/id/eprint/588.

20 Schultze-Lutter F, Ruhrmann S, Klosterkötter J: Can schizophrenia be predicted phenomenologically?; in Johannessen JO, Martindale B, Cullberg J (eds): Evolving Psychosis. Different Stages, Different Treatments. London, Routledge, 2006, pp 104–123.

21 Fusar-Poli P, Borgwardt S, Bechdolf A, Addington J, Riecher-Rössler A, Schultze-Lutter F, Keshavan M, Wood SJ, Ruhrmann S, Seidman LJ, Valmaggia L, Cannon T, Velthorst E, De Haan L, Cornblatt B, Bonoldi I, Birchwood M, McGlashan TH, Carpenter W, McGorry P, Klosterkötter J, McGuire P, Yung AR: The psychosis high-risk state: a comprehensive state-of-the-art review. JAMA Psychiatry 2013;70: 107–120.

22 Schultze-Lutter F, Michel C, Schmidt SJ, Benno G, Schimmelmann BG, Maric NP, Salokangas RKR, Riecher-Rössler A, van der Gaag M, Nordentoft M, Raballo A, Meneghelli A, Marshall M, Morrison A, Ruhrmann S, Klosterkötter J: EPA guidance on the early detection of clinical high risk states of psychosis. Eur Psychiatry 2015;30:405–416.

23 Phillips LJ, Yung AR, McGorry PD: Identification of young people at risk of psychosis: validation of Personal Assessment and Crisis Evaluation Clinic intake criteria. Aust NZ J Psychiatry 2000;34(suppl):S164–S169.

24 Chapman LJ, Chapman JP: Scales for rating psychotic and psychotic-like experiences as continua. Schizophr Bull 1980;6:477–489.

25 Debanné M, Eliez S, Badoud D, Conus P, Flückiger R, Schultze-Lutter F: Developing psychosis and its risk states through the lens of schizotypy. Schizophr Bull, DOI: 10.1093/schbul/sbu176.

26 Ruhrmann S, Paruch J, Bechdolf A, Pukrop R, Wagner M, Berning J, Schultze-Lutter F, Janssen B, Gaebel W, Möller HJ, Maier W, Klosterkötter J: Reduced subjective quality of life in persons at risk for psychosis. Acta Psychiatr Scand 2008;117:357–368.

27 Olesen J, Gustavsson A, Svensson M, Wittchen HU, Jönsson B; CDBE2010 Study Group; European Brain Council: The economic cost of brain disorders in Europe. Eur J Neurol 2012;19:155–162.

28 Gore FM, Bloem PJ, Patton GC, Ferguson J, Joseph V, Coffey C, Sawyer SM, Mathers CD: Global burden of disease in young people aged 10–24 years: a systematic analysis. Lancet 2011;377:2093–2102.

29 Campion J, Bhui K, Bhugra D; European Psychiatric Association: European Psychiatric Association (EPA) guidance on prevention of mental disorders. Eur Psychiatry 2012;27:68–80.

30 Schmidt SJ, Schultze-Lutter F, Schimmelmann BG, Maric NP, Salokangas RKR, Riecher-Rössler A, van der Gaag M, Meneghelli A, Nordentoft M, Marshall M, Morrison A, Raballo A, Klosterkötter J, Ruhrmann S: EPA guidance on the early intervention in clinical high-risk states of psychoses. Eur Psychiatry 2015;30:388–404.

31 Häfner H, Maurer K, Ruhrmann S, Bechdolf A, Klosterkötter J, Wagner M, Maier W, Bottlender R, Möller HJ, Gaebel W, Wölwer W: Early detection and secondary prevention of psychosis: facts and visions. Eur Arch Psychiatry Clin Neurosci 2004;254:117–128.

32 Ruhrmann S, Schultze-Lutter F, Klosterkötter J: Early detection and intervention in the initial prodromal phase of schizophrenia. Pharmacopsychiatry 2003;36(suppl 3):162–167.

33 Bechdolf A, Wagner M, Ruhrmann S, Harrigan S, Putzfeld V, Pukrop R, Brockhaus-Dumke A, Berning J, Janssen B, Decker P, Bottlender R, Maurer K, Möller HJ, Gaebel W, Häfner H, Maier W, Klosterkötter J: Preventing progression to first-episode psychosis in early initial prodromal states. Br J Psychiatry 2012;200:22–29.

34 Schultze-Lutter F, Ruhrmann S, Berning J, Maier W, Klosterkötter J: Basic symptoms and ultrahigh risk criteria: symptom development in the initial prodromal state. Schizophr Bull 2010;36:182–191.

35 Gaebel W, Möller HJ: European guidance: a project of the European Psychiatric Association. Eur Psychiatry 2012;27:65–67.

36 Fusar-Poli P, Bechdolf A, Taylor MJ, Bonoldi I, Carpenter WT, Yung AR, McGuire P: At risk for schizophrenic or affective psychoses? A meta-analysis of DSM/ICD diagnostic outcomes in individuals at high clinical risk. Schizophr Bull 2013;39:923–932.

37 Ruhrmann S, Schultze-Lutter F, Salokangas RKR, Heinimaa M, Linszen D, Dingemans P, Birchwood M, Patterson P, Juckel G, Heinz A, Morrison A, Lewis S, Graf von Reventlow H, Klosterkötter J: Prediction of psychosis in adolescents and young adults – results from the Prospective European Multicenter Study (EPOS). Arch Gen Psychiatry 2010;67:241–251.

38 Schultze-Lutter F, Klosterkötter J, Ruhrmann S: Improving the clinical prediction of psychosis by combining ultra-high risk criteria and cognitive basic symptoms. Schizophr Res 2014;154:100–106.

39 Michel C, Ruhrmann S, Schimmelmann BG, Klosterkötter J, Schultze-Lutter F: A stratified model for psychosis prediction in clinical practice. Schizophr Bull 2014;40:1533–1542.

40 Marshall M, Johnson C, Neelam K, Drake R: Predicting psychosis in clinical practice: outcome of patients seen in an NHS Prodrome Clinic. Eur Arch Psychiatry Clin Neurosci 2013;63(suppl 1):S14.

41 McGlashan TH, Walsh B, Woods S: The Psychosis-Risk Syndrome. Handbook for Diagnosis and Follow-Up. New York, Oxford University Press, 2010.

42 Schimmelmann BG, Schultze-Lutter F: Early detection and intervention of psychosis in children and adolescents: urgent need for studies. Eur Child Adolesc Psychiatry 2012;21:239–241.

43 Ziermans TB, Schothorst PF, Sprong M, van Engeland H: Transition and remission in adolescents at ultra-high risk for psychosis. Schizophr Res 2011;126:58–64.

44 Cornblatt BA, Lencz T, Smith CW, Olsen R, Auther AM, Nakayama E, Lesser ML, Tai JY, Shah MR, Foley CA, Kane JM, Correll CU: Can antidepressants be used to treat the schizophrenia prodrome? Results of a prospective, naturalistic treatment study of adolescents. J Clin Psychiatry 2007;68:546–557.

45 Schimmelmann BG, Michel C, Martz-Irngartinger A, Linder C, Schultze-Lutter F: Age matters in the prevalence and clinical significance of ultra-high-risk for psychosis symptoms and criteria in the general population: findings from the BEAR and BEARS-Kid studies. World Psychiatry 2015;14:189–197.

46 Kelleher I, Keeley H, Corcoran P, Lynch F, Fitzpatrick C, Devlin N, Molloy C, Roddy S, Clarke MC, Harley M, Arseneault L, Wasserman C, Carli V, Sarchiapone M, Hoven C, Wasserman D, Cannon M: Clinicopathological significance of psychotic experiences in non-psychotic young people: evidence from four population-based studies. Br J Psychiatry 2012; 201:26–32.

47 Brandizzi M, Schultze-Lutter F, Masillo A, Lanna A, Curto M, Lindau JF, Solfanelli A, Listanti G, Patanè M, Kotzalidis G, Gebhardt E, Meyer N, Di Pietro D, Leccisi D, Girardi P, Fiori Nastro P: Self-reported attenuated psychotic-like experiences in help-seeking adolescents and their association with age, functioning and psychopathology. Schizophr Res 2014;160: 110–117.

48 Fux L, Walger P, Schimmelmann BG, Schultze-Lutter F: The Schizophrenia Proneness Instrument, Child and Youth version (SPI-CY): practicability and discriminative validity. Schizophr Res 2013;146: 69–78.

49 Daneault JG, Stip E; Refer-O-Scope Group: Genealogy of instruments for prodrome evaluation of psychosis. Front Psychiatry 2013;4:25.

50 Meng H, Schimmelmann BG, Koch E, Bailey B, Parzer P, Günter M, Mohler B, Kunz N, Schulte-Markwort M, Felder W, Zollinger R, Bürgin D, Resch F: Basic symptoms in the general population and in psychotic and non-psychotic adolescents. Schizophr Res 2009;111:32–38.

Prof. Frauke Schultze-Lutter
University Hospital of Child and Adolescent Psychiatry and Psychotherapy, University of Bern
Bolligenstrasse 111, Haus A
CH–3000 Bern 60 (Switzerland)
E-Mail frauke.schultze-lutter@kjp.unibe.ch

Riecher-Rössler A, McGorry PD (eds): Early Detection and Intervention in Psychosis: State of the Art and Future Perspectives. Key Issues Ment Health. Basel, Karger, 2016, vol 181, pp 42–54 (DOI: 10.1159/000440913)

Psychosis High-Risk States in Adolescents

Andor E. Simon

Department of Psychiatry, Specialized Early Psychosis Outpatient Service for Adolescents and Young Adults, Bruderholz, Department of Psychiatry and Psychotherapy (UPK), University of Basel, Basel, and University Hospital of Psychiatry, University of Bern, Bern, Switzerland

Abstract

The increasing availability of early psychosis services has led to a much broader diagnostic spectrum now being seen in these services. Especially in adolescent age, mental state may meet psychosis risk on a purely psychometric basis, yet may be the phenotypical expression of another underlying mental disorder or a merely transient phenomenon. Five groups of symptoms and clinical features that are frequently reported by individuals with suspected psychosis risk states, yet share strong commonalities with other mental disorders and conditions and thus can be conceptualized as being part of diagnostic spectra, each reaching from nonpsychotic to psychotic symptom formation, are reviewed: isolated hallucinations; unusual bodily perceptions, hypochondriatic fears and cenesthetic psychotic symptoms; depersonalization; obsessive-compulsive, overvalued, and delusional ideas; and autism spectrum disorders. Of the 639 individuals so far assessed in the Bruderholz Early Psychosis Outpatient Service for Adolescents and Young Adults, 230 (36%) met ultra-high-risk criteria, 206 (89.6%) of whom suffered from one of the five symptom groups mentioned above. The present chapter highlights that with a purely psychometric approach, the above-mentioned diagnostic spectra may wrongly be attributed to a psychosis risk state. The final conclusion of a clinical assessment should take into account the *gestalt* of these particular symptoms and clinical features and consider the age-specific *landscape* on which the latter were able to develop. However, the appraisal of the diagnostic spectra and their overlapping symptoms constitute a tremendous challenge in the clinical assessment of each referred individual.   © 2016 S. Karger AG, Basel

In recent years, transition rates to psychosis in at-risk individuals have substantially declined across different early psychosis centres in the world [1, 2]. Large proportions of at-risk individuals do not convert to psychosis [3] or even remit from an ultra-high-risk (UHR) state [4]. Terms such as 'clinical high risk' or 'at-risk mental state' thus gradually replaced the term 'UHR', as risk could no longer be considered 'ultra-high' [5].

What are the reasons for the declining transition rates to psychosis? These can be summarized as follows: development of more appropriate and tailored intervention models that prevent conversion to psychosis [1, 2]; potential lead-time bias [4, 6]; effects of promoting early intervention to both health professionals [7] and the general population [8]; less selective referrals, often occurring with the aim to rule out psychosis risk, thus including individuals with isolated and/or transient attenuated psychotic symptoms [9], and tapping a more 'extended psychosis phenotype' [10].

The last two factors are particularly noteworthy as it must be kept in mind that initial findings were obtained from clinical observations of individuals with more severe symptom levels who had passed through various filters of help-care resulting in an enrichment of high-risk subjects. In comparison, assessments in specialized early psychosis services today cover a large continuum reaching from benign subclinical, i.e. attenuated, psychotic symptoms in some healthy individuals to severe and disabling psychotic symptoms in others. If the early intervention of psychosis is promoted on a large scale, it must be expected that a non-negligible proportion of referrals occur to rule out psychosis risk and to primarily allay the fears and concerns of individuals and their relatives. This is the case particularly in adolescence, a lifespan where individuals undergo multitudinous changes in behaviour, develop diversity of contextual thinking, and experience frequent emotional turmoil, which may resemble phenomena often seen in emerging psychosis. We must keep in mind, however, that the age of onset of psychosis coincides with the age of onset of the majority of other mental disorders [11]. Thus, adolescence represents the age group with a general risk to develop any type of mental disorder. Adolescence also parallels the increasing incidence of many physical illnesses such as cardiovascular [12] or cancerous diseases [13], as well as the peak incidence of divorce [14] in the middle-aged groups, i.e. the adolescents' parents, and the increased risk of mortality in elderlies, i.e. the adolescents' grandparents. Thus, adolescents are embedded in a lifespan where they face the challenge of often dramatic life events and developmental changes. The phenomena that come along with such age-specific developmental changes are often wrongly interpreted as risk for psychosis if the *gestalt* of these phenomena is not appropriately considered and an exclusively psychometric approach applied to assess these adolescents.

The present chapter is an appraisal of symptoms and clinical features that are frequently reported by individuals with suspected psychosis risk states, yet share strong commonalities with other mental disorders and conditions and thus can be conceptualized as being part of diagnostic spectra, each reaching from non-psychotic to psychotic symptom formation. Historical and phenomenological issues of the various diagnostic spectra are discussed, and the terms that constitute the cornerstones along the above-mentioned spectra are reviewed.

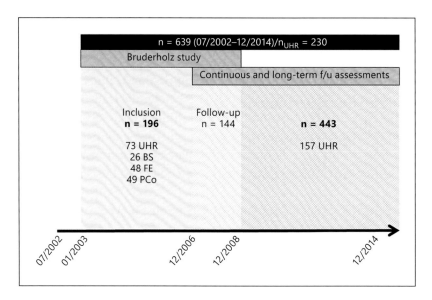

Fig. 1. Patient sample of the Bruderholz Early Psychosis Outpatient Service for Adolescents and Young Adults. This service was established in July 2002. The prospective Bruderholz study was conducted between January 1, 2003 and December 31, 2008, with patient inclusions until December 31, 2006 and follow-up assessments continued until December 31, 2008. As of January 1, 2007, the service provides continuous assessment of referred individuals including long-term follow-up assessments. UHR = Ultra-high risk; BS = basic symptoms (at-risk state); FE = first episode of psychosis; PCo = patient controls; f/u = follow-up.

Methods and Study Sample

Five groups of symptoms and clinical features that show considerable overlap along various diagnostic spectra were chosen: isolated hallucinations; unusual bodily perceptions, hypochondriatic fears, and cenesthetic psychotic symptoms; depersonalization; obsessive-compulsive, overvalued, and delusional ideas; and autism spectrum disorders (ASDs). Symptoms of any of these five groups may meet formal, i.e. psychometric, UHR criteria. These five symptom groups were chosen on the basis of the clinical experience that was gathered between July 2002 and December 2014 in 639 patients assessed in the Bruderholz Early Psychosis Outpatient Service for Adolescents and Young Adults (fig. 1). This service was established in 2002 in North-Western Switzerland as a clinical research facility [15–17].

Of the 639 patients, 230 (36%) met formal UHR criteria according to the Structured Interview for Prodromal Syndromes (SIPS) [18]. The first 196 ($n_{UHR} = 73$) of the 639 patients were included in the Bruderholz study between January 1, 2003 and December 31, 2006, and were prospectively examined for 2 years in terms of clinical and cognitive outcome [16, 17]. Of the 443 patients who were assessed between January 1, 2007 and December 31, 2014, a further 157 patients met formal UHR criteria according to the SIPS.

Table 1. Age and gender of the UHR study sample (n = 206)

	Hallucinations (n = 92)	Cenesthopathies (n = 29)	Depersonalization (n = 32)	OCS/delusions (n = 46)	Autism spectrum (n = 7)
Mean age, years	18.0	20.0	18.7	18.8	14.1
Gender (male/female), n	21/71	21/8	24/8	37/9	7/0

Of the 639 patients assessed and of the 230 meeting UHR criteria, 206 (36% and 89.6%, respectively) suffered from one of the five above-mentioned symptom groups. As shown in table 1, all groups revealed a preponderance of the male gender, with the exception of isolated hallucinations which were far more common in female adolescents.

Symptom Groups and Diagnostic Spectra

Isolated Hallucinations

One of the most common misdiagnoses in adolescent psychiatry is to ascribe isolated hallucinations to schizophrenia [19]. The diagnostic validity of isolated hallucinations in young populations that reach criterion A, but not criterion B, of DSM-IV [American Psychiatric Association (APA), 1994] and DSM-5 (2013) schizophrenia, constitutes a major diagnostic challenge. Also in classical psychiatry, hallucinations have not been conceptualized uniformly. In 1911, Eugen Bleuler [20] described auditory verbal hallucinations as accessory and therefore non-fundamental symptoms of schizophrenia, while in 1959, Kurt Schneider [21] assigned voices of arguing, discussing, or commenting character to the first-rank symptoms, essentially influencing the formal diagnostic criteria for schizophrenia to this day. Indeed, no other clinical phenomena are as likely to be attributed to schizophrenia as hallucinations, yet no other clinical phenomenon common to schizophrenia is as widely spread across numerous other states and disorders.

In adolescents, hallucinations are often transitory phenomena and show considerable rates of discontinuation [22]. They have been reported in a vast array of non-psychotic disorders such as depressive and anxiety disorders [23], attention deficit-hyperactivity disorder [24], conduct disorders [25], borderline personality disorders [26], or DSM-5 separation anxiety disorder and schizotypal personality disorder. They have also been reported in various mental states such as emotional distress and bereavement [27], family disruptions, parental separation, and persistent incriminating family settings [28], i.e. so-called 'type II' trauma. For the latter, the term 'complex post-traumatic stress disorder' was introduced [29]. Auditory verbal hallucinations, including the Schneiderian first-rank types, may occur in complex post-traumatic stress disorder [30] as well as following so-called 'type I' trauma in post-traumatic stress disorder and show no significant difference in quality and intensity when compared to schizophrenia [31]. It is agreed upon that hallucinations occurring in the context of traumatic experiences are considered dissociative phenomena [32].

The majority of studies report that subthreshold hallucinations are of limited prognostic value for later psychosis [33, 34]. Further, none of the recent prospective studies of patients at initial risk for psychosis found hallucinations to be a single predictor for transition to psychosis [2, 35–37]. In contrast, in the German Cologne Early Recognition (CER) study, acoustic and visual perception disturbances were reported to be predictive of later psychosis in a patient sample that was highly selective [38].

Unusual Bodily Perceptions, Hypochondriatic Fears, and Cenesthetic Psychotic Symptoms

One of the most fascinating yet challenging phenomena in adolescents are unusual bodily perceptions and repeated somatic complaints with no associated medical cause. Such unusual bodily perceptions, spreading from age-specific insecurities and fears about physical health and appearance, through hypochondriasis, to an actual psychotic dimension underlying these phenomena, may thus occur on a diagnostic spectrum of considerable width.

In no further period of life do physical changes occur as dramatically as in adolescence. This increases awareness in these young people of their physical appearance and their concern as to personal physical health and well-being. The latter arises when unexpected and previously not experienced symptoms evolve, in particular in association with organs to which higher fragility or vital importance are attributed, e.g. the brain, the eyes, or the heart. A sudden episode of intense anxiety that precedes novel bodily perceptions is not unusual in these young individuals [39]. The French psychiatrists Dupre and Camus [40] introduced the term 'cenesthopathy' for states of disordered cenesthesia [41], i.e. pathological bodily perceptions.

It is of particular importance that adolescent cenesthopathy more often affects anxiety-prone, socially insecure, and shy individuals, and predominantly young males [42]. Anxiety-prone adolescents with disturbed narcissistic regulation may react with a catastrophic appraisal of normally transient symptoms following an initial episode of intense anxiety [43]. If such catastrophic appraisal persists, the differentiation between cenesthopathy and hypochondriasis becomes a challenging task, as the essential part of any definition of hypochondriasis is a morbid preoccupation with one's body or state of health, either mental or physical [44]. Bleuler [20] may have been the first to emphasize the clinical importance of bodily complaints among schizophrenia patients and suggested that the majority of (treatment-resistant) hypochondriacs were schizophrenia patients who may have stagnated at the initial stage of the disease process and therefore may belong to the category of latent schizophrenia. Terms referring to both diagnostic dimensions, e.g. 'hypochondriacal paraphrenia' [45] or 'hypochondriacal psychosis' [46], provide historical evidence for the difficulty to distinguish hypochondriasis from psychosis.

Gerd Huber [47] first described patients with cenesthetic schizophrenia as a sub-type of schizophrenia that is characterized by peculiar disturbances of bodily perceptions, but that remained often unidentified as a psychotic disorder due to its longstanding hypochondriacal features. Cenesthetic schizophrenia has never been incorporated in DSM and appears undefined in ICD-10 among other schizophrenia without having been identified in previous ICD editions. Huber claimed a close resemblance to Bleuler's [20] latent schizophrenia. He suggested that this was a type of schizophrenia that comes to a standstill after one or a few short psychotic episodes. However, it is well recognized that cenesthetic disturbances also occur in a large percentage of other schizophrenia subtypes and in emerging schizophrenia [48].

Depersonalization

Depersonalization is another fascinating psychological phenomenon. As it is a particular type of dissociation involving a disrupted integration of self-perceptions and constitutes a condition that many clinicians have never encountered, it is most commonly misdiagnosed as psychosis. DSM-5 depersonalization disorder is classified as a dissociative disorder, whereas ICD-10 classifies it as an independent neurotic condition labeled as 'depersonalization-derealization syndrome'. Depersonalization occurs along a spectrum of severity with short-lasting episodes (normal depersonalization) to severe and disabling forms (depersonalization disorder) [49]. In about two thirds of these patients, depersonalization persists, and in one third of patients it runs an episodic course, with each episode usually lasting from a few days to a few months [50].

Whereas patients with psychosis experience their symptoms as real, most of the patients with depersonalization disorder typically struggle to describe the experience. They allude to a variety of metaphors and commonly use the prefix 'as if' to describe their symptoms [50, 51]. In two recent factor analytical studies, the following factors emerged: anomalous body experience and body distortion, emotional numbing, anomalous subjective recall, and alienation from surroundings (i.e. derealization) [52, 53].

Depersonalization is more likely to manifest in pre-psychotic states than in established schizophrenia [47]. Indeed, phenomena related to anomalous body experience and body distortion as well as a derealization feature among the basic symptoms, as do difficulties in discriminating between different emotions [54]. Also, derealization was reported to be predictive of later psychosis [38]. In contrast, just as is the case with isolated hallucinations, depersonalization and derealization have been reported in a multitude of non-psychotic disorders, in particular in anxiety disorders including panic disorders and social phobia, but also avoidant-insecure personality disorders as well as in patients with mood disorders and borderline or obsessive-compulsive personality disorders [50]. Importantly, they are also reported in various mental states such as in individuals with childhood trauma, especially emotional, physical, and sexual abuse [55]. Sustained parental conflict is a common psychosocial constant in individuals with depersonalization and derealization. Similar to cenesthopathic symptoms, it predominantly affects anxiety-prone, socially insecure, and shy young males [49].

Obsessive-Compulsive, Overvalued, and Delusional Ideas
Accounts of patients with both psychotic and obsessive-compulsive symptoms (OCS) have occurred in the literature since the 19th century [56]. OCS and obsessive-compulsive disorder (OCD) co-occur at substantial rates in schizophrenia patients [57, 58]. Also, OCS has been reported to occur in about one fifth of UHR subjects [59].

The considerable co-occurrence of OCS and obsessive-compulsive disorder, respectively, and schizophrenia suggest that obsessive ideas in the sense of a neurotic phenomenon and psychotic delusional ideas mark the two opposing poles of a continuum. Overvalued ideas [60], i.e. unreasonable and sustained beliefs that are maintained with less than delusional intensity, are thus conceptually situated somewhere between these two opposing poles. Bleuler [20] suggested that the entire obsessive-compulsive syndrome may be a prodrome or a latent variant of schizophrenia and OCS and therefore be considered accessory symptoms of schizophrenia. Also, Karl Leonhard [45] described pronounced OCS in subtypes of schizophrenia which he termed 'verschrobene Hebephrenie (eccentric hebephrenia)' and 'manirierte Katatonie (manneristic catatonia)'.

In clinical practice, the differentiation between obsessive and delusional ideas, i.e. between non-psychotic and psychotic thought content, however, presents one of the most difficult and demanding tasks, and is another pitfall for erroneous diagnoses. This is unintentionally mirrored in DSM-IV and DSM-5 where the specifier 'with poor insight' is allowed for the diagnosis of obsessive-compulsive disorder, and even more so in DSM-5 which has implemented the – rather inapt – additional specifier 'with absent insight/delusional belief'. According to Karl Jaspers [61], obsession in the strict sense means assessing the contents of consciousness as being unfounded, nonsensical, and incomprehensible (i.e. ego-dystonic). In some cases of long-standing neurosis, however, obsessive ideas are integrated into one's own experience and may acquire an ego-syntonic character. Further, an ego-syntonic and even bizarre character may also emerge in anxiety-driven compulsive acts when these are performed to prevent the occurrence of catastrophic or fatal events. However, whereas the patient with an obsession in the strict sense is in general able to reflect upon himself and to evaluate his own thoughts as nonsensical, this is not the case in patients with delusional ideation. Here, self-reflexivity collapses and the ego can no longer keep up an evaluating distance from his thought contents, but is completely seized by them (i.e. ego-syntonic).

To disentangle between obsessive and delusional, i.e. psychotic, thought content, the core aspects of the phenomenological analysis of the delusional *gestalt*, presented by German psychiatrist Klaus Conrad in 1958 [62] and to date considered as one of the most impressive descriptions ever written on early schizophrenia [63, 64], need to be examined carefully in each of these cases. Conrad highlighted that once a psychotic dimension is reached, patients are unable to shift the 'frame of reference'. He provides a phenomenological stage model with a prodromal delusional mood preceding the onset of delusion formation: the patient experiences an increasingly oppressive tension and a feeling of expectation that something very important is about to happen ('Trema'), similar to what Jaspers termed 'Wahnstimmung' when patients explain that 'something is in the air'. The patient then draws attention to irrelevant stimuli and thoughts ('Wahnwahrnehmung'), which now become a potential threat. This threat then spreads to the entire perceptual field and prepares the basis for subsequent delusion formation. Finally, the inner world is also contaminated and first-rank symptoms appear. Such phenomenological stages would not be experienced by patients with mere obsessive thought contents.

Autism Spectrum Disorders

The final spectrum that I wish to discuss is composed of two spectra in itself, e.g. ASDs and psychosis or schizophrenia spectrum disorders. Contrary to what specialists of either spectrum may posit, a clear-cut delineation between these two spectra is not – and has never been – an obvious task in all instances, as a brief historical retrospective underlines.

The term autism is a reduction of the term autoerotism which was first used by British scientist Havelock Ellis in 1898 in his description of sexual behaviour in infants and was adopted by Sigmund Freud to define the relationship between the infant's sexual thrive and object [65]. It was Eugen Bleuler who coined the term 'autism', which he first mentioned in his work on negativism in schizophrenia in 1910 [66] and a year later in more depth in his seminal monograph [20], distancing himself from the strong sexual connotation of the term 'autoerotism'. For Bleuler, autism represented the prime fundamental symptom of schizophrenia [67]. He described autism as a gap between the patient's fantasy world and his inhabited reality. In the course of time, Bleuler's concept of autism was adapted on various occasions in German psychiatry, e.g. Karl Leonhard [45] who posited that disturbed contact with their environment was particularly prominent in patients with the autistic hebephrenia subtype of schizophrenia. While autism as a specific term thus emerged in adult psychiatry, it was applied to paediatric populations far earlier than when Leo Kanner published his work in 1943 [68]. Descriptions of characteristic autistic traits have been found in paediatric populations since the late 19th century [69]. Russian paediatric neurologist Grunja Ssucharewa, whose work only became known to a broader readership when it was translated into English in 1996, published a small case series of children in 1926 in a German publication and highlighted their autistic attitude, supplying further work in the following years on heavily autistic behaviour in young patients with childhood schizophrenia [70]. Subsequently, the term 'autism' became a hallmark in defining childhood schizophrenia, and for many decades to come, autism would be considered inseparable from childhood-onset schizophrenia by most mental health professionals [71]. Thus, by the time Leo Kanner used the term 'infantile autism' in 1943 to describe children who exhibited limited interest in and impaired social response to others from infancy onward, and Hans Asperger [72] described a similar group of male children in 1944, autism had already been described by other authors in paediatric populations.

When DSM-II appeared in 1968, autism was referred to as schizophrenia, childhood type, and was characterized by 'atypical and withdrawn behaviour'. Thus, DSM-II autism was nothing else than childhood-onset schizophrenia, which is defined by an onset of psychosis before age 13 years. However, post-DSM-II work conducted by Kolvin [73] and Rutter [74] was influential in distinguishing between childhood-onset schizophrenia and autism in terms of clinical characteristics. In 1980, DSM-III (1980) introduced a new category of 'pervasive developmental disorders' which included 'infantile autism' that was now separated from schizophrenia. The 1987 revisions in DSM-III-R changed the diagnostic label to 'autistic disorder'. The pervasive developmental disorder category was maintained in DSM-IV and replaced by a separate chapter on ASDs in DSM-5 which subsumes all autism subtypes.

However, the question whether autism and schizophrenia spectrum disorders can be considered distinct diagnostic spectra, or whether both spectra overlap, and if, to what degree they overlap, has been the focus of an increasing number of studies and reviews in more recent years [69]. Some of the symptom overlaps are as follows: impairments in social interaction and communication as well as restricted interests and thinking, defined as the typical triad for ASD, can be found in adolescents with emerging psychosis, and similarly, deficits in social interaction and communication have been shown in home video analyses as well as in genetic high-risk and birth cohort studies [75] of patients who later developed schizophrenia; depression and anxiety occur at high prevalence rates in both spectra [76]; impaired theory of mind is found in both spectra [77], in some instances appearing as overvalued ideas or even as delusional thoughts in ASD patients due to misinterpretation and insecurity in social situations; social withdrawal, one of the clinical expressions of Bleuler's autism, is a core phenomenon in adolescents with emerging psychosis [78], while social withdrawal may be misinterpreted as negative psychotic symptom in ASD patients; and finally, even if in a clear minority, auditory verbal hallucinations may occur in adolescents with ASD [79].

Conclusions

The classification of symptoms with psychometric equality constitutes a challenging task that reaches far beyond mere comorbidity [76] or 'clinical noise' [2]. Symptoms that are common to adolescents with potential risk for psychosis are also found in other mental disorders and conditions and thus constitute a considerable overlap along various diagnostic spectra, reaching from benign, normal developmental, and transient features to severe and disabling psychotic symptoms. Adolescents frequently present as diagnostic conundrums and may not be assigned to one specific diagnostic category. Although such an approach is at odds with the traditional concept of classifying mental health disorders into single categories, diagnoses may overlap in terms of symptoms with no necessary *clear water* between single categories [69]. While most mental states typically emerge in adolescence [11] and a proportion of young people continue to be at risk of developing psychosis, we must keep in mind that multitudinous changes in behaviour and physical development as well as experience of frequent emotional turmoil are typical in this age group. It is also the age group which is paralleled by potential and dramatic shifts and changes in the family system, with increased incidence of physical diseases and mortality in the parents and grandparents of these adolescents, and with parental divorce reaching peak incidence. It is within this developmental context that mental phenomena must be understood. Obviously, an exclusively psychometric approach does not suffice to capture such contextual understanding, e.g. the *gestalt* of a symptom. The comprehension of the *gestalt*, however, provides us with the indispensable key to better understand whether a specific symptom actually mirrors psychosis risk or whether it occurs only transiently.

Acknowledgements

I should like to thank Daniel Umbricht for his longstanding friendship and his invaluable help and collaboration. I should also like to thank the following collaborators for their indispensable contributions at the Bruderholz Early Psychosis Outpatient Service for Adolescents and Young Adults (in alphabetical order): Mara Aeschbacher, Dima Arbach, Michelle Bürgisser, Diane Dvorsky, Kerstin Gruber, Emanuel Isler, Jasmine Ouertani, Binia Roth, Kathrin Stöcklin, Milena Ulrich, Alexander Zimmer, and Solange Zmilacher.

References

1 Fusar-Poli P, Bonoldi I, Yung AR, Borgwardt S, Kempton MJ, Valmaggia L, Barale F, Caverzasi E, McGuire P: Predicting psychosis: meta-analysis of transition outcomes in individuals at high clinical risk. Arch Gen Psychiatry 2012;69:220–229.

2 Nelson B, Yuen HP, Wood SJ, Lin A, Spiliotacopoulos D, Bruxner A, Broussard C, Simmons M, Foley DL, Brewer WJ, Francey SM, Amminger GP, Thompson A, McGorry PD, Yung AR: Long-term follow-up of a group at ultra-high risk ('prodromal') for psychosis: the PACE 400 study. JAMA Psychiatry 2013;70:793–802.

3 Simon AE, Velthorst E, Nieman DH, Linszen D, Umbricht D, de Haan L: Ultra high-risk state for psychosis and non-transition: a systematic review. Schizophr Res 2011;132:8–17.

4 Simon AE, Borgwardt S, Riecher-Rössler A, Velthorst E, de Haan L, Fusar-Poli P: Moving beyond transition outcomes: meta-analysis of remission rates in individuals at high clinical risk for psychosis. Psychiatry Res 2013;209:266–272.

5 Fusar-Poli P, Borgwardt S, Bechdolf A, Addington J, Riecher-Rössler A, Schultze-Lutter F, Keshavan M, Wood S, Ruhrmann S, Seidman LJ, Valmaggia L, Cannon T, Velthorst E, De Haan L, Cornblatt B, Bonoldi I, Birchwood M, McGlashan T, Carpenter W, McGorry P, Klosterkötter J, McGuire P, Yung A: The psychosis high-risk state: a comprehensive state-of-the-art review. JAMA Psychiatry 2013;70:107–120.

6   Yung AR, Yuen HP, Berger G, Francey S, Hung TC, Nelson B, Phillips L, McGorry P: Declining transition rate in ultra-high risk (prodromal) services: dilution or reduction of risk? Schizophr Bull 2007;33: 673–681.

7   Simon AE, Theodoridou A, Schimmelmann B, Schneider R, Conus P: The Swiss Early Psychosis Project SWEPP: a national network. Early Interv Psychiatry 2012;6:106–111.

8   Joa I, Johannessen JO, Auestad B, Friis S, McGlashan T, Melle I, Opjordsmoen S, Simonsen E, Vaglum P, Larsen TK: The key to reducing duration of untreated first psychosis: information campaigns. Schizophr Bull 2008;34:466–472.

9   Kelleher I, Murtagh A, Molloy C, Roddy S, Clarke MC, Harley M, Cannon M: Identification and characterization of prodromal risk syndromes in young adolescents in the community: a population-based clinical interview study. Schizophr Bull 2012;38: 239–246.

10 van Os J, Linscott RJ: Introduction: the extended psychosis phenotype – relationship with schizophrenia and with ultrahigh risk status for psychosis. Schizophr Bull 2012;38:227–230.

11 Paus T, Keshavan M, Giedd JN: Why do many psychiatric disorders emerge during adolescence? Nat Rev Neurosci 2008;9:947–957.

12 American Heart Association. http://www.heart.org.

13 UK Cancer Research. http://www.cancerresearchuk.org.

14 Bundesamt für Statistik. http://www.bfs.admin.ch.

15 Simon AE, Dvorsky DN, Boesch J, Roth B, Isler E, Schueler P, Petralli C, Umbricht D: Defining patients at risk for psychosis: a comparison of two approaches. Schizophr Res 2006;81:83–90.

16 Simon AE, Cattapan-Ludewig K, Zmilacher S, Arbach D, Gruber K, Dvorsky DN, Roth B, Isler E, Zimmer A, Umbricht D: Cognitive functioning in the schizophrenia prodrome. Schizophr Bull 2007;33: 761–771.

17 Simon AE, Grädel M, Cattapan-Ludewig K, Gruber K, Ballinari P, Roth B, Umbricht D: Cognitive functioning in at-risk mental states for psychosis and 2-year clinical outcome. Schizophr Res 2012;142: 108–115.

18 McGlashan TH, Miller TJ, Woods SW, Hoffman RE, Davidson L: Structured Interview for Prodromal Syndromes (Version 3.0, unpublished manuscript). New Haven, PRIME Research Clinic, Yale School of Medicine, 2001.

19 Berenson CK: Frequently missed diagnoses in adolescent psychiatry. Psychiatr Clin North Am 1998; 21:917–926,

20 Bleuler E: Dementia Praecox oder die Gruppe der Schizophrenien. Leipzig, Deuticke, 1911.

21 Schneider K: Clinical Psychopathology, ed 5. New York, Grune & Stratton, 1959.

22 Escher S, Romme M, Buiks A, Delespaul P, van Os J: Formation of delusional ideation in adolescent hearing voices: a prospective study. Am J Med Genet 2002;114:913–920.

23 Apter A, Bleich A, Tyano S: Affective and psychotic psychopathology in hospitalized adolescents. J Am Acad Child Adolesc Psychiatry 1988;27:116–120.

24 McGee R, Williams S, Poulton R: Hallucinations in nonpsychotic children. J Am Acad Child Adolesc Psychiatry 2000;39:12–13.

25 Garralda ME: Hallucinations in children with conduct and emotional disorders: I. The clinical phenomena. Psychol Med 1984;14:589–596.

26 Yee L, Korner AJ, McSwiggan S, Meares RA, Stevenson J: Persistent hallucinosis in borderline personality disorder. Compr Psychiatry 2005;46:147–154.

27 Yates TT, Bannard JR: The 'haunted' child: grief, hallucinations, and family dynamics. J Am Acad Child Adolesc Psychiatry 1988;27:573–581.

28 Best NT, Mertin P: Correlates of auditory hallucinations in nonpsychotic children. Clin Child Psychol Psychiatry 2007;12:611–623.

29 Herman JL: Complex PTSD: a syndrome in survivors of prolonged and repeated trauma. J Trauma Stress 1992;5:377–391.

30 van der Hart O, Nijenhuis ER, Steele K: Dissociation: an insufficiently recognized major feature of complex posttraumatic stress disorder. J Trauma Stress 2005;18:413–423.

31 Scott JG, Nurcombe B, Sheridan J, McFarland M: Hallucinations in adolescents with post-traumatic stress disorder and psychotic disorder. Australas Psychiatry 2007;15:44–48.

32 Nurcombe B, Mitchell W, Begtrup R, Tramontana M, LaBarbera J, Pruitt J: Dissociative hallucinosis and allied conditions; in Volkmar FR (ed): Psychoses and Pervasive Developmental Disorders of Childhood and Adolescence. Washington, American Psychiatric Press, 1996.

33 Dhossche D, Ferdinand R, Van der Ende J, Hofstra MB, Verhulst F: Diagnostic outcome of self-reported hallucinations in a sample of adolescents. Psychol Med 2002;32:619–627.

34 Simon AE, Cattapan-Ludewig K, Gruber K, Ouertani J, Zimmer A, Roth B, Isler E, Umbricht D: Subclinical hallucinations in adolescent outpatients: an outcome study. Schizophr Res 2009;108:265–271.

35 Cannon TD, Cadenhead K, Cornblatt B, Woods SW, Addington J, Walker E, Seidman LJ, Perkins D, Tsuang M, McGlashan TH, Heinssen R: Prediction of psychosis in youth at high clinical risk: a multisite study in North America. Arch Gen Psychiatry 2008;65:28–37.

36 Riecher-Rössler A, Pflueger MO, Aston J, Borgwardt SJ, Brewer WJ, Gschwandtner U, Stieglitz RD: Efficacy of using cognitive status in predicting psychosis: a 7-year follow-up. Biol Psychiatry 2009;66: 1023–1030.

37 Ruhrmann S, Schultze-Lutter F, Salokangas RK, Hein-imaa M, Linszen D, Dingemans P, Birchwood M, Pat-terson P, Juckel G, Heinz A, Morrison A, Lewis S, von Reventlow HG, Klosterkötter J: Prediction of psycho-sis in adolescents and young adults at high risk: results from the prospective European prediction of psycho-sis study. Arch Gen Psychiatry 2010;67:241–251.

38 Klosterkötter J, Hellmich M, Steinmeyer EM, Schul-tze-Lutter F: Diagnosing schizophrenia in the initial prodromal phase. Arch Gen Psychiatry 2001;58:158–164.

39 Roth M: The phobic anxiety-depersonalization syn-drome. Proc R Soc Med 1959;52:587–595.

40 Dupre E, Camus P: Les Cenestopathies. L'Encephale 1907;2:616–631.

41 Reil JC: Gesammelte kleine physiologische Schriften. Wien, Gesellschaft angehender Ärzte, 1811.

42 Watanabe H, Takahashi T, Tonoike T, Suwa M, Aka-hori K: Cenesthopathy in adolescence. Psychiatry Clin Neurosci 2003;57:23–30.

43 Schilder P: Selbstbewusstsein und Persönlichkeits-bewusstsein. Eine psychopathologische Studie. Ber-lin, Springer, 1914.

44 Kenyon FE: Hypochondriacal states. Br J Psychiatry 1976;129:1–14.

45 Leonhard K: Die Aufteilung der endogenen Psycho-sen. Berlin, Akademie-Verlag, 1957.

46 Mayer-Gross W: Die Klinik der Schizophrenie; in Bumke O (ed): Handbuch der Geisteskrankheiten. Berlin, Springer, 1932, pp 377–382.

47 Huber G: Cenesthetic schizophrenia. Fortschr Neu-rol Psychiatr 1957;25:491–520.

48 Stanghellini G, Ballerini M, Fusar-Poli P, Cutting J: Abnormal bodily experiences may be marker if early schizophrenia. Curr Pharm Des 2012;18:392–398.

49 Michal M, Wiltink J, Subic-Wrana C, Zwerenz R, Tuin I, Lichy M, Brähler E, Beutel ME: Prevalence, correlates and predictors of depersonalization expe-riences in the German general population. J Nerv Ment Dis 2009;197:499–506.

50 Simeon D, Knutelska M, Nelson D, Guralnik O: Feeling unreal: a depersonalization disorder update of 117 cases. J Clin Psychiatry 2003;64:990–997.

51 Sierra M: Depersonalization: A New Look at a Ne-glected Syndrome, ed 1. New York, Cambridge Uni-versity Press, 2009.

52 Sierra M, Baker D, Medford N, David AS: Unpacking the depersonalization syndrome: an exploratory fac-tor analysis on the Cambridge Depersonalization Scale. Psychol Med 2005;35:1523–1532.

53 Simeon D, Kozin DS, Segal K, Lerch B, Dujour R, Giesbrecht T: De-constructing depersonalization: further evidence for symptom clusters. Psychiatry Res 2008;157:303–306.

54 Gross G, Huber G, Klosterkötter J, Linz M: Bonn Scale for the Assessment of Basic Symptoms – BSABS. Ber-lin/Heidelberg/New York, Springer, 1987.

55 Simeon D, Guralnik O, Schmeidler J, Sirof B, Knu-telska M: The role of childhood interpersonal trauma in depersonalization disorder. Am J Psychiatry 2001;158:1027–1033.

56 Berrios GE: Obsessive-compulsive disorder: its con-ceptual history in France during the 19th century. Compr Psychiatry 1989;30:283–295.

57 Frommhold K: Obsessive-compulsive disorder and schizophrenia. A critical review (in German). Fortschr Neurol Psychiatr 2006;74:32–48.

58 Hagen K, Hansen B, Joa I, Larsen TK: Prevalence and clinical characteristics of patients with obsessive-compulsive disorder in first-episode psychosis. BMC Psychiatry 2013;13:156.

59 Fontenelle LF, Lin A, Pantelis C, Wood SJ, Nelson B, Yung AR: A longitudinal study of obsessive-compul-sive disorder in individuals at ultra-high risk for psy-chosis. J Psychiatr Res 2011;45:1140–1145.

60 Wernicke C: Grundriss der Psychiatrie in klinischen Vorlesungen. Leipzig, Thieme, 1900.

61 Jaspers K: Allgemeine Psychopathologie. Berlin, Springer, 1946.

62 Conrad K: Die beginnende Schizophrenie. Stuttgart, Georg Thieme Verlag, 1958.

63 Hambrecht M, Häfner H: 'Trema, apophany, apoca-lypse' – is Conrad's phase model empirically found-ed (in German)? Fortschr Neurol Psychiatr 1993;61:418–423.

64 Mishara AL: Klaus Conrad (1905–1961): delusional mood, psychosis, and beginning schizophrenia. Schizophr Bull 2010;36:9–13.

65 Freud S: Drei Abhandlungen zur Sexualtheorie. Leipzig, Deuticke, 1915.

66 Bleuler E: Zur Theorie des schizophrenen Negativis-mus. Psychiatr Neurolog Wochenschr 1910;19:184–187.

67 Parnas J: A disappearing heritage: the clinical core of schizophrenia. Schizophr Bull 2011;37:1121–1130.

68 Kanner L: Autistic disturbances of affective contact. Nerv Child 1943;2:217–250.

69 Shorter E, Wachtel LE: Childhood catatonia, autism and psychosis past and present: is there an 'iron tri-angle'? Acta Psychiatr Scand 2013;128:21–33.

70 Ssucharewa GE: Die schizoiden Psychopathien im Kindesalter. Monatsschr Psychiatr Neurol 1926;60:235–261.

71 Tidmarsch L, Volkmar FR: Diagnosis and epidemi-ology of autism spectrum disorders. Can J Psychiatry 2003;48:517–525.

72 Asperger H: Die 'Autistischen Psychopathen' im Kindesalter. Arch Psychiatr Nervenkr 1944;117:76–136.

73 Kolvin I: Studies in childhood psychoses. I. Diagnos-tic criteria and classification. Br J Psychiatry 1971;118:381–384.

74 Rutter M: Childhood schizophrenia reconsidered. J Autism Child Schizophr 1972;2:315–337.

75 Hallerbäck MU, Lugnegard T, Gillberg C: Is autism spectrum disorder common in schizophrenia? Psychiatry Res 2012;198:12–17.

76 Fusar-Poli P, Nelson B, Valmaggia L, Yung AR, McGuire PK: Comorbid depressive and anxiety disorders in 509 individuals with an at-risk mental state: impact on psychopathology and transition to psychosis. Schizophr Bull 2014;40:120–131.

77 Korkmaz B: Theory of mind and neurodevelopmental disorders of childhood. Pediatric Res 2011;69: 1001–1108.

78 Häfner H, Löffler W, Maurer K, Hambrecht M, van der Heiden W: Depression, negative symptoms, social stagnation and social decline in the early course of schizophrenia. Acta Psychiatr Scand 1999;100: 105–118.

79 Cochran DM, Dvir Y, Frazier JA: 'Autism plus' spectrum disorders. Intersection with psychosis and the schizophrenia spectrum. Child Adolesc Psychiatr Clin N Am 2013;22:609–627.

PD Dr. med. Andor E. Simon
Department of Psychiatry, Psychiatric Outpatient Services
Specialized Early Psychosis Outpatient Clinic for Adolescents and Young Adults
CH–4101 Bruderholz (Switzerland)
E-Mail andor.simon@bluewin.ch

Riecher-Rössler A, McGorry PD (eds): Early Detection and Intervention in Psychosis: State of the Art and Future Perspectives. Key Issues Ment Health. Basel, Karger, 2016, vol 181, pp 55–68 (DOI: 10.1159/000440914)

The Psychosis High-Risk State

Grazia Rutigliano · Merrie Manalo · Paolo Fusar-Poli

Department of Psychosis Studies, Institute of Psychiatry, Psychology and Neuroscience, King's College London, London, UK

Abstract

The disabling nature and costly impact of mental disorders, such as schizophrenia, can cause significant burden to both person and society. It is also indicated that the negative outcomes associated with psychosis may, in part, be due to the delayed detection and initiation of treatment. Preventative interventions in several arenas of medicine have advanced, but have only come to the fore in psychiatry in the last two decades. It was long known that a preclinical phase preceded psychosis, now commonly termed as 'ultra-high-risk (UHR)' status. The advent of specialized early intervention services provided the cornerstone in taking a preventative and timely endeavor to maximize the chance of positive outcomes in psychosis. Despite the potential, the current state of the UHR concept lacks consensus in how at-risk individuals should be approached. This chapter aims to provide an overview of how preventative medicine can intersect with psychiatry by focusing on the psychosis high-risk state. It describes the current criteria and screening procedures used to prospectively detect UHR individuals and discusses the validity of these tools. While advocating the benefits of focused interventions, this chapter also recognizes current challenges and the controversy that leaves the psychosis high-risk state on fertile ground for wavering opinions. The chapter concludes with an exploration and discussion that proposes an improved conceptualization of the high-risk state and how this can direct intervention, as well as suggests future lines of research in this area.

© 2016 S. Karger AG, Basel

Over the past couple of decades, preventative approaches in several medical fields have flourished and developed. In fact, in the industrialized countries, the last century has seen an *epidemiological shift* occur from infectious to chronic diseases, hence from premature death to years lived with disability, as the main concern for health-related professions [1]. As a consequence, the major goal of health policies became to preserve individuals in full health for the standard life expectancy by means of preventative interventions.

The Institute of Medicine defines three categories of preventative interventions, according to their target population's level of risk:

(1) Universal preventive interventions target 'the general population that has not been identified on the basis of individual risk' [2], hence they are usually implemented in schools, whole communities, or workplaces.

(2) Selective preventive interventions target 'population sub-groups with a significantly higher risk than the wider population' [2]. They aim at preventing the emergence of a given disorder, by addressing biological, psychological, or social risk factors known to be more prominent among high-risk groups.

(3) Indicated preventive interventions target 'high-risk individuals who are identified as having minimal but detectable signs or symptoms foreshadowing a given disorder' [2]. Interventions focus on the immediate risk and protective factors present in the environments surrounding individuals.

Until two decades ago, the field of psychiatry had remained excluded from preventative approaches, particularly for interventions in schizophrenia. Psychiatric interventions were confined to address the acute phase of illness where positive and negative symptoms were florid, or the more chronic stage where functional decline was evident [3]. Over the past two decades, however, the availability of psychometric instruments to prospectively identify subjects at high clinical risk for psychosis has triggered the development of preventative diagnoses and interventions in psychosis.

Clinical Relevance and Impact of Delayed Treatment

Recent surveys into the morbidity burden in Europe have reported disorders of the brain and mental disorders as contributing 26.6% of the total cause burden (30.1% in females and 23.4% in males; fig. 1), as measured by disability-adjusted life years (DALYs), which is the sum of the years of life lost due to premature mortality and years lived with disability [4]. Mental disorders are extremely disabling and costly, as indicated by the amount of work loss days, loss of work productivity, early retirement, and quality of life. Moreover, compared to other chronic diseases, they exert their load mainly on young adult men from 15 to 39 years of age, who represent the most economically active fraction of the population [5] (fig. 1). Among disorders of the brain, schizophrenia ranks as the 8th most common cause of DALYs in Europe [4]. Worldwide, a disturbingly high gap exists between the prevalence of those with mental disorders and those who receive treatment, particularly in low-middle income countries. It has emerged that only about 35–50% of all subjects with mental disorders receive any professional help [6]. Moreover, even once provided, there is often a notable treatment delay. A recent prospective study has estimated that the duration of untreated psychosis (DUP), defined as the time of onset of the first psychotic symptom to the initiation of adequate treatment [7], has a median value of 25.7 weeks, ranging from 2 weeks up to 182 weeks [8]. A significant correlation has

Rutigliano · Manalo · Fusar-Poli

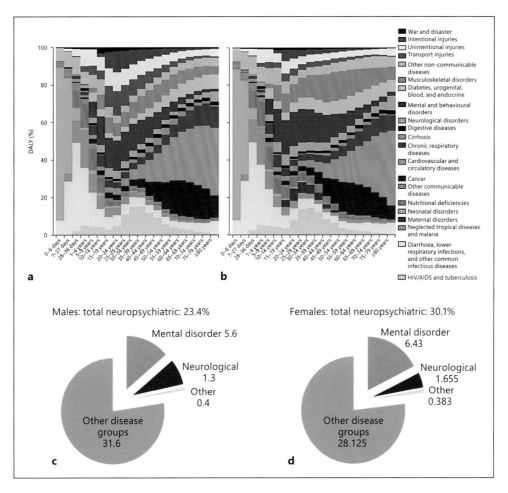

Fig. 1. Percentage of global DALYs by age, sex, and cause in 2010 worldwide. Distribution of DALYs for male individuals (**a**) and female individuals (**b**) [5]. Morbidity burden of disorders of the brain and mental disorders in the EU for male (**c**) and female (**d**) individuals [4].

been consistently observed between long lapses of DUP and outcome [9]. A long DUP has been found to be associated with more severe positive and negative symptoms [10–12], longer length of first hospitalization [13], poorer remission status, and higher risk of relapse and rehospitalization [8, 11, 13, 14]. Such negative outcomes can lead to further consequences, such as increased burden and expressed emotion in the family [15]; reduced compliance to treatment [16, 17]; lower treatment response rates [18–22]; increased risk of depression, suicide, and self-harming behavior [23–25]; higher risk of violence, aggression, and delinquent behavior [26–28], and eventually greater impairment in general functioning, social functioning, and quality of life [11, 14, 29, 30].

Early detection and intervention services serve as potential means of the timely recognition and initiation of treatment for psychosis. Indeed, evidence has shown that the introduction of such services is consistently followed by a reduction in the DUP, an increase in the proportion of patients treated within 6 months of onset, and a significant improvement in short-term clinical outcome, in terms of rates of hospitalization and compulsory admission [31, 32].

Delaying treatment to the point where acute and disturbing psychotic symptoms have manifested may potentially place the individual at a vulnerable stage along the continuum of schizophrenia, which is a slippery slope down towards the classically described deterioration syndrome [30].

Detectable Preclinical Phase

The existence of early symptoms predating the onset of schizophrenia has long been recognized [33, 34], and these were initially named 'prodromal' in 1932 by Mayer-Gross [35]. The research field regarding psychotic antecedents was launched in 1989 with the work of Huber and Gross [36], who investigated the chance of those presenting with basic disturbances transitioning to full-blown psychosis. Later, the ABC (Age, Begin, and Course) Schizophrenia Study, a representative study of a large group of patients, of whom 232 suffered from first-episode psychosis, provided more robust evidence that psychotic symptoms are already present before the first hospitalization for schizophrenia – on average for 1 year and up to 5 years in up to 73% of all patients [37–39]. The earliest signs of a mental disorder in the sense of prodromal symptoms had occurred an average 5–6 years before first hospitalization and 4–5 years before the first psychotic symptoms [37–40].

Despite the concept being widely known, the prodromal phase still lacked univocal definition until two decades ago. This was due to the difficulty in unambiguously marking whether or when an individual's experience or behavior has crossed the boundary from eccentric or unusual into the psychotic. A further challenge was the blurred and pleiotropic nature of prodromal symptoms, which lay mainly in the domain of depressive mood, negative symptoms, and functional impairment [41], rather than in that of the more dramatic positive psychotic symptoms, such as hallucinations and delusions [37, 42] (fig. 2).

A reliable and accurate detection of the preclinical phase of schizophrenia requires adequate frameworks and instruments. Over the past two decades two major trains of research have been developed for and applied to young help-seeking individuals at specialized services. The former, which was pioneered by the Melbourne Group of the Personal Assessment and Crisis Evaluation (PACE) Clinic [43, 44], gave rise to ultra-high-risk (UHR) [45], clinical high-risk [46], or at-risk mental state (ARMS) status [47]; the latter, based on the investigations of Klosterkötter et al. [48] (1996), focused on basic symptoms (BS).

The preliminary investigations put forth the operationalized high-risk diagnostic criteria below:

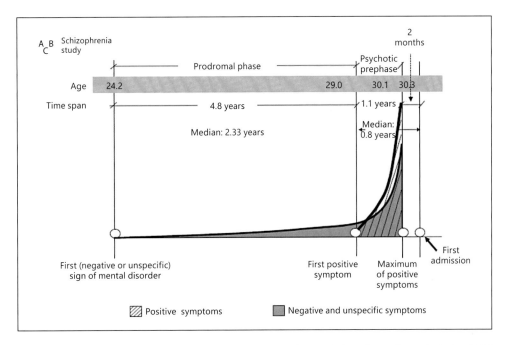

Fig. 2. The early stages of schizophrenia from first sign of mental disorder to first admission [ABC first-episode sample n = 232; (108 men, 124 women)] [38].

- Attenuated psychotic symptoms (APS), which encompasses young people experiencing psychotic symptoms at subthreshold intensity – not severe enough – or subthreshold frequency – not occurring often enough to meet a diagnosis of schizophrenia
- Brief limited intermittent psychotic symptoms (BLIPS), defined as the presence of a psychotic episode of less than 7 days which remit spontaneously with no medication or hospitalization
- Genetic risk and deterioration syndrome (GRD), which includes young people at-risk of psychosis due to the combination of trait vulnerability (i.e. family history of psychosis in a first-degree relative or schizotypal personality disorder in the identified patient) and a significant deterioration in mental state and/or functioning
- Cognitive perceptive BS, which identifies at-risk persons on the basis of subtle cognitive and perceptive alterations; BS are subjective disturbances of different domains, including perception, thought processing, language, and attention that are distinct from classical psychotic symptoms. They are independent of abnormal thought content and reality testing, and insight into the symptoms' psychopathologic nature is intact [49].

The APS criterion is the most prevalent within the ARMS. For example, it resulted in the most represented diagnostic group (70%) followed by APS + genetic risk and deterioration syndrome (11%) and BLIPS (9%) in a 10-year survey (2001–2011) of the Outreach and Support in South London (OASIS) service [50].

The Screening Procedures

The assessment of young help-seeking subjects is performed via different semistructured psychometric interviews, which operationalize the abovementioned criteria. Similar, yet not exactly alike, instruments have been developed and prospectively validated for the UHR/clinical high-risk/ARMS state. The first psychometric instrument, the Comprehensive Assessment of At-Risk Mental State (CAARMS), was proposed by Yung et al. [51] on the basis of the work of the Melbourne Group of PACE [52], whose goal was to determine the reliability of the prodromal symptoms in first-episode patients.

In the following years, three further semistructured interviews were developed: the Structured Interview for Prodromal Symptoms (SIPS) [including the companion Scale of Prodromal Symptoms (SOPS)] [53], the Early Recognition Inventory for the Retrospective Assessment of the Onset of Schizophrenia (ERIraos) [54], and the Basel Screening Instrument for Psychosis (BSIP) [55]. Additionally, a self-rating prodromal screening questionnaire (PQ) was developed and validated [56].

Regarding BS, they were originally assessed using the Bonn Scale for the Assessment of Basic Symptoms (BSABS) [57] and, more recently, the Schizophrenia Proneness Instrument, Adult version (SPI-A) [58]. Besides a variety of subjective disturbances in affect, drive, stress tolerance, and body perception, these instruments focus on self-perceived cognitive and perceptual changes, ultimately clustered in 2 subsets relating to the COPER (10 cognitive-perceptive BS) and the COGDIS (the 9 cognitive BS that are the most predictive of later psychosis) criteria [see the chapter by Schultze-Lutter, this vol., pp. 29–41].

Positive Predictive Value

Although summary results of the diagnostic accuracy of the UHR criteria are still lacking, data from different research groups carrying out psychosis preventative interventions are available and informative. A recent retrospective evaluation in patients with first-episode psychosis found the UHR construct to be highly sensitive. Up to 98.4% of patients reported prodromal symptoms predating the onset of full-blown psychosis [59].

As for positive predictive value, a meta-analysis calculated that on average 29.2% of subjects in a high-risk state transitioned to a full psychotic episode within 24 months. The transition risk progressively increased over time, ranging from 17.7% at 6 months up to a peak of 35.8% at 36 months [60].

The transition risk following a UHR diagnosis was significantly higher in subjects meeting the criteria compared to help-seeking subjects who screened as negative (30 vs. 2%) [61].

Epidemiology of Ultra-High-Risk Symptoms

In order to further support the validity of the 'attenuated psychotic syndrome' criteria currently listed in section III of the fifth revision of the Diagnostic and Statistical Manual for Mental Disorders (DSM-5) [62], its prevalence and clinical significance in the general population needs to be elucidated. The epidemiological validity of the UHR state remains a major issue. In fact, the psychosis high-risk criteria achieved validity only in help-seeking subjects. Furthermore, the UHR syndrome did not show epidemiological stability over time, as a decline in transition rates has been observed over recent years. Different explanations were proposed for the reported trend. Firstly, local communities are becoming more familiar with the high-risk state, thus referring younger clients at earlier and less severe stages of the prodrome, which could require longer follow-up periods to transition. Secondly, more recent studies have recruited subjects who are also offered active treatments, and this clinical engagement can potentially impact on the transition risk [60]. Some studies have investigated non-help-seeking community-based adolescents. In these samples, UHR criteria, as operationalized by the aforementioned psychometric instruments, were met by 2–8% of the participants, without applying the criterion of a 30% drop in functioning in the last year. The latter decreased the figure to 0–0.9% [63, 64]. Another study in the general population found that 0.3% of young adults (age range: 16–40 years) met current 'attenuated psychosis syndrome' criteria, after having excluded the criterion for an onset or worsening of the APS within the past year [62]. It has been proposed to revise the latter in order to capture the differential diagnosis between APS and schizotypal traits (i.e. to 'not always having been present in its current severity') rather than the progression towards frank psychosis [65], in line with the proposed reconceptualization of APS as a self-contained rather than an at-risk syndrome [66].

The epidemiological studies conducted in the general population are affected by several limitations. Telephone interviews are generally preferred to face-to-face interviews because of their assumed larger response rate. However, they may introduce some selection bias given to unequally distributed availability of telephone numbers or language skill exclusion criterion. On the other hand, face-to-face interviews may lead to ascertainment bias, as persons with family history might be more willing to participate, thus enriching the rates of the condition under study. Besides these caveats, future studies in the general population should compare the risks using different time and functioning deficit criteria in order to identify an optimal threshold to reliably distinguish between at-risk and non-at-risk persons [63–65].

Focused Interventions

The care provided by early intervention services has been shown to reduce the DUP as well as improve short-term clinical outcomes, such as the rates of hospitalization and compulsory admission [32].

Table 1. Treatment guidelines for the psychosis high-risk state

Organization	Recommendations
American Psychiatric Association	'Careful assessment and frequent monitoring'
Canadian Psychiatric Association	'Should be offered monitoring' 'May be offered supportive therapy and symptomatic treatment'
International Early Psychosis Association	'Antipsychotic medications not usually indicated' unless 'rapid deterioration' or 'severe suicidal risk and treatment of depression has proven ineffective' or 'aggression and hostility are increasing and pose a risk to others' If antipsychotics are considered, they 'may be continued' up to 2 years, and then 'attempt to withdraw the medication should be made'
Royal Australian and New Zealand College of Psychiatrists	'Antipsychotic medication not normally prescribed' unless 'symptoms are directly associated with risk of self-harm or aggression'
Italian National Institute of Health	'Use of antipsychotic medication' is 'doubtful'; behavioral cognitive treatment is recommended
German Association for Psychiatry, Psycho-therapy, and Neurology	'Continuous care and follow-up. If relevant symptoms reaching disorder level occur, CBT and sociotherapy should be offered. If psychotic symptoms emerge, antipsychotics should be offered'

CBT = Cognitive behavioral therapy.

Although the implementation of early intervention services leads to a great economic burden compared to the costs of standard care in the first years, the apparent economic loss due to direct costs (diagnostic measures, treatment, and care) [4] is largely compensated in the following years by a substantial reduction of the disproportionally high indirect cost burden (disability, quality of life) of psychosis. A meta-analysis has further confirmed the cost-effectiveness of early detection and early intervention services [67].

Treatment guidelines proposed by different international organizations are depicted in table 1. A recent meta-analysis of 11 trials including 1,246 participants showed that focused interventions can halve the risk of psychosis onset (RR = 0.5) [68]. Treatments that have demonstrated efficacy include cognitive therapy [69], cognitive behavioral therapy [70], antipsychotic drugs [71], combined psychological and pharmacological interventions (risperidone + cognitive behavioral therapy) [72], nutritional interventions (omega-3 fatty acids) [73], and integrated psychological interventions (cognitive therapy, social skills training, psychoeducation for family, and cognitive remediation) [74]. However, the evidence collected from these trials is not to be considered conclusive but rather preliminary [68]. Moreover, since the

Table 2. Psychosis prevention compared to common preventative approaches in clinical medicine

At-risk population	Outcome	Transition risk	Risk-focused treatment	Placebo	RRR	ARR	NNT
Psychosis high-risk state	Psychosis	17–28% (1 year) [68]	CBT 7% (1 year) [68]	Supportive counselling 14% (1 year) [68]	0.5 (1 year) [68]	0.07 (1 year) [68]	14 (1 year) [68]
			CBT + risperidone 17% (1 year) [68]	CBT + placebo 28% (1 year) [68]	0.39 (1 year) [68]	0.11 (1 year) [68]	9 (1 year) [68]
			Omega 3 FA 7.2% (1 year) [68]	Supportive counselling 40% (1 year) [68]	0.82 (1 year) [68]	0.33 (1 year) [68]	3 (1 year) [68]
Prediabetes	Diabetes	5–19% (1 year) [87]	Metformin 21.7% (3 years) [79]	Placebo 28.9% (3 years) [79]	0.25 (3 years) [87]	0.07 (3 years) [79]	14 (3 years) [79]
			Lifestyles 14.4% (3 years) [79]	Placebo 28.9% (3 years) [79]	0.5 (3 years) [87]	0.14 (3 years) [79]	7 (3 years) [79]
Cardiovascular high-risk patients[a]	Serious cardiovascular events[b]	1.5% [88]	Antiplatelet therapy 9.9% (2 years) [80]	Placebo 14% (2 years) [80]	0.35 (2 years) [80]	0.04 (2 years) [80]	25 (2 years) [80]

[a] High-risk patients defined as subjects with stable angina. [b] Serious cardiovascular events defined as nonfatal myocardial infarction, nonfatal stroke, or death from a vascular cause. ARR = Absolute risk reduction; CBT = cognitive behavioral therapy; FA = fatty acids.

treatment is biased toward attenuated positive psychotic symptoms, it is scarcely tailored to negative symptoms and early deficits, which are among the main complaints of high-risk subjects and best correlate with loss of functioning and a worse prognosis [75, 76]. Until better alternative interventions specifically targeting this medical condition are identified, the safest approach is recommended with careful consideration of the risk-benefit ratio of treatment.

Comparison with Other Preventative Approaches in Somatic Medicine

The goodness of psychosis prevention can be expressed through statistical indexes and so directly compared with other established preventative approaches in somatic medicine. Preventative cognitive behavioral therapies in psychosis are associated with a 0.5 RRR (relative risk reduction) and a NNT (number of subjects who need to be treated to prevent one additional bad outcome) of 14 [77, 78]. These values are comparable to those calculated for metformin in the prevention of diabetes (NNT = 14) [79] and even superior to those found for statins in preventing cardiovascular serious events (NNT = 25), although these were computed in the longer term [80] (table 2).

Risk Syndrome or Mental Disorder

The preparation of the DSM-5 raised a debate about the inclusion of a risk syndrome for psychosis, which is like the diagnosis of each grade of cervical dysplasia included in ICD-10. The main objections to its inclusion pointed towards the potential stigma associated with a diagnosis of schizophrenia as well as the overtreatment of subjects falsely classified as positive, i.e. who will never go on to develop psychosis. Indeed, UHR individuals, by definition, already experience changes in thinking, perception, affect, and behavior, as well as significant decline in psychosocial functioning and quality of life. The formal evidence that high-risk subjects are 'probably at risk but certainly ill' [66] derives from a meta-analysis which demonstrated that high-risk subjects are as impaired as psychotic patients in quality of life and global functioning at a level that is lower than healthy controls [81]. Moreover, the level of global functioning seems to predict later conversion to psychosis [81]. Therefore, it has been proposed that the currently defined 'at-risk state' be conceptualized as an independent disorder in its own right [82]. Consequently, the emphasis would move from prediction and prevention to symptom improvement.

Nonetheless, the observations above only provide support for the conceptual validity of the high-risk state, i.e. correctly distinguishing between disorder and normality. There is still much to be done in order to fulfill construct validity, i.e. correctly distinguishing between the actual and other disorders, which will be needed in order to bring a new APS syndrome in the DSM-5.1 main text [83]. In particular, the syndrome should additionally demonstrate biological plausibility, such as laboratory and instrumental correlates, epidemiological validity and sociodemographic consistency, and diagnostic stability, in terms of delineation of one disorder from another and predictability of the course of illness [84]. With regard to diagnostic stability, it should be noted that UHR is usually an aggregate of comorbid disorders. Since psychopathological boundaries are not so well-defined, patients at-risk for psychosis may fulfill diagnostic criteria for depression, anxiety, substance abuse, personality disorders, and developmental disorders [70]. More importantly, the construct holds the characteristic of pluripotency, in terms of heterogeneity of longitudinal outcomes. Among nontransitioning patients, about 46% appear to remit [85], some persist in ongoing attenuated psychotic symptoms, and others progress to other disorders, mainly bipolar disorder, depression, and anxiety [70]. A meta-analysis performed on a database of 2,182 high-risk subjects revealed that the available high-risk criteria, in particular the BS criteria, are strongly biased toward the identification of early prodromal phases of schizophrenic psychosis (73%) rather than affective psychosis (11%) [86]. In conclusion, the pluripotent model of the psychosis high-risk state encompasses different types of cases with attenuated psychotic experiences, each associated with a different evolution. Some of the baseline psychopathology may reflect the emergence of an underlying core psychotic process prodromal for schizophrenia or another psychotic disorder (true prodromal); some may be associated with a nonpsychotic clinical condition such as depression (clinical noise), and some may represent normal variation in the general population (incidental psychosis).

Conclusions and Future Directions

The past two decades have seen a great interest and rise in the importance of the prodromal phase of psychosis. This has been achieved by shifting the traditional negative views of schizophrenia as a disorder with an unpredictable onset and that may be progressive in nature with disabling outcomes (dementia praecox) to a disorder that can be delayed, if not prevented, through recognition of those at imminent risk. In this chapter, the evidence advocating this category as the possible target of focused interventions has been summarized. Moreover, its role as a new diagnosis in its own right in DSM-5 has been discussed, and a shift of the focus from an uncertain future outcome to current psychopathology and needs has been proposed. However, further research is warranted since many questions remain unanswered. First, it is not clear whether the validity of UHR as used by specialized services can be generalized to general psychiatry/psychology and primary care. It has been argued that the diagnosis of APS in general practice may lead to excessive therapeutics doing more harm than good as well as adding a significant burden, in terms of stigma, to persons experiencing attenuated psychotic symptoms. However, greater attention should be paid to impairments in self, autonomy, personhood, and emotional regulation that people meeting criteria for APS already present. Second, because APS is a broad-based concept, interventions aimed at secondary prevention of psychosis could be tailored on which psychotic disorder vulnerability is present (i.e. schizophrenia spectrum disorder, bipolar disorder, or mood disorder). Third, reliable markers are needed in order to stratify the high-risk population according to the prediction of outcome; thus, broader and better validated longitudinal studies would be recommended, comparing high-risk subjects to healthy individuals as well as to people suffering from comorbid diagnoses. Finally, effective interventions should be developed and tested that address the specific needs of at-risk people. Therapeutic discovery should be more focused on functional outcomes or methods for enhancing resiliency or for reducing risk factors such as stress, with less emphasis placed on psychosis prevention. To date, the treatments that have been proven to be effective in frank psychosis have largely focused on positive symptoms; however, there is increasing evidence to suggest that negative symptoms as well as cognitive and social functioning meaningfully restrict the prognosis. For example, therapies aimed at ameliorating emotion recognition or exerting a neuroprotective effect may have potential benefits. APS may serve as a platform for future research and clinical work.

References

1 McLeroy KR, Crump CE: Health promotion and disease prevention: a historical perspective. Generations 1994;18:9–17.

2 National Research Council and Institute of Medicine of the National Academies: Preventing Mental, Emotional, and Behavioral Disorders among Young People: Progress and Possibilities. Washington, National Academy Press, 2009.

3 Marshall M, Lockwood A: Early Intervention for psychosis. Cochrane Database Syst Rev 2004;2: CD004718.

4 Wittchen HU, et al: The size and burden of mental disorders and other disorders of the brain in Europe 2010. Eur Neuropsychopharmacol 2011;21:655–679.

5 Murray CJL, et al: Disability-adjusted life years (DALYs) for 291 diseases and injuries in 21 regions, 1990–2010: a systematic analysis for the Global Burden of Disease Study 2010. Lancet 2012;380:2197–2223.

6 Rebello TJ, et al: Innovative strategies for closing the mental health treatment gap globally. Curr Opin Psychiatry 2014;27:308–314.

7 Norman RMG, Malla AK: Duration of untreated psychosis: a critical examination of the concept and its importance. Psychol Med 2001;31:381–400.

8 Tang JY, et al: Prospective relationship between duration of untreated psychosis and 13-year clinical outcome: a first-episode psychosis study. Schizophr Res 2014;153:1–8.

9 Riecher-Rössler A, et al: Early detection and treatment of schizophrenia: how early? Acta Psychiatr Scand 2006;113:73–80.

10 Boonstra N, et al: Duration of untreated psychosis and negative symptoms – a systematic review and meta-analysis of individual patient data. Schizophr Res 2012;142:12–19.

11 Hill M, et al: Prospective relationship of duration of untreated psychosis to psychopathology and functional outcome over 12 years. Schizophr Res 2012; 141:215–221.

12 Haas GL, Garratt LS, Sweeney JA: Delay to first antipsychotic medication in schizophrenia: impact on symptomatology and clinical course of illness. J Psychiatr Res 1998;32:151–159.

13 Penttila M, et al: Association between the duration of untreated psychosis and short- and long-term outcome in schizophrenia within the Northern Finland 1966 Birth Cohort. Schizophr Res 2013;143:3–10.

14 Fraguas D, et al: Duration of untreated psychosis predicts functional and clinical outcome in children and adolescents with first-episode psychosis: a 2-year longitudinal study. Schizophr Res 2014;152:130–138.

15 Alvarez-Jimenez M, et al: Differential predictors of critical comments and emotional over-involvement in first-episode psychosis. Psychol Med 2010;40:63–72.

16 Dassa D, et al: Factors associated with medication non-adherence in patients suffering from schizophrenia: a cross-sectional study in a universal coverage health-care system. Aust NZ J Psychiatry 2010; 44:921–928.

17 Hill M, et al: Nonadherence to medication four years after a first episode of psychosis and associated risk factors. Psychiatr Serv 2010;61:189–192.

18 Zhang HX, et al: Predictors of response to second generation antipsychotics in drug naive patients with schizophrenia: a 1 year follow-up study in Shanghai. Psychiatry Res 2014;215:20–25.

19 Pelayo-Teran JM, et al: Trajectories of symptom dimensions in short-term response to antipsychotic treatment in patients with a first episode of non-affective psychosis. Psychol Med 2014;44:37–50.

20 Schennach-Wolff R, et al: Predictors of response and remission in the acute treatment of first-episode schizophrenia patients – is it all about early response? Eur Neuropsychopharmacol 2011;21:370–378.

21 Gunduz-Bruce H, et al: Duration of untreated psychosis and time to treatment response for delusions and hallucinations. Am J Psychiatry 2005;162:1966–1969.

22 Ucok A, et al: Duration of untreated psychosis may predict acute treatment response in first-episode schizophrenia. J Psychiatr Res 2004;38:163–168.

23 Mauri MC, et al: Suicide attempts in schizophrenic patients: clinical variables. Asian J Psychiatry 2013;6:421–427.

24 Sonmez N, et al: Depressive symptoms in first episode psychosis: a one-year follow-up study. BMC Psychiatry 2013;13:106.

25 Challis S, et al: Systematic meta-analysis of the risk factors for deliberate self-harm before and after treatment for first-episode psychosis. Acta Psychiatr Scand 2013;127:442–454.

26 Humphreys MS, et al: Dangerous behaviour preceding first admissions for schizophrenia. Br J Psychiatry 1992;161:501–505.

27 Latalova K: Violence and duration of untreated psychosis in first-episode patients. Int J Clin Pract 2014; 68:330–335.

28 Richard-Devantoy S, et al: Homicide, schizophrenia and substance abuse: a complex interaction (in French). Rev Epidemiol Sante Publique 2013;61:339–350.

29 Loebel AD, et al: Duration of psychosis and outcome in first-episode schizophrenia. Am J Psychiatry 1992; 149:1183–1188.

30 Penttila M, et al: Duration of untreated psychosis as predictor of long-term outcome in schizophrenia: systematic review and meta-analysis. Br J Psychiatry 2014;205:88–94.

31 Marshall M, et al: Impact of early intervention services on duration of untreated psychosis: data from the National EDEN prospective cohort study. Schizophr Res 2014;159:1–6.

32 Valmaggia LR, et al: Duration of untreated psychosis and need for admission in patients who engage with mental health services in the prodromal phase. Br J Psychiatry 2015;207:130–134.

33 Bleuler E: Dementia praecox oder Gruppe der Schizophrenien; in Aschaffenburg G (ed): Handbuch der Psychiatrie. Leipzig, Deuticke, 1911, pp 1–420.

34 Kraepelin E: Psychiatrie. Ein Lehrbuch für Studierende und Aerzte, ed 4. Leipzig, Barth, 1893.

35 Mayer-Gross W: Die Klinik der Schizophrenie; in Bumke O (ed): Handbuch der Geisteskrankheiten. Berlin, Springer, 1932.

36 Huber G, Gross G: The concept of basic symptoms in schizophrenic and schizoaffective psychoses. Recenti Prog Med 1989;80:646–652.

37 Häfner H, et al: The influence of age and sex on the onset and early course of schizophrenia. Br J Psychiatry 1993;162:80–86.

38 Häfner H, et al: The ABC Schizophrenia Study: a preliminary overview of the results. Soc Psychiatry Psychiatr Epidemiol 1998;33:380–386.

39 Riecher A, et al: Schizophrenia – a disease of young single males – preliminary-results from an investigation on a representative cohort admitted to hospital for the 1st time. Eur Arch Psychiatry Clin Neurosci 1989;239:210–212.

40 Häfner H, et al: Sex differences in schizophrenic diseases (in German). Fortschr Neurol Psychiatr 1991; 59:343–360.

41 Häfner H, et al: Early detection and secondary prevention of psychosis: facts and visions. Eur Arch Psychiatry Clin Neurosci 2004;254:117–128.

42 Browne S, et al: Determinants of quality of life at first presentation with schizophrenia. Br J Psychiatry 2000;176:173–176.

43 Phillips LJ, Yung AR, McGorry PD: Identification of young people at risk of psychosis: validation of Personal Assessment and Crisis Evaluation Clinic intake criteria. Aust NZ J Psychiatry 2000;34:S164–S169.

44 Yung AR, et al: Prediction of psychosis – a step towards indicated prevention of schizophrenia. Br J Psychiatry 1998;172:14–20.

45 Yung AR: Commentary: The schizophrenia prodrome: a high-risk concept. Schizophr Bull 2003;29:859–865.

46 Cornblatt BA, et al: The schizophrenia prodrome revisited: a neurodevelopmental perspective. Schizophr Bull 2003;29:633–651.

47 Yung AR, et al: Monitoring and care of young people at incipient risk of psychosis. Schizophr Bull 1996; 22:283–303.

48 Klosterkötter J, et al: Diagnostic validity of basic symptoms. Eur Arch Psychiatry Clin Neurosci 1996; 246:147–154.

49 Schultze-Lutter F: Subjective symptoms of schizophrenia in research and the clinic: the basic symptom concept. Schizophr Bull 2009;35:5–8.

50 Fusar-Poli P, et al: Outreach and Support in South London (OASIS), 2001–2011: ten years of early diagnosis and treatment for young individuals at high clinical risk for psychosis. Eur Psychiatry 2013;28: 315–326.

51 Yung AR, et al: Mapping the onset of psychosis: the comprehensive assessment of at-risk mental states. Aust NZ J Psychiatry 2005;39:964–971.

52 Jackson HJ, McGorry PD, McKenzie D: The reliability of DSM-III prodromal symptoms in first-episode psychotic-patients. Acta Psychiatr Scand 1994;90: 375–378.

53 Miller TJ, et al: Interview for prodromal syndromes and the scale of prodromal symptoms: predictive validity, interrater reliability, and training to reliability. Schizophr Bull 2003;29:703–715.

54 Häfner H, et al: IRAOS – an instrument for the assessment of onset and early course of schizophrenia. Schizophr Res 1992;6:209–223.

55 Riecher-Rössler A, et al: The Basel Screening Instrument for Psychosis (BSIP): development, structure, reliability and validity (in German). Fortschr Neurol Psychiatr 2008;76:207–216.

56 Loewy RL, et al: The prodromal questionnaire (PQ): preliminary validation of a self-report screening and psychotic measure for prodromal syndromes. Schizophr Res 2005;79:117–125.

57 Klosterkötter J, et al: Evaluation of the 'Bonn Scale for the Assessment of Basic Symptoms BSABS' as an instrument for the assessment of schizophrenia proneness: a review of recent findings. Neurol Psychiatry Brain Res 1997;5:137–150.

58 Schultze-Lutter F, et al: Schizophrenia Proneness Instrument, Adult Version (SPI-A). Rome, Giovanni Fioriti Editore, 2007.

59 Schultze-Lutter F, et al: Basic symptoms and ultra-high risk criteria: symptom development in the initial prodromal state. Schizophr Bull 2010;36:182–191.

60 Fusar-Poli P, et al: Predicting psychosis meta-analysis of transition outcomes in individuals at high clinical risk. Arch Gen Psychiatry 2012;69:220–229.

61 Woods SW, et al: Validity of the Prodromal Risk Syndrome for First Psychosis: findings from the North American Prodrome Longitudinal Study. Schizophr Bull 2009;35:894–908.

62 Diagnostic and Statistical Manual of Mental Disorders (DSM-5), ed 5. Arlington, American Psychiatric Association, 2013.

63 Kelleher I, et al: Identification and characterization of prodromal risk syndromes in young adolescents in the community: a population-based clinical interview study. Schizophr Bull 2012;38:239–246.

64 Schimmelmann BG, et al: What percentage of people in the general population satisfies the current clinical at-risk criteria of psychosis? Schizophr Res 2011;125: 99–100.

65 Schultze-Lutter F, et al: Prevalence and clinical significance of DSM-5-attenuated psychosis syndrome in adolescents and young adults in the general population: the Bern Epidemiological At-Risk (BEAR) study. Schizophr Bull 2014;40:1499–1508.

66 Ruhrmann S, Schultze-Lutter F, Klosterkötter J: Probably at-risk, but certainly ill – advocating the introduction of a psychosis spectrum disorder in DSM-V. Schizophr Res 2010;120:23–37.

67 Valmaggia LR, et al: Economic impact of early detection and early intervention of psychosis. Curr Pharm Des 2012;18:592–595.

68 Stafford MR, et al: Early interventions to prevent psychosis: systematic review and meta-analysis. BMJ 2013;346:f185.

69 Morrison AP, et al: Cognitive therapy for the prevention of psychosis in people at ultra-high risk – randomised controlled trial. Br J Psychiatry 2004;185:291–297.

70 Addington J, et al: A randomized controlled trial of cognitive behavioral therapy for individuals at clinical high risk of psychosis. Schizophr Res 2011;125: 54–61.

71 McGlashan TH, et al: Randomized, double-blind trial of olanzapine versus placebo in patients prodromally symptomatic for psychosis. Am J Psychiatry 2006;163:790–799.

72 McGorry PD, et al: Randomized controlled trial of interventions designed to reduce the risk of progression to first-episode psychosis in a clinical sample with subthreshold symptoms. Arch Gen Psychiatry 2002;59:921–928.

73 Amminger GP, et al: Long-chain omega-3 fatty acids for indicated prevention of psychotic disorders: a randomized, placebo-controlled trial. Arch Gen Psychiatry 2010;67:146–154.

74 Bechdolf A, et al: Rationale and baseline characteristics of PREVENT: a second-generation intervention trial in subjects at-risk (prodromal) of developing first-episode psychosis evaluating cognitive behavior therapy, aripiprazole, and placebo for the prevention of psychosis. Schizophr Bull 2011;37:S111–S121.

75 Green MF: What are the functional consequences of neurocognitive deficits in schizophrenia? Am J Psychiatry 1996;153:321–330.

76 Green MF, et al: Neurocognitive deficits and functional outcome in schizophrenia: are we measuring the 'right stuff'? Schizophr Bull 2000;26:119–136.

77 Wiffen PJ, Moore RA: Demonstrating effectiveness – the concept of numbers-needed-to-treat. J Clin Pharm Ther 1996;21:23–27.

78 Fusar-Poli P, et al: The psychosis high-risk state: a comprehensive state-of-the-art review. JAMA Psychiatry 2013;70:107–120.

79 Knowler WC, et al: Reduction in the incidence of type 2 diabetes with lifestyle intervention or metformin. N Engl J Med 2002;346:393–403.

80 Antithrombotic Trialists' Collaboration: Collaborative meta-analysis of randomised trials of antiplatelet therapy for prevention of death, myocardial infarction, and stroke in high risk patients. BMJ 2002;324: 71–86.

81 Fusar-Poli P, Rocchetti M, Sardella A, Avila A, Brandizzi M, Caverzasi E, Politi P, Ruhrmann S, McGuire P: Disorder, not just state of risk: meta-analysis of functioning and quality of life in people at high risk of psychosis. Br J Psychiatry 2015;207:198–206.

82 Fusar-Poli P, et al: Attenuated psychosis syndrome: ready for DSM-5.1? Annu Rev Clin Psychol 2014;10: 155–192.

83 Wakefield JC: Wittgenstein's nightmare: why the RDoC grid needs a conceptual dimension. World Psychiatry 2014;13:38–40.

84 Epperson CN, et al: Premenstrual dysphoric disorder: evidence for a new category for DSM-5. Am J Psychiatry 2012;169:465–475.

85 Lin A, et al: Outcomes of nontransitioned cases in a sample at ultra-high risk for psychosis. Am J Psychiatry 2015;172:249–258.

86 Fusar-Poli P, et al: At risk for schizophrenic or affective psychoses? A meta-analysis of DSM/ICD diagnostic outcomes in individuals at high clinical risk. Schizophr Bull 2013;39:923–932.

87 Tabak AG, et al: Prediabetes: a high-risk state for diabetes development. Lancet 2012;379:2279–2290.

88 Daly CA, et al: Predicting prognosis in stable angina – results from the Euro heart survey of stable angina: prospective observational study. BMJ 2006;332:262–267.

Dr. Paolo Fusar-Poli
Department of Psychosis Studies
Institute of Psychiatry, Psychology and Neuroscience
King's College London
PO63, De Crespigny Park
London SE58AΓ (UK)
E-Mail paolo.fusar-poli@kcl.ac.uk

Riecher-Rössler A, McGorry PD (eds): Early Detection and Intervention in Psychosis: State of the Art and Future Perspectives. Key Issues Ment Health. Basel, Karger, 2016, vol 181, pp 69–82 (DOI: 10.1159/000440915)

Early Detection of Psychosis – Helpful or Stigmatizing Experience for Those Concerned?

Martina Uttinger[a] · Martina Papmeyer[a, b] · Anita Riecher-Rössler[a]

[a]Center for Gender Research and Early Detection, University of Basel Psychiatric Clinics, Basel, and [b]Division of Systems Neuroscience of Psychopathology, Translational Research Center, University Hospital of Psychiatry, University of Bern, Bern, Switzerland

Abstract

This chapter provides an overview of the literature on early detection of psychosis concerning stigma and discrimination in individuals with an at-risk mental state (ARMS) for psychosis. Extended surveys about stigma and psychosis/schizophrenia show that these patients belong to the most stigmatized patient groups. Therefore, ARMS individuals are conceivably affected by stigma and its consequences. In response to the recent scientific debate concerning potential stigma associated with an ARMS for psychosis, a small but growing number of studies on the topic have been carried out. The following two questions are addressed in this chapter: (1) do ARMS individuals experience stigma – and if so, what kind of stigma, and (2) are early detection centers contributing to stigma in any form or is the support offered rather experienced as helpful? Special emphasis is placed on the subjective perspective of ARMS individuals. Research reviewed in this chapter suggests that ARMS individuals fear stigma rather than having experienced it. They suffer from fear of negative reactions from peers, leading to concealment of mental issues, social withdrawal and delayed help-seeking. According to the literature reviewed, early detection services help individuals coping with symptoms, social isolation and potential stigma instead of enhancing or causing the latter. More emphasis should be placed on the subjective experiences and perspectives of those concerned in future research. Potential stigma including self-stigmatization should be assessed and included into treatment recommendations for individuals with an ARMS.

© 2016 S. Karger AG, Basel

Psychosis is commonly preceded by nonspecific symptoms such as difficulties concentrating, depressed mood, social withdrawal, lack of energy, and motivation or sleeping problems. Some patients already experience attenuated psychotic symptoms (e.g. subthreshold auditory hallucinations or delusions) in this early phase [1–3]. These attenuated psychotic symptoms can precede transition to psychosis by up to several years and clearly necessitate clinical attention as well as intervention. Early detection and intervention is thought to prevent numerous negative consequences such as a chronic course of illness and loss of quality of life [4]. Therefore, specialized early detection and early intervention services have been developed worldwide.

Since the emergence of the concept of psychosis early detection, one of the most common criticisms has been that informing individuals about their risk of developing psychosis potentially causes stigma. Especially the high rates of at-risk mental state (ARMS) individuals without transition to psychosis – on average 64% [5, 6] – have raised concerns that early detection centers seem to capture a high proportion of 'false positives' and lead to unnecessary fear, treatment and stigma [7, 8]. There were heated debates preceding the decision not to include the attenuated psychosis syndrome as a new category in the main body of the fifth edition of the Diagnostic and Statistical Manual (DSM-5), but instead in the research section [7, 9]. The inclusion in the DSM-5 was suggested since ARMS individuals frequently suffer from symptoms that need clinical attention which are not fully covered by any diagnostic category in the fourth edition of the Diagnostic and Statistical Manual (DSM-IV) [7]. However, one of the arguments amongst others contributing to the noninclusion of the attenuated psychosis syndrome in the DSM-5 were concerns that being informed about having an ARMS may lead to harmful stigma [10]. Given the serious consequences of stigma in addition to a mental health issue [11], there has been growing interest in research about the subjective perspective of those concerned as well as stigma in the recent years [12].

The literature reviewed in this chapter is based on a systematic literature search using PubMed, Web of Science and Medline with the keywords: (Stigma* OR Discrimination) AND (ARMS OR 'clinical high risk' OR 'ultra high risk' OR 'psychosis risk'). The references of relevant papers were additionally screened for further studies on the topic.

The main focus of this chapter concerns two questions. Do ARMS individuals experience any stigma – and if so what kind? And are early detection centers contributing to stigma in any form or is the support offered by early detection centers experienced as helpful? Special emphasis is placed on the subjective perspective of those concerned.

General concepts and definitions of different aspects of stigma will be introduced first. Second, a brief literature review on stigma and schizophrenia/psychosis will be provided. Third, a literature review on stigma in ARMS will be presented, focusing on public stigma, internalized stigma and stigma stress. Fourth, helpful aspects as well as potentially stigmatizing ones will be described. Fifth, promising ways of how stigma could be addressed in ARMS individuals will be presented. Finally, conclusions will be drawn.

General Concepts of Stigma and Labeling

Stigma is commonly defined as 'an attribute that is deeply discrediting and that reduces the bearer from a whole and usual person to a tainted, discounted one' [13] as well as 'the negative attitude (based on prejudice and misinformation) that is triggered by a marker of illness' [14]. In psychiatry, the most investigated aspect of stigma is public stigma – the opinion of the general public about those affected by a mental illness. This is usually measured with questionnaires such as Link's Devaluation-Discrimination Scale [15] and incorporates measures of desired social distance from those affected by mental illness. This questionnaire is able to capture stereotypes reliably as it allows respondents to imagine those affected by mental illness according to socially determined stereotypes in the absence of appropriate knowledge. Public stigma has been found to be relatively stable if not even slightly increasing in the last decade [16].

Mental health services are possibly contributing to stigma by labeling a help-seeking individual as a 'psychiatric patient' at first contact and later on using a diagnosis such as 'schizophrenia'. Labeling is defined as 'when people distinguish a human difference as significant and assign it to a label' [11]. In the case of psychosis risk, the label consists of the ARMS. The labeling theory is further elaborated in the literature elsewhere [17].

Since individuals concerned about mental health issues are part of the society like everyone else, they are also affected themselves by stereotypes about mental illness as these are developed during socialization [18]. As they enter psychiatric services and get diagnosed, the extent of their own identification with those stereotypes determines if and how strongly they experience stigma. The process of 'becoming aware of negative stereotypes associated with the label and identifying oneself with them' is referred to as self-stigmatization or internalized stigma [11]. This has been associated with low self-esteem, depression, reduced help-seeking and poor prognosis [19–22].

Stigma in Those Affected by Psychosis/Schizophrenia

Extended surveys within the general population found that schizophrenia patients are the most stigmatized among psychiatric patient groups [11, 23, 24]. There are fewer studies focusing on the topic from the subjective perspective of schizophrenia patients, but they come to the same conclusion [25]. Furthermore, it has been shown that stigmatization is already evident at the first episode of psychosis [12, 26]. Concerning internalized stigma in patients with schizophrenia, there is evidence that it has a mediating role between insight and depression. Illness insight is therefore more likely to contribute to depression when internalized stigma is high and patients identify themselves with negative stereotypes [27]. This again points to the importance of taking aspects of stigma into account that pertain to the subjective perspective of those concerned. For those diagnosed with schizophrenia, it has been shown that stigma stress – the perceived relevance of personal stigma as a stressor – may arise as part of developing illness insight [28].

Stigma in Individuals with an At-Risk Mental State for Psychosis

One review analyzing the theoretical and empirical literature on stigma in ARMS individuals concluded that there was an urgent need for further research and adaptation of systematic measures to assess stigma in those concerned [9]. The few existing studies came to similar conclusions – stating that stigma carries potentially negative consequences for those concerned and that more research was needed. However, practical advice in dealing with stigma seems to be lacking – not just in the field of psychosis early detection [29]. Research has also predominantly focused on public stigma instead of the subjective experiences of those concerned. Fortunately, in the last years, this situation has started to change. However, there is still a very small but growing number of studies investigating potential stigma in these individuals.

A recent review, entitled 'Diagnosis telling in people with psychosis' by Milton and Mullan [30], dedicates a paragraph to articles on ARMS individuals and first-episode psychosis patients – including four studies with ARMS individuals. The authors state that there is still a lack of research on communication of risk information [31], but that the available evidence can be used to derive some recommendations for communicating the risk status to ARMS individuals. Another review came to the same conclusion [31]. Since the subject of diagnosis telling is fundamentally linked to the issue of stigma, there are some suggestions concerning stigma in the review which will be elaborated further in the course of this chapter.

Public Stigma in Those with an ARMS for Psychosis

Studies on public stigma in ARMS individuals were mostly using vignettes – written descriptions of typical affected individuals and their behavior – when investigating labeling and aspects such as stereotypes (e.g. perceived dangerousness, fear) or desired social distance. These short vignettes were shown to participants followed by a number of questions or items investigating the subject of interest. A study that examined spontaneous labeling among peers in that manner suggested that the majority of respondents did not use diagnostic labels spontaneously when asked to describe the presented individual [32]. However, the most frequently used label was 'paranoid' – a characteristic symptom of psychosis. Participants using this label were also more likely to describe fear in response to the vignette character than those that used labels such as 'weird' or 'troubled'. This points to the risk of stigma due to unusually altered behavior of those affected without necessarily being labelled with a psychiatric diagnosis or being in contact with a psychiatric center. A previous vignette study which used a priori diagnosis showed greater stigma in the context of a psychosis-related than mood-related diagnosis [33]. Therefore, the authors suspect that an ARMS diagnosis could lead to greater stigma in peers than the manifestation of altered behavior on its own [33]. However, since altered perception and behavior are apparent prior to first contact with the health care system [10], their contribution towards stigma in ARMS individuals should not be underestimated [18].

Accordingly, there is evidence that both the unusually altered behavior as well as the psychosis-related labels may subject ARMS individuals to considerable stigma. The presence of common stereotypes about psychosis and schizophrenia in the minds of ARMS individuals combined with a lack of knowledge about the disease also seems to promote self-stigmatization. However, most studies so far have not researched how individuals subjectively perceive stigma.

Besides labeling and self-labeling, there are other aspects suspected to be linked with proneness to stigma in ARMS individuals. Potential misinterpretation of the ARMS as being equivalent to schizophrenia [9, 34] would be an example of such a factor. Another factor possibly enhancing stigma would be that the age group mostly affected by the onset of psychotic-like symptoms (i.e., adolescence and young adulthood) shows especially high levels of negative stereotyping related to mental illness [9]. There is, however, no evidence so far for either one of these two aspects. One qualitative study showed that ARMS individuals were aware of common stereotypes about psychosis, but no differences between the age groups were observed [35]. However, the sample size of the aforementioned qualitative study was too small to draw firm conclusions, as it consisted of 11 individuals only, aged between 20 and 42 years. Further, ARMS individuals seem to be keen on getting information about their condition and psychoeducation has been found to be one of the most accepted forms of intervention [30, 35, 36]. Young age groups seem to be especially open and interested in being informed about their condition.

The literature reviewed in this paragraph generates rather heterogeneous results concerning public stigma in ARMS individuals. While the altered behavior as well as psychosis-related labels and stereotypes seem to be an issue in ARMS individuals, no study has investigated the effect of the ARMS label on individuals after they had received psychoeducation. Existing findings must also be interpreted with caution as they have not been replicated thoroughly. Nevertheless, these results point to the importance of the subjective side of how the public stigma is perceived and endorsed respectively by those concerned. This is enforced by studies that suggest that stigma stress in ARMS individuals mediates help-seeking behavior and the attitude of those concerned [37, 38].

Studies with ARMS individuals suggest that the perceived public stigma, shame and self-labelling of ARMS were independently associated with an increase in stigma stress [37]. The next sections of this chapter are therefore dedicated to different aspects of internalized stigma reported in research on ARMS individuals.

Internalized Stigma in Those with an ARMS for Psychosis
Studies have shown that internalized stigma in ARMS individuals is associated with a number of negative consequences such as depression, social anxiety and decreased well-being [21, 38]. Qualitative studies with ARMS individuals could elaborate several aspects that pertain to internalized stigma in ARMS.

The concerns about potential stigma that are prominent in critics of early detection are also found in those affected by the ARMS. Unlike other conditions, the ARMS is –

as most other psychiatric diseases up to a certain stage of illness – invisible to others. This enables individuals affected to conceal their problem. Besides the advantages of maintaining a seemingly normal façade, it may have negative consequences or even come at tremendous costs for the individual such as having to play a role at all times and not being able to talk openly even to close friends.

Accordingly, ARMS individuals experience insecurities and fear regarding the disclosure of their problems as well as the ARMS diagnosis to others close to them. This theme has been found consistently throughout several qualitative studies [35, 39, 40]. Patients frequently find it hard to admit to themselves that they do have issues and even harder to admit this to others. Seeking treatment is delayed because getting help implies disclosure about one's problems. Accordingly, stigma stress has been found to delay help-seeking in ARMS individuals [37]. Individuals withdraw socially and isolate themselves out of fear that others might discover they have issues. They often also feel incapable of dealing with social contact due to symptoms like paranoid thoughts or social anxiety [41].

One reason for withholding information on problems in ARMS individuals are rooted in stereotypes and the fear of 'going mad' [39, 41]. ARMS individuals are concerned that if others discovered they had issues, they would react in a negative way and/or distance themselves from the affected individual. Some ARMS individuals clearly perceive that there is something wrong with them, but do not know what it is. This induces fear and keeping problems a secret [35, 41]. Disclosure of problems to a mental health professional therefore has a special importance as will be described in a later section of this chapter [41].

Also, there seems to be a difference between disclosing problems and the ARMS state. In one qualitative study that interviewed ARMS individuals, many had disclosed their problems or parts of them to peers and relatives using watered-down versions, but fewer also disclosed that they had been given an ARMS diagnosis [35]. Reasons for this included that it was uncertain that they would actually develop psychosis, and that they found it too complicated or did not feel up to the task to explain to someone that they had a risk of developing something that they did not fully understand at that time. Many of them also stated that the previously mentioned fear of how others would react stopped them from disclosing the ARMS. However, from those that had talked about their problems and their ARMS, none experienced negative reactions from their peers or family. This is in line with the results of another qualitative study [40]. It highlights once again the existing gap between the fear of disclosing their problems that causes patients to withdraw and the actual support and acceptance they experience in real life if they are able to overcome the fear. Offering knowledge and support to help facilitate the latter in early detection services therefore plays an important role for those concerned.

In one qualitative study, several patients reported 'not being taken seriously' or 'being perceived as lazy or lacking motivation' by their social environment [35]. This includes friends thinking they were skipping school out of laziness as well as family

Uttinger · Papmeyer · Riecher-Rössler

doctors giving a few days of sick leave without the requested referral to a mental health professional. Therefore, they felt relieved to be finally perceived as having a mental health condition during their contact with the early detection center.

In conclusion, internalized stigma in ARMS individuals seems to be rooted in stereotypes about mental illness in combination with the insight that there is something wrong with them. Not knowing what is wrong, the fear of 'going mad' and interpersonal relationships are contributing factors to delayed help-seeking and stigma. There seems to be a certain amount of internalized stigma before individuals enter early detection services. The next section will cover the contribution of early detection services in dealing with stigma in their patients.

Contribution of Early Detection Services to Stigma in ARMS Individuals
So far, qualitative studies have shown that ARMS individuals are able to distinguish clearly between the ARMS and actual schizophrenia and that they take the uncertainty of prognosis into account when dealing with the information about the ARMS [35, 40]. The literature reviewed suggests that early detection services help individuals coping with symptoms, social isolation and potential stigma instead of enhancing or causing the latter.

One qualitative study revealed some relevant aspects of stigma [35]. First of all, the individuals interviewed were aware of the common stereotypes about psychosis. Nevertheless, they did not seem to endorse the stereotypes but instead distanced themselves from them and thus from internalized stigma. Concerning the question about whether early detection centers contribute to stigma in ARMS, patient statements revealed no evidence of such additional stigma. This is in accordance with a previous study by Welsh and Tiffin [40]. The findings summarized above suggest that the support offered by early detection centers helps alleviate stigma. This is further underlined by patients' reports of generally positive experiences with the early detection clinic [21].

And even if mentioning the terms psychosis risk may at first be disconcerting or even lead to some internalized stigma [35], the benefits of the help ARMS individuals receive in early detection centers far outweighs any harmful effects it may have at first. This is especially the case in the light of the severe consequences of no or greatly delayed treatment [2]. The following section explains these helpful aspects in detail.

Helpful Aspects of Support Offered in Early Detection Services

Early detection clinics intend to identify patients meeting the ARMS criteria in order to monitor their symptoms and to offer treatment if necessary. They mainly focus on the immediate presenting problems and try to reduce the risk of transition by dealing with immediate issues of stress, etc. They do not catastrophize about the possibility of transition, but instead educate in an optimistic way about the current possibilities of treatment and course. In doing so, they aim at counteracting numerous negative consequences of eventual emerging psychotic disorders such as the chronic course of illness or loss of social relationships [42]. Recommended treatment for ARMS individuals includes cognitive behavioral therapy in early stages and pharmacological interventions in cases not responding to the former [42].

Early treatment is thus thought to be a crucial protecting factor against stigmatization resulting from harmful consequences of prodromal symptoms [43, 44] [for reviews, see 1, 42]. The following paragraphs summarize several helpful aspects that ARMS individuals have emphasized so far. These are based mostly on the qualitative research available.

Information About the ARMS Is Helpful and Wanted
One study investigated psychology undergraduate students' responses regarding the news of being at enhanced risk of psychosis. The study showed that the news about the risk of developing schizophrenia was on par with the anticipated impact of news about the risk of developing cancer, but less desirable than the risk for depression. Higher anticipated stigmatization was one of the predicting factors for the anticipated negative impact of news on the psychosis risk [44]. In a second study, the participants were told they had a risk of developing schizophrenia, depression and cancer, respectively, based on a bogus saliva test. Participants were told they had an enzyme which was linked to an enhanced risk of developing one of the conditions outlined. Interestingly, there was no difference in the level of stress response between the news about different risk states and the control group that was told about the presence of the enzyme, without relating it to a specific illness risk. Anticipated stigmatization also did not alter the stress response to the news about the risk of developing schizophrenia [44]. So while the first study suggests that there seems to be an anticipated higher stress response, evidence from the second study suggests that there is no such response given the actual information. How do these results investigating healthy psychology students transfer to individuals with an actual ARMS?

Qualitative studies have shown that patients clearly demand to be informed about their condition [35, 40]. Further, being able to name their condition proved to be relieving and helpful [35, 40]. There is no evidence for long-lasting negative consequences of the information about having an ARMS for affected individuals. Short-term effects reported by one qualitative study include being shocked at first as well as a strong need to discuss further questions and insecurities with the staff of the early detection center [35]. This is in line with evidence from studies assessing the psychological impact of at-risk states for other illnesses (e.g. cardiovascular risk, risk of cancer, etc.). These have shown that information about an at-risk status was related to anxiety, depression and distress in the short term only [45].

Also, modern medicine usually regards the autonomy of patients and their right to know about their condition as very important, and this should also be considered in the case of ARMS individuals [30]. It needs to be researched as to whether this need for information is necessarily only covered by using the attenuated psychosis syndrome or the ARMS, or if better suited notions that capture the condition exist [46]. Analogously, there were also considerations in the literature about the possible impact of changing the term 'schizophrenia' and instead using a notion less attached to stigma [47, 48].

The Helpful Nature of Social Contact with Mental Health Professionals

Disclosure of problems to mental health professionals was experienced as helpful and relieving in many ways [39]. This has been shown in several qualitative studies [35, 49, 50]. The relief was particularly strong in patients who were either lacking interpersonal relationships with family members or friends to feel comfortable enough to disclose their problems or were afraid of negative reactions – as described above.

The most beneficial aspect, however, for many individuals seems to be interpersonal contact with the staff of an early detection clinic [39]. The importance of social contact in ARMS has consistently been emphasized in several studies about ARMS individuals [41, 50]. It is noteworthy that the majority of individuals interviewed in one study expressed interest in sharing experiences with other individuals affected by ARMS [35]. These findings support the crucial role of early detection clinics in providing social contact with mental health professionals and other affected individuals, possibly in the form of group therapy or guided self-help groups. Offering a neutral, nonjudging environment encourages individuals to address stigma. Normalizing experiences such as conversations using informal everyday language and noncatastrophic reactions to disclosure of unusual experiences are helpful as well [31, 49].

Focus of Treatment on Normalizing and Everyday Life

ARMS individuals tend to favor informal and accepting ways of communication as well as use of common language. Treatment approaches conveying normalization of unusual psychological experiences and treatment as collaboration were stated as being especially helpful [41]. This includes adequate information, building an alliance between patient and therapist, and shared decision-making as far as possible. Another need expressed by ARMS individuals is support concerning their everyday problems [35]. For example, this can be achieved by offering supportive psychotherapy or cognitive behavioral therapy, case management, social work, etc.

Stigma-Free and Youth Friendly Culture of Care

Furthermore, early detection services should be accessible for everyone and placed in a nonstigmatizing environment. Centrally located buildings with a loose or no visible association to psychiatry (e.g. not in the same building as acute psychiatric wards) would be best suited for that matter. Low-threshold support in the form of counselling with a professional could reduce the fear of stigma and foster the confidence to talk openly about one's problems. Flyers or newspaper articles featuring information about early detection services should be created in a readable manner suited to the needs of young people. Specialized early detection centers should be well connected with all centers that are part of providing services to young people (e.g. schools, general counselling centers) in order to offer quick and low-threshold help for individuals in need. The FePsy Clinic in Basel, Switzerland (www.fepsy.ch) as well as the Australian headspace centers (www.headspace.org.au) [51, 52] are examples fulfilling these criteria.

Possible Interventions Regarding Stigma in Those Affected by an ARMS

Traditionally, psychotic symptoms are treated with antipsychotic medication. Since psychopharmacological treatment of psychotic symptoms is associated with potentially harmful side effects, it is recommended only to implement it when transition to frank psychosis happens. Psychosocial interventions are the favored treatment in ARMS [42, 52]. Additionally, since it has been proven to be an issue for those concerned, stigma should also be considered when treating ARMS individuals.

Qualitative studies have shown that the needs of ARMS individuals concerning support as well as the aspects they found helpful are highly dependent on the individual [35, 41]. Therefore, treatment guidelines for ARMS individuals should be flexible enough to be able to incorporate individual needs of patients concerning stigma. Nevertheless, there is a need for standardized guidelines to address stigma when treating ARMS individuals.

Shift in Attitude of Professionals Towards ARMS Individuals
Studies have shown that mental health professionals are also affected by stigma and stereotypes related to mental illness [53]. Early treatment of patients with beginning psychosis often consists of erroneously either failing to diagnose them or diagnosing them with psychosis already and treating them with neuroleptics. Either way, ARMS individuals are possibly not receiving adequate support. Since these individuals in many cases are in desperate need of help, psychiatrists, psychologists, family doctors and any other health professionals involved should be increasingly sensitive to the condition and refer patients to specialized early detection and early intervention services for assessment and treatment. If these services are not available, patients should be supported with the help available. A change in attitude of mental health professionals towards ARMS individuals to a supportive and understanding way of treating them is very urgently due in order to break the cycle of helplessness.

Standardized Assessment of Stigma in ARMS Individuals
Standardized assessment of stigma should be part of any clinical assessment for psychosis risk. This could be done with a short questionnaire [21] or additionally with questions embedded in the clinical interview used to assess the risk criteria. The focus should be on internalized stigma and the presence and endorsement of negative

stereotypes regarding psychosis or mental health services. Such assessment could later be used to personalize the information about the risk status and psychoeducation by placing special emphasis on correcting stereotypes in patients who identify themselves strongly with negative stereotypes.

Psychoeducation

There has been a general controversy whether information about mental health conditions is helpful or if it encourages further stigma. This has been referred to as the insight paradox in the literature [22, 27]. Nevertheless, psychoeducation is one of the most accepted forms of intervention in ARMS individuals [30]. As described above, patients want to know about their condition [35, 40]. Furthermore, information is essential to conquer false beliefs and stereotypes that are present in ARMS individuals. Actively addressing stigma by correcting false beliefs about psychosis is especially important as patients do not tend to bring these subjects up spontaneously. In order to overcome the fear of others' negative reactions and talk about their problems and their condition, ARMS individuals benefit greatly from the information and the support offered in early detection centers [41]. Normalizing unusual psychological experiences has been found to be very important in that matter [39]. Empowering individuals to become experts of their own condition could help to alleviate the fear of rejection.

Cognitive Behavioral Therapy

Recommended treatment for ARMS individuals includes cognitive behavioral therapy in early stages and additional pharmacological interventions in cases not responding to the former [42]. Psychosocial interventions are well accepted [54] and as opposed to pharmacological treatment have a considerably lower risk of side effects. Besides evidence that cognitive behavior therapy so far seemed to reduce rates of transition to psychosis [4, 54], there is also evidence for reduced severity of symptoms in individuals treated with psychotherapy [54].

However, similar to psychoeducation, there have also been concerns that cognitive behavioral therapy may increase stigma in ARMS individuals instead of alleviating it [54]. There has been only one study by Morrison et al. [43] that investigated the effects of cognitive behavioral therapy on internalized stigma in ARMS individuals. Their results suggest that cognitive behavioral therapy in individuals meeting ARMS criteria does not increase but rather seems to reduce negative appraisals of unusual cognitive experiences over a time period of 12–24 months.

Methods to Cope with Stigma Stress

Besides addressing stigma, methods to cope with stigma-related stress should be considered. There was a study showing good results for individuals with psychosis using a pre-/posttest evaluation of an intervention offered in a day clinic setting [55]. Another qualitative study showed promising results in an outpatient setting with psychosis patients [56], and one part of a manual used in that study covers internalized stigma. Therefore, it seems likely that ARMS individuals could also benefit from such an intervention and that the manual could be adapted for this purpose.

Group Therapy/Self-Help Groups
To the best of our knowledge, there is no established manual available for group therapy or self-help groups with ARMS individuals. So far, the wish for exchange of experiences with other individuals affected has been shown in one qualitative study [35]. Other studies also point to the importance of social contact – an area in which ARMS individuals are often lacking [41]. The knowledge that they are not the only ones affected by this condition seems to be relieving to many patients. Therefore, it is to be expected that some of them would benefit from an exchange of experiences with other individuals affected by the same condition. All of these possible interventions require further testing in randomized controlled studies with ARMS individuals.

Conclusions

With respect to stigma in ARMS, there seems to be a gap between what is generally expected and what is experienced by those concerned. This bias is found in critics of early detection as well as in students investigated in studies and in ARMS individuals themselves.

Qualitative research has yielded new insights to our understanding of the effect of being informed about having an ARMS. Individuals were able to provide detailed and meaningful descriptions of their experiences [41]. Patients seem to benefit from sharing their personal view including that on eventual stigma. Since ARMS individuals are affected by stigma in terms of stereotype awareness and self-stigmatization, early detection centers play an important role in counteracting and preventing stigma by sharing knowledge and adjusting stereotypes. Any treatment manual used in ARMS individuals should include standardized assessment of stigma as well as interventions actively addressing stereotypes, internalized stigmatization and associated coping skills. Qualitative studies can serve as a base for further investigations on this topic.

References

1 Riecher-Rössler A, Pflueger MO, Aston J, et al: Efficacy of using cognitive status in predicting psychosis: a 7-year follow-up. Biol Psychiatry 2009;66: 1023–1030.

2 Riecher-Rössler A, Gschwandtner U, Borgwardt S, et al: Early detection and treatment of schizophrenia: how early? Acta Psychiatr Scand Suppl, 2006, pp 73–80.

3 Yung AR, McGorry PD: The prodromal phase of first-episode psychosis: past and current conceptualizations. Schizophr Bull 1996;22:353–370.

4 van der Gaag M, Smit F, Bechdolf A, et al: Preventing a first episode of psychosis: meta-analysis of randomized controlled prevention trials of 12 month and longer-term follow-ups. Schizophr Res 2013; 149:56–62.

5   Fusar-Poli P, Borgwardt S, Bechdolf A, et al: The psychosis high-risk state: a comprehensive state-of-the-art review. JAMA Psychiatry 2013;70:107–120.

6   Simon AE, Borgwardt S, Riecher-Rössler A, et al: Moving beyond transition outcomes: meta-analysis of remission rates in individuals at high clinical risk for psychosis. Psychiatry Res 2013;209:266–272.

7   Yung AR, Woods SW, Ruhrmann S, et al: Whither the attenuated psychosis syndrome? Schizophr Bull 2012;38:1130–1134.

8   Simon AE, Velthorst E, Nieman DH, et al: Ultra high-risk state for psychosis and non-transition: a systematic review. Schizophr Res 2011;132:8–17.

9   Yang LH, Wonpat-Borja AJ, Opler MG, et al: Potential stigma associated with inclusion of the psychosis risk syndrome in the DSM-V: an empirical question. Schizophr Res 2010;120:42–48.

10 Shrivastava A, McGorry PD, Tsuang M, et al: 'Attenuated psychotic symptoms syndrome' as a risk syndrome of psychosis, diagnosis in DSM-V: the debate. Indian J Psychiatry 2011;53:57–65.

11 Link BG, Struening EL, Neese-Todd S, et al: On describing and seeking to change the experience of stigma. Psychiatr Rehabil Skills 2002;6:201–231.

12 Gerlinger G, Hauser M, De Hert M, et al: Personal stigma in schizophrenia spectrum disorders: a systematic review of prevalence rates, correlates, impact and interventions. World Psychiatry 2013;12:155–164.

13 Goffman E: Stigma Notes on the Management of Spoiled Identity. New York, Simon and Schuster, 1986.

14 Sartorius N: Stigma and mental health. Lancet 2007; 370:810–811.

15 Link BG, Yang LH, Phelan JC, et al: Measuring mental illness stigma. Schizophr Bull 2004;30:511–541.

16 Thornicroft G, Brohan E, Rose D, et al: Global pattern of experienced and anticipated discrimination against people with schizophrenia: a cross-sectional survey. Lancet 2009;373:408–415.

17 Link BG, Cullen FT, Struening E, et al: A modified labeling theory approach to mental disorders: an empirical assessment. Am Soc Rev 1989;54:400–423.

18 van Zelst C: Stigmatization as an environmental risk in schizophrenia: a user perspective. Schizophr Bull 2009;35:293–296.

19 Ritsher JB, Phelan JC: Internalized stigma predicts erosion of morale among psychiatric outpatients. Psychiatry Res 2004;129:257–265.

20 Ruhrmann S, Paruch J, Bechdolf A, et al: Reduced subjective quality of life in persons at risk for psychosis. Acta Psychiatr Scand 2008;117:357–368.

21 Pyle M, Stewart SL, French P, et al: Internalized stigma, emotional dysfunction and unusual experiences in young people at risk of psychosis. Early Interv Psychiatry 2015;9:133–140.

22 Schrank B, Amering M, Hay AG, et al: Insight, positive and negative symptoms, hope, depression and self-stigma: a comprehensive model of mutual influences in schizophrenia spectrum disorders. Epidemiol Psychiatr Sci 2014;23:271–279.

23 Gaebel W, Baumann A, Witte AM, et al: Public attitudes towards people with mental illness in six German cities: results of a public survey under special consideration of schizophrenia. Eur Arch Psychiatry Clin Neurosci 2002;252:278–287.

24 van Zelst C: Which environments for G × E? A user perspective on the roles of trauma and structural discrimination in the onset and course of schizophrenia. Schizophr Bull 2008;34:1106–1110.

25 Mestdagh A, Hansen B: Stigma in patients with schizophrenia receiving community mental health care: a review of qualitative studies. Soc Psychiatry Psychiatr Epidemiol 2014;49:79–87.

26 Harris K, Collinson C, das Nair R: Service-users' experiences of an early intervention in psychosis service: an interpretative phenomenological analysis. Psychol Psychother 2012;85:456–469.

27 Bouvet C, Bouchoux A: Exploring the relationship between internalized stigma, insight and depression for inpatients with schizophrenia (in French). Encephale 2014, Epub ahead of print.

28 Pruss L, Wiedl KH, Waldorf M: Stigma as a predictor of insight in schizophrenia. Psychiatry Res 2012;198: 187–193.

29 Norman RM, Windell D, Manchanda R: Examining differences in the stigma of depression and schizophrenia. Int J Soc Psychiatry 2012;58:69–78.

30 Milton AC, Mullan BA: Diagnosis telling in people with psychosis. Curr Opin Psychiatry 2014;27:302–307.

31 Welsh P, Tiffin PA: Attitudes of patients and clinicians in relation to the at-risk state for psychosis. Early Interv Psychiatry 2013;7:361–367.

32 Anglin DM, Greenspoon MI, Lighty Q, et al: Spontaneous labelling and stigma associated with clinical characteristics of peers 'at-risk' for psychosis. Early Interv Psychiatry 2014;8:247–252.

33 Yang LH, Anglin DM, Wonpat-Borja AJ, et al: Public stigma of the psychosis risk syndrome in a college population: implications for peer intervention. Psychiatr Serv 2013;64:284–288.

34 Yang LH, Lo G, Wonpat-Borja AJ, et al: Effects of labeling and interpersonal contact upon attitudes towards schizophrenia: implications for reducing mental illness stigma in urban China. Soc Psychiatry Psychiatr Epidemiol 2012;47:1459–1473.

35 Uttinger M, Koranyi S, Papmeyer M, et al: Early detection of psychosis – helpful or stigmatizing experience? A qualitative study. Early Interv Psychiatry 2015, Epub ahead of print.

36 Welsh P, Brown S: 'I'm not insane, my mother had me tested': the risk and benefits of being labelled 'at-risk' for psychosis. Health Risk Soc 2013;15:648–662.

37 Rüsch N, Heekeren K, Theodoridou A, et al: Attitudes towards help-seeking and stigma among young people at risk for psychosis. Psychiatry Res 2013;210:1313–1315.

38 Rüsch N, Müller M, Heekeren K, et al: Longitudinal course of self-labeling, stigma stress and well-being among young people at risk of psychosis. Schizophr Res 2014;158:82–84.

39 Byrne R, Morrison AP: Young people at risk of psychosis: a user-led exploration of interpersonal relationships and communication of psychological difficulties. Early Interv Psychiatry 2010;4:162–168.

40 Welsh P, Tiffin PA: Observations of a small sample of adolescents experiencing an at-risk mental state (ARMS) for psychosis. Schizophr Bull 2012;38:215–218.

41 Hardy KV, Dickson JM, Morrison AP: Journey into and through an early detection of psychosis service: the subjective experience of persons at risk of developing psychosis. Early Interv Psychiatry 2009;3:52–57.

42 McGorry PD, Nelson B, Amminger GP, et al: Intervention in individuals at ultra-high risk for psychosis: a review and future directions. J Clin Psychiatry 2009;70:1206–1212.

43 Morrison AP, Birchwood M, Pyle M, et al: Impact of cognitive therapy on internalised stigma in people with at-risk mental states. Br J Psychiatry 2013;203:140–145.

44 Alder RG, Young JL, Russell EI, et al: The impact and desirability of news of risk for schizophrenia. PLoS One 2013;8:e62904.

45 Shaw C, Abrams K, Marteau TM: Psychological impact of predicting individuals' risks of illness: a systematic review. Soc Sci Med 1999;49:1571–1598.

46 Koren D: Early detection and intervention in psychiatry in the post-DSM-5 publication era: is it time to rethink the trees we bark up? Early Interv Psychiatry 2013;7:235–237.

47 Tranulis C, Lecomte T, El-Khoury B, et al: Changing the name of schizophrenia: patient perspectives and implications for DSM-V. PLoS One 2013;8:e55998.

48 Sartorius N, Chiu H, Heok KE, et al: Name change for schizophrenia. Schizophr Bull 2014;40:255–258.

49 Byrne RE, Morrison AP: Young people at risk of psychosis: their subjective experiences of monitoring and cognitive behaviour therapy in the early detection and intervention evaluation 2 trial. Psychol Psychother 2014;87:357–371.

50 Welsh P, Tiffin PA: Experience of child and adolescent mental health clinicians working within an at-risk mental state for psychosis service: a qualitative study. Early Interv Psychiatry 2012;6:207–211.

51 McGorry PD, Goldstone SD, Parker AG, et al: Cultures for mental health care of young people: an Australian blueprint for reform. Lancet Psychiatry 2014;1:559–568.

52 Rickwood DJ, Telford NR, Parker AG, et al: headspace – Australia's innovation in youth mental health: who are the clients and why are they presenting? Med J Aust 2014;200:108–111.

53 Sartorius N, Gaebel W, Cleveland HR, et al: WPA guidance on how to combat stigmatization of psychiatry and psychiatrists. World Psychiatry 2010;9:131–144.

54 Stafford MR, Jackson H, Mayo-Wilson E, et al: Early interventions to prevent psychosis: systematic review and meta-analysis. BMJ 2013;346:f185.

55 Sibitz I, Provaznikova K, Lipp M, et al: The impact of recovery-oriented day clinic treatment on internalized stigma: preliminary report. Psychiatry Res 2013;209:326–332.

56 Sibitz I, Amering M, Gössler R, et al: Patients' perspective on what works in psychoeducational groups for schizophrenia: a qualitative study. Soc Psychiatry Psychiatr Epidemiol 2007;42:909–915.

Prof. Anita Riecher-Rössler
Center for Gender Research and Early Detection, University of Basel Psychiatric Clinics
Kornhausgasse 7
CH–4051 Basel (Switzerland)
E-Mail anita.riecher@upkbs.ch

Riecher-Rössler A, McGorry PD (eds): Early Detection and Intervention in Psychosis: State of the Art and Future Perspectives. Key Issues Ment Health. Basel, Karger, 2016, vol 181, pp 83–94 (DOI: 10.1159/000440916)

Structural and Functional MRI in the Prediction of Psychosis

Dominic B. Dwyer · Philip McGuire

Institute of Psychiatry, Psychology, and Neuroscience, Department of Psychosis Studies, King's College London, London, UK

Abstract

It is difficult to predict whether an individual who is at high risk for psychosis will go on to develop the disorder using clinical and behavioural measures alone. This chapter describes findings from neuroimaging research that may be useful in helping to predict outcomes in this group. The main methods employed will be reviewed and the potential for translating research findings into clinical practice will be discussed.   © 2016 S. Karger AG, Basel

The Rationale of Finding Predictive Markers Using Neuroimaging

The notion that early detection and treatment provides the best opportunity for recovery is well established across medical fields [1]. The application of this approach to psychosis has led to the characterisation of clinical and behavioural features that are associated with an increased risk of psychosis [see 2, 3] and the definition of a clinical syndrome [4–6] associated with a high probability of developing psychosis in 3 years [4, 7]. However, within a sample of people at high risk, it is difficult to predict which individuals will go on to develop psychosis on the basis of their specific clinical features. As a result, at present, potentially preventative clinical interventions are usually offered to all those at risk, even though most will not subsequently become psychotic and some will recover without any treatment. This represents an inefficient use of clinical resources and raises ethical questions. Thus, there is a clear clinical need for biomarkers that could be used to identify the individuals who are most likely to become psychotic so that preventative interventions could be selectively provided to this subgroup.

The search for predictors of outcomes in those at high risk for psychosis is not a new endeavour, and a number of behavioural assessments that provide an indirect measure of brain functioning have been examined, including tests of olfactory processing [8] and cognitive performance [7, 9]. However, neuroimaging permits a more direct assessment of the structure and functioning of the brain in vivo, and thus has particular potential to identify biomarkers that may be used to predict clinical outcomes.

Structural MRI of the High-Risk State

To date, the most commonly used neuroimaging method used to identify predictors in high-risk subjects has been structural magnetic resonance imaging (MRI). These studies have ranged from a priori, hypothesis-driven investigations of a specific brain region of interest [e.g., 10], to largely hypothesis-free exploratory investigations of the whole brain [e.g., 11].

Manual Tracing Methods
Lawrie et al. [12] manually traced brain regions implicated in schizophrenia in young adults with a first-degree relative with schizophrenia. They demonstrated that the combined volume of the amygdala and hippocampus in high-risk individuals was lower than in control subjects, but higher than in patients with first-episode psychosis. Manual tracing methods have also been used to identify differences between subjects at ultra- (or 'clinical') high-risk and controls. These have found reductions in the thickness of the anterior cingulate cortex [13] and in the volume of the superior temporal gyrus [14], the insula [15], and the pars triangularis [16]. Additionally, other region of interest based studies have investigated the folding of the brain into sulci and gyri to find associations between transition to psychosis and patterns of orbitofrontal folding [17] and the depth of the olfactory sulcus [18].

While some follow-up studies of high-risk samples have found that decreased hippocampal volume at baseline was associated with a later transition to psychosis [18–22], others have not [10, 20, 23–25]. These mixed results may reflect the complexity in measuring brain regions using structural MRI data. Although manual tracing produces reliable and sensitive findings, the regional boundaries are often defined separately by each study, limiting the possibility of independent replication. Indeed, even in the same sample, the application of different tracing methods can yield different results [10, 20]. Other research suggests that group differences are specific to particular hippocampal subregions that may or may not be distinguishable using different methods [21].

Whole-Brain Analyses

A complementary approach is to examine changes across the entire brain using automated or semi-automated methods, such as voxel-based morphometry [26, 27]. This approach is appealing because the same algorithms can be applied across different studies, which increases convergent validity while also allowing the valid aggregation of results from different centres in quantitative meta-analyses [28–30]. A further advantage is that one can examine the entire brain, rather than be limited to a small number of regions of interest [26]. Pantelis et al. [11] conducted the first voxel-based morphometry analysis of MRI data from high-risk individuals. They found that at baseline, subjects who later transitioned to psychosis had less grey matter in areas of the medial/lateral temporal cortices, prefrontal cortex, cingulate cortex, and basal ganglia than those who did not. Longitudinal analyses also indicated that in the subjects who later developed psychosis there was a reduction in the volume of the parahippocampal gyrus, as well as in the cingulate, orbitofrontal and fusiform gyri, and the cerebellum. Subsequent studies have also reported smaller volumes in limbic, paralimbic, and neocortical areas in high-risk individuals who later developed psychosis compared to those who did not [31–35]. Whole-brain changes in MRI data can also be examined at the level of the cortical surface [35–37], and one study reported a retraction in the surface of the dorsolateral prefrontal cortex in high-risk subjects who later transitioned to psychosis. However, some studies have failed to find MRI features that were specific to the later onset of psychosis [31, 38]. These differences may be partly due to the use of small samples, especially when groups are subdivided by outcome into smaller subgroups. A further factor may be variation in the age of the high-risk subjects across studies, with different investigations involving subjects at quite different stages of neurodevelopment.

Meta-analyses of data from multiple studies provide a means of overcoming the limitations of small sample sizes, and identifying the most robust among a variety of different findings [28, 29, 39]. Using this approach, Fusar-Poli et al. [29] found that in comparison to controls, high-risk individuals showed reductions of grey matter in the medial temporal lobe, insula cortex, superior temporal gyrus, inferior frontal gyrus, posterior cingulate/precuneus, and the medial frontal lobe (fig. 1a). Within high-risk samples, reductions in the inferior frontal gyrus and the superior temporal gyrus were associated with the later transition to psychosis (fig. 1b).

Overall, the literature suggests that within the set of structural MRI findings associated with the high-risk state, there is a subset of findings that are specifically associated with the later onset of psychosis.

Using Structural Neuroimaging for Prediction

The structural MRI studies discussed thus far have used inferential statistical methods to detect statistically significant group differences. This implies that the results are meaningful within a population of individuals at risk for psychosis, rather than in an individual subject. In addition, because most of the techniques used in these studies

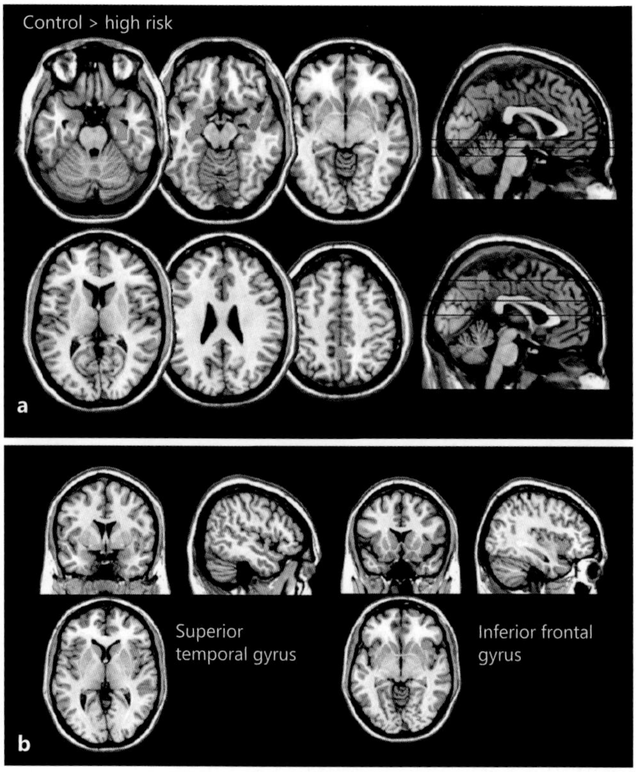

Fig. 1. Meta-analysis of voxel-based morphometry MRI studies in clinical high-risk individuals. **a** High-risk subjects had smaller grey matter volumes than healthy volunteers in the frontal, temporal, and medial parietal cortices. **b** High-risk individuals who subsequently developed psychosis had smaller superior temporal and inferior frontal volumes than high-risk subjects who did not become psychotic. Adapted with permission from Elsevier [29].

are fundamentally univariate, they cannot detect shared relationships between brain regions that become dysfunctional together – as proposed in neural network models of psychotic disorders [40, 41]. There has thus been increasing interest in the application of multivariate methods that permit classification at the individual subject level [42]. This shift has mainly involved the use of machine learning approaches that mathematically model distributed brain pathology in samples of individuals and then generalise these models to new patients [34, 42–47]. For example, a set of algorithms (i.e., a 'machine') can be applied to data from a high-risk sample to identify a complex pattern of MRI abnormalities that best distinguishes subjects that do and do not subsequently develop psychosis. MRI data from an individual subject can then be examined with respect to this neurobiological signature, and the subject can be classified as belonging to one or the other outcome subgroups.

Although there are many machine learning methods (e.g., artificial neural networks, decision trees, Gaussian process classification), support vector machine learning has been the most widely used. Using this approach, Koutsouleris et al. [34] reported that the likelihood that an individual at high risk would later develop psychosis could be predicted with an accuracy of 88%. Application of the same method in an independent sample yielded a classification accuracy of ~84% [43]. However, these findings were derived from small samples, and the brain areas that discriminated be-

Dwyer · McGuire

tween transitions and non-transitions were diffusely distributed in a pattern that was very different from that seen in the univariate comparisons. However, more recently the same group has reported that the later onset of psychosis is associated with reduced volumes in prefrontal, cingulate, striatal, and cerebellar brain regions [46]. Other research using machine learning with MRI data has described a classification rate of 63% in separating high-risk individuals from controls [47]. This suggests that the predictive accuracy may vary, depending on the clinical and demographic characteristics of the high-risk sample, and rate of transition in each sample.

Functional MRI in People at High Risk

Task-Based Neuroimaging
Functional imaging studies investigating vulnerability to psychosis began with samples of individuals at familial high risk who were assessed using executive functioning tasks [reviewed in 48]. A review of studies in this literature found medium to large effect sizes for differences in prefrontal activation between controls and those with a high familial risk [48]. Early studies in subjects at clinical high risk examined responses to executive functioning [49], working memory [50], and during a visual oddball task [51]. These studies reported that clinical high-risk subjects showed a level of activation in the prefrontal and anterior cingulate cortex that was intermediate between that in controls and patients with psychosis. Subsequent studies have found differential responses in clinical high-risk groups compared to controls during other tasks of executive function [52–60] and memory [61, 62], as well as during movement generation [50] and language production [63–65]. Some of these studies found that the clinical high risk was associated with increased activation, while others found the opposite. The direction of the group difference in response may depend on the nature of the task being examined. For example, high-risk subjects may show greater prefrontal activation during tasks involving language/executive function, but decreased prefrontal activation during tasks involving episodic and working memory [66].

Task-based functional MRI studies have also investigated the relationship between longitudinal changes in activation and clinical or functional outcomes. Reductions in symptoms and improvement in daily functioning following presentation have been associated with a normalisation of activation in the occipitoparietal [57], lateral prefrontal [58], and anterior cingulate cortices [67]. To date, only one functional imaging study has reported an association between the pattern of activation at baseline and later transition to psychosis. Allen et al. [53] found that increased activation in the prefrontal and hippocampal cortices and in the midbrain during a verbal fluency task was associated with the onset of psychosis in the 18 months after scanning (fig. 2).

Collectively, these findings suggest that the high-risk state is associated with altered regional activation during a range of cognitive tasks. There is also evidence that these functional abnormalities are related to alterations in brain structure and chemistry in

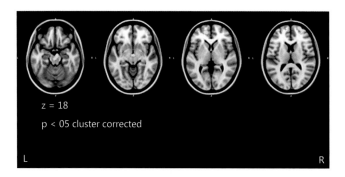

Fig. 2. Functional activation differences during a verbal fluency task between high-risk individuals who later developed psychosis and those who did not. The former subgroup showed greater activation at baseline in the prefrontal and medial temporal cortex, and in the midbrain. Adapted with permission from Oxford University Press [53].

high-risk subjects. One study found that a reduction in thalamic glutamate was associated with altered prefrontal, hippocampal, and temporal function in high-risk individuals during a verbal fluency task [67]. Additionally, both hippocampal and prefrontal activation have been linked to the level of striatal and midbrain dopamine functioning [53, 59, 61, 62, 68], and to thalamic and hippocampal glutamate levels [52, 56, 69].

Connectivity Analyses
Psychotic disorders are thought to involve a dysconnectivity between brain regions [see 40]. The first study to investigate connectivity in clinical high-risk subjects was by Crossley et al. [55], who used dynamic causal modelling to examine causal relationships (i.e., the influence of one brain region over another) during a working memory task. They found that the magnitude of connectivity between the superior temporal gyrus and the middle frontal gyrus in high-risk individuals was intermediate to that in controls and patients with first-episode psychosis. A similar pattern of group differences was evident in a dynamic causal modelling study of a working memory task, although in this case the connections were from the middle frontal gyrus to the parietal lobe [70]. A study of different working memory paradigms identified deficits in hippocampal-prefrontal connectivity in high-risk subjects that were comparable to those in first-episode patients [71].

Connectivity in high-risk subjects has also been investigated during the 'resting state' [72–75]. These studies have reported connectivity differences within and between large-scale brain networks (e.g., the default-mode network) [74, 75], in addition to specific differences in striatal connectivity [72]. One study reported that connectivity abnormalities of anterior cingulate cortex were particularly marked in the subgroup which later developed psychosis [73]. Taken together, the findings from task and resting-state connectivity studies are consistent with the results from structural

Dwyer · McGuire

and functional imaging studies in high-risk subjects, as the connectivity findings involve alterations in similar regions (e.g., striatum, superior temporal gyrus, and anterior cingulate cortex).

Looking ahead, functional neuroimaging studies in high-risk subjects are likely to involve increasing use of resting-state paradigms to probe network dysfunction, as in other areas of psychiatric research [76]. Resting-state protocols also have the advantage of being relatively easy to implement and being language-independent, making them particularly suitable for large-scale multi-centre studies. Research using multi-modal imaging is likely to continue to advance the field by linking functional changes to alterations in brain structure and chemistry. The use of multi-centre studies that can recruit large samples of high-risk subjects, combined with analytical approaches like machine learning, is likely to facilitate studies of functional imaging predictors of clinical outcomes.

Limitations and Future Directions

A major limitation of most structural and functional imaging work in high-risk subjects to-date is that such studies have been conducted in relatively small samples. This largely reflects the fact that high-risk subjects are difficult to recruit, especially if there is no specialised clinical service for this group. Another potential limitation is that most of the studies have been conducted in individuals who are at high-risk for psychosis, as opposed to other disorders: much less is known about the brain changes in people at risk for bipolar disorder, depression, anxiety, and obsessive compulsive disorder. The extent to which the findings reviewed here are specific to the risk for psychosis, as opposed to other disorders or mental illness more generally is thus unclear. For example, although there is a large body of literature reporting hippocampal differences in individuals at risk for psychosis, there is also evidence for hippocampal changes in depression, post-traumatic stress, substance use, and personality disorders [77–81]. A further consideration is that diagnostic categories, such as schizophrenia or psychosis, may be neurobiologically heterogenous, comprising a variety of conditions with differing aetiologies. It may thus be unlikely that there will be a single neuroimaging feature that predicts transition to psychosis in every high-risk subject.

In light of the current limitations, there has thus been a move towards the establishment of research consortia (e.g., NAPLS, EU-GEI, PSYSCAN, and PRONIA) that can recruit large samples of high-risk individuals across multiple sites. Most of these consortia have been formed relatively recently, and the first data from multi-centre neuroimaging studies in high-risk subjects have only begun to be published [e.g., 32, 82]. Many of these studies also aim to use machine learning to enhance predictive accuracy at the level of each individual with the combination of brain imaging measures with clinical, demographic, cognitive, and genomic data.

Conclusions

Neuroimaging research has shown that there are structural and functional brain differences between those at high risk for psychosis and controls, and differences between high-risk subjects who will later develop psychosis and those who will not. However, whether the best predictor of outcomes in this group will involve a single brain region, a network of regions, or inter-regional interactions at a whole brain level is still an open question. Some of the outstanding issues may be addressed through large, multi-site studies involving state-of-the-art methods to facilitate the translation of findings from neuroimaging research into tools that could allow clinicians to predict outcomes and personalise intervention.

References

1 Cannon TD, Cadenhead K, Cornblatt B, Woods SW, Addington J, Walker E, Seidman LJ, Perkins D, Tsuang M, McGlashan T, Heinssen R: Prediction of psychosis in youth at high clinical risk: a multisite longitudinal study in North America. Arch Gen Psychiatry 2008;65:28–37.

2 McGlashan TH, Johannessen JO: Early detection and intervention with schizophrenia: rationale. Schizophr Bull 1996;22:201–222.

3 Yung AR, McGorry PD: The prodromal phase of first-episode psychosis: past and current conceptualizations. Schizophr Bull 1996;22:353–370.

4 Klosterkötter J, Hellmich M, Steinmeyer EM, Schultze-Lutter F: Diagnosing schizophrenia in the initial prodromal phase. Arch Gen Psychiatry 2001;58: 158–164.

5 McGorry PD, Yung AR and Phillips LJ: The 'close-in' or ultra high-risk model: a safe and effective strategy for research and clinical intervention in prepsychotic mental disorder. Schizophr Bull 2003;29: 771–790.

6 Yung AR, Phillips LJ, McGorry PD, McFarlane CA, Francey S, Harrigan S, Patton GC, Jackson HJ: Prediction of psychosis. A step towards indicated prevention of schizophrenia. Br J Psychiatry Suppl 1998; 172:14–20.

7 Fusar-Poli P, Borgwardt S, Bechdolf A, Addington J, Riecher-Rössler A, Schultze-Lutter F, Keshavan M, Wood S, Ruhrmann S, Seidman LJ, Valmaggia L, Cannon T, Velthorst E, De Haan L, Cornblatt B, Bonoldi I, Birchwood M, McGlashan T, Carpenter W, McGorry P, Klosterkötter J, McGuire P, Yung A: The psychosis high-risk state: a comprehensive state-of-the-art review. JAMA Psychiatry 2013;70.107–120.

8 Brewer WJ, Wood SJ, McGorry PD, Francey SM, Phillips LJ, Yung AR, Anderson V, Copolov DL, Singh B, Velakoulis D, Pantelis C: Impairment of olfactory identification ability in individuals at ultra-high risk for psychosis who later develop schizophrenia. Am J Psychiatry 2003;160:1790–1794.

9 Seidman LJ, Giuliano AJ, Meyer EC, Addington J, Cadenhead KS, Cannon TD, McGlashan TH, Perkins DO, Tsuang MT, Walker EF, Woods SW, Bearden CE, Christensen BK, Hawkins K, Heaton R, Keefe RSE, Heinssen R, Cornblatt BA; North American Prodrome Longitudinal Study (NAPLS) Group: Neuropsychology of the prodrome to psychosis in the NAPLS consortium: relationship to family history and conversion to psychosis. Arch Gen Psychiatry 2010;67:578–588.

10 Velakoulis D, Wood SJ, Wong MTH, McGorry PD, Yung A, Phillips L, Phillips L, Smith D, Brewer W, Proffitt TM, Desmond P, Pantelis C: Hippocampal and amygdala volumes according to psychosis stage and diagnosis. Arch Gen Psychiatry 2006;63:139–149.

11 Pantelis C, Velakoulis D, McGorry PD, Wood SJ, Suckling J, Phillips LJ, Yung AR, Bullmore ET, Brewer W, Soulsby B, Desmond P, McGuire PK: Neuroanatomical abnormalities before and after onset of psychosis: a cross-sectional and longitudinal MRI comparison. Lancet 2003;361:281–288.

12 Lawrie SM, Whalley HC, Abukmeil SS, Kestelman JN, Donnelly L, Miller P, Best JJK, Cunningham Owens DG, Johnstone EC: Brain structure, genetic liability, and psychotic symptoms in subjects at high risk of developing schizophrenia. Biol Psychiatry 2001;49:811–823.

13 Fornito A, Yung AR, Wood SJ, Phillips LJ, Nelson B, Cotton S, Velakoulis D, McGorry PD, Pantelis C, Yücel M: Anatomic abnormalities of the anterior cingulate cortex before psychosis onset: an MRI study of ultra-high-risk individuals. Biol Psychiatry 2008;64:758–765.

14 Takahashi T, Wood SJ, Yung AR, Soulsby B, McGorry PD, Suzuki M, Kawasaki Y, Phillips LJ, Velakoulis D, Pantelis C: Progressive gray matter reduction of the superior temporal gyrus during transition to psychosis. Arch Gen Psychiatry 2009;66:366–376.

15 Takahashi T, Wood SJ, Yung AR, Phillips LJ, Soulsby B, McGorry PD, Tanino R, Zhou S-Y, Suzuki M, Velakoulis D, Pantelis C: Insular cortex gray matter changes in individuals at ultra-high-risk of developing psychosis. Schizophr Res 2009;111:94–102.

16 Iwashiro N, Suga M, Takano Y, Inoue H, Natsubori T, Satomura Y, Koike S, Yahata N, Murakami M, Katsura M, Gonoi W, Sasaki H, Takao H, Abe O, Kasai K, Yamasue H: Localized gray matter volume reductions in the pars triangularis of the inferior frontal gyrus in individuals at clinical high-risk for psychosis and first episode for schizophrenia. Schizophr Res 2012;137:124–131.

17 Lavoie S, Bartholomeuz CF, Nelson B, Lin A, McGorry PD, Velakoulis D, Whittle SL, Yung AR, Pantelis C, Wood SJ: Sulcogyral pattern and sulcal count of the orbitofrontal cortex in individuals at ultra high risk for psychosis. Schizophr Res 2014;154:93–99.

18 Takahashi T, Wood SJ, Yung AR, Nelson B, Lin A, Yücel M, Phillips LJ, Nakamura Y, Suzuki M, Brewer WJ, Proffitt TM, McGorry PD, Velakoulis D, Pantelis C: Altered depth of the olfactory sulcus in ultra high-risk individuals and patients with psychotic disorders. Schizophr Res 2014;153:18–24.

19 Bechdolf A, Wood SJ, Nelson B, Velakoulis D, Yucel M, Takahashi T, Yung AR, Berk M, Wong MT, Pantelis C, McGorry PD: Amygdala and insula volumes prior to illness onset in bipolar disorder: a magnetic resonance imaging study. Psychiatry Res 2012;201:34–39.

20 Phillips LJ, Velakoulis D, Pantelis C, Wood S, Yuen HP, Yung AR, Desmond P, Brewer W, McGorry PD: Non-reduction in hippocampal volume is associated with higher risk of psychosis. Schizophr Res 2002;58:145–158.

21 Witthaus H, Mendes U, Brune M, Ozgurdal S, Bohner G, Gudlowski Y, Kalus P, Andreasen N, Heinz A, Klingebiel R, Juckel G: Hippocampal subdivision and amygdalar volumes in patients in an at-risk mental state for schizophrenia. J Psychiatry Neurosci 2010;35:33–40.

22 Wood SJ, Kennedy D, Phillips LJ, Seal ML, Yucel M, Nelson B, Yung AR, Jackson G, McGorry PD, Velakoulis D, Pantelis C: Hippocampal pathology in individuals at ultra-high risk for psychosis: a multi-modal magnetic resonance study. Neuroimage 2010;52:62–68.

23 Buehlmann E, Berger GE, Aston J, Gschwandtner U, Pflueger MO, Borgwardt SJ, Radue EW, Riecher-Rössler A: Hippocampus abnormalities in at risk mental states for psychosis? A cross-sectional high resolution region of interest magnetic resonance imaging study. J Psychiatr Res 2010;44:447–453.

24 Stone JM, Day F, Tsagaraki H, Valli I, McLean MA, Lythgoe DJ, O'Gorman RL, Barker GJ, McGuire PK: Glutamate dysfunction in people with prodromal symptoms of psychosis: relationship to gray matter volume. Biol Psychiatry 2009;66:533–539.

25 Wood SJ, Yücel M, Velakoulis D, Phillips LJ, Yung AR, Brewer W, McGorry PD, Pantelis C: Hippocampal and anterior cingulate morphology in subjects at ultra-high-risk for psychosis: the role of family history of psychotic illness. Schizophr Res 2005;75:295–301.

26 Wright IC, Ellison ZR, Sharma T, Friston KJ, Murray RM, McGuire PK: Mapping of grey matter changes in schizophrenia. Schizophr Res 1999;35:1–14.

27 Wright IC, McGuire PK, Poline JB, Travere JM, Murray RM, Frith CD, Frackowiak RS, Friston KJ: A voxel-based method for the statistical analysis of gray and white matter density applied to schizophrenia. Neuroimage 1995;2:244–252.

28 Chan RCK, Di X, McAlonan GM, Gong Qy: Brain anatomical abnormalities in high-risk individuals, first-episode, and chronic schizophrenia: an activation likelihood estimation meta-analysis of illness progression. Schizophr Bull 2010;37:177–188.

29 Fusar-Poli P, Borgwardt S, Crescini A, Deste G, Kempton MJ, Lawrie S, Guire PM, Sacchetti E: Neuroanatomy of vulnerability to psychosis: a voxel-based meta-analysis. Neurosci Biobehav Rev 2011;35:1175–1185.

30 Smieskova R, Fusar-Poli P, Allen P, Bendfeldt K, Stieglitz RD, Drewe J, Radue EW, McGuire PK, Riecher-Rössler A, Borgwardt SJ: Neuroimaging predictors of transition to psychosis: a systematic review and meta-analysis. Neurosci Biobehav Rev 2010;34:1207–1222.

31 Borgwardt SJ, Riecher-Rössler A, Dazzan P, Chitnis X, Aston J, Drewe M, Gschwandtner U, Haller S, Pflüger M, Rechsteiner E, D'Souza M, Stieglitz RD, Radü EW, McGuire PK: Regional gray matter volume abnormalities in the at risk mental state. Biol Psychiatry 2007;61:1148–1156.

32 Cannon TD, Chung Y, He G, Sun D, Jacobson A, van Erp TGM, McEwen S, Addington J, Bearden CE, Cadenhead K, Cornblatt B, Mathalon DH, McGlashan T, Perkins D, Jeffries C, Seidman LJ, Tsuang M, Walker E, Woods SW, Heinssen R; North American Prodrome Longitudinal Study Consortium: Progressive reduction in cortical thickness as psychosis develops: a multisite longitudinal neuroimaging study of youth at elevated clinical risk. Biol Psychiatry 2015;77:147–157.

33 Job DE, Whalley HC, Johnstone EC, Lawrie SM: Grey matter changes over time in high risk subjects developing schizophrenia. Neuroimage 2005;25: 1023–1030.

34 Koutsouleris N, Meisenzahl EM, Davatzikos C, Bottlender R, Frodl T, Scheuerecker J, Schmitt G, Zetzsche T, Decker P, Reiser M, Möller H-J, Gaser C: Use of neuroanatomical pattern classification to identify subjects in at-risk mental states of psychosis and predict disease transition. Arch Gen Psychiatry 2009;66:1–13.

35 Sun D, Phillips L, Velakoulis D, Yung A, McGorry PD, Wood SJ, van Erp TGM, Thompson PM, Toga AW, Cannon TD, Pantelis C: Progressive brain structural changes mapped as psychosis develops in 'at risk' individuals. Schizophr Res 2009;108:85–92.

36 Jung WH, Kim JS, Jang JH, Choi JS, Jung MH, Park JY, Han JY, Choi CH, Kang DH, Chung CK, Kwon JS: Cortical thickness reduction in individuals at ultra-high-risk for psychosis. Schizophr Bull 2011;37: 839–849.

37 Ziermans TB, Durston S, Sprong M, Nederveen H, van Haren NEM, Schnack HG, Lahuis BE, Schothorst PF, van Engeland H: No evidence for structural brain changes in young adolescents at ultra high risk for psychosis. Schizophr Res 2009;112:1–6.

38 Meisenzahl E, Koutsouleris N, Gaser C, Bottlender R, Schmitt G, McGuire P, Decker P, Burgermeister B, Born C, Reiser M: Structural brain alterations in subjects at high-risk of psychosis: a voxel-based morphometric study. Schizophr Res 2008;102:150–162.

39 Fusar-Poli P, Bonoldi I, Yung AR, Borgwardt S, Kempton MJ, Valmaggia L, Barale F, Caverzasi E, McGuire P: Predicting psychosis: meta-analysis of transition outcomes in individuals at high clinical risk. Arch Gen Psychiatry 2012;69:220–229.

40 McGuire PK, Frith CD: Disordered functional connectivity in schizophrenia. Psychol Med 1996;26: 663–667.

41 Modinos G, Allen P, Grace AA, McGuire P: Translating the MAM model of psychosis to humans. Trends Neurosci 2015;38:129–138.

42 Orrù G, Pettersson-Yeo W, Marquand AF, Sartori G, Mechelli A: Using support vector machine to identify imaging biomarkers of neurological and psychiatric disease: a critical review. Neurosci Biobehav Rev 2012;36:1140–1152.

43 Koutsouleris N, Borgwardt S, Meisenzahl EM, Bottlender R, Moller HJ, Riecher-Rössler A: Disease prediction in the at-risk mental state for psychosis using neuroanatomical biomarkers: results from the FePsy Study. Schizophr Bull 2012;38:1234–1246.

44 Koutsouleris N, Davatzikos C, Borgwardt S, Gaser C, Bottlender R, Frodl T, Falkai P, Riecher-Rössler A, Moller HJ, Reiser M, Pantelis C, Meisenzahl E: Accelerated brain aging in schizophrenia and beyond: a neuroanatomical marker of psychiatric disorders. Schizophr Bull 2014;40:1140–1153.

45 Koutsouleris N, Gaser C, Bottlender R, Davatzikos C, Decker P, Jäger M, Schmitt G, Reiser M, Möller H-J, Meisenzahl EM: Use of neuroanatomical pattern regression to predict the structural brain dynamics of vulnerability and transition to psychosis. Schizophr Res 2010;123:175–187.

46 Koutsouleris N, Riecher-Rossler A, Meisenzahl EM, Smieskova R, Studerus E, Kambeitz-Ilankovic L, von Saldern S, Cabral C, Reiser M, Falkai P, Borgwardt S: Detecting the psychosis prodrome across high-risk populations using neuroanatomical biomarkers. Schizophr Bull 2015;41:471–482.

47 Pettersson-Yeo W, Benetti S, Marquand AF, Dell Acqua F, Williams SCR, Allen P, Prata D, McGuire P, Mechelli A: Using genetic, cognitive and multimodal neuroimaging data to identify ultra-high-risk and first-episode psychosis at the individual level. Psychol Med 2013;43:2547–2562.

48 Fusar-Poli P, Perez J, Broome M, Borgwardt S, Placentino A, Caverzasi E, Cortesi M, Veggiotti P, Politi P, Barale F, McGuire P: Neurofunctional correlates of vulnerability to psychosis: a systematic review and meta-analysis. Neurosci Biobehav Rev 2007;31:465–484.

49 Broome MR, Matthiasson P, Fusar-Poli P, Woolley JB, Johns LC, Tabraham P, Bramon E, Valmaggia L, Williams SCR, Brammer MJ, Chitnis X, McGuire PK: Neural correlates of executive function and working memory in the 'at-risk mental state'. Br J Psychiatry 2008;194:25–33.

50 Broome MR, Fusar-Poli P, Matthiasson P, Woolley JB, Valmaggia L, Johns LC, Tabraham P, Bramon E, Williams SCR, Brammer MJ, Chitnis X, Zelaya F, McGuire PK: Neural correlates of visuospatial working memory in the 'at-risk mental state'. Psychol Med 2010;40:1987–1999.

51 Morey RA, Inan S, Mitchell TV, Perkins MD, Lieberman JA, Belger A: Implications of normal brain development for the pathogenesis of schizophrenia. Arch Gen Psychiatry 2005;62:254–262.

52 Allen P, Chaddock CA, Egerton A, Howes OD, Barker G, Bonoldi I, Fusar-Poli P, Murray R, McGuire P: Functional outcome in people at high risk for psychosis predicted by thalamic glutamate levels and prefronto-striatal activation. Schizophr Bull 2015; 41:429–439.

53 Allen P, Luigjes J, Howes OD, Egerton A, Hirao K, Valli I, Kambeitz J, Fusar-Poli P, Broome M, McGuire P: Transition to psychosis associated with prefrontal and subcortical dysfunction in ultra high-risk individuals. Schizophr Bull 2012;38:1268–1276.

54 Benetti S, Pettersson-Yeo W, Hutton C, Catani M, Williams SCR, Allen P, Kambeitz-Ilankovic LM, McGuire P, Mechelli A: Elucidating neuroanatomical alterations in the at risk mental state and first episode psychosis: a combined voxel-based morphometry and voxel-based cortical thickness study. Schizophr Res 2013;150:505–511.

55 Crossley NA, Mechelli A, Fusar-Poli P, Broome MR, Matthiasson P, Johns LC, Bramon E, Valmaggia L, Williams SCR, McGuire PK: Superior temporal lobe dysfunction and frontotemporal dysconnectivity in subjects at risk of psychosis and in first-episode psychosis. Hum Brain Mapp 2009;30:4129–4137.

56 Fusar-Poli P, Stone JM, Broome MR, Valli I, Mechelli A, McLean MA, Lythgoe DJ, O'Gorman RL, Barker GJ, McGuire PK: Thalamic glutamate levels as a predictor of cortical response during executive functioning in subjects at high risk for psychosis. Arch Gen Psychiatry 2011;68:881–890.

57 Fusar-Poli P, Broome MR, Matthiasson P, Woolley JB, Johns LC, Tabraham P, Bramon E, Valmaggia L, Williams SC, McGuire P: Spatial working memory in individuals at high risk for psychosis: longitudinal fMRI study. Schizophr Res 2010;123:45–52.

58 Fusar-Poli P, Broome MR, Matthiasson P, Woolley JB, Mechelli A, Johns LC, Tabraham P, Bramon E, Valmaggia L, Williams SC, McGuire P: Prefrontal function at presentation directly related to clinical outcome in people at ultrahigh risk of psychosis. Schizophr Bull 2010;37:189–198.

59 Fusar-Poli P, Howes OD, Allen P, Broome M, Valli I, Asselin M-C, Grasby PM, McGuire PK: Abnormal frontostriatal interactions in people with prodromal signs of psychosis. Arch Gen Psychiatry 2010;67:1–9.

60 Smieskova R, Allen P, Simon A, Aston J, Bendfeldt K, Drewe J, Gruber K, Gschwandtner U, Klarhoefer M, Lenz C, Scheffler K, Stieglitz R-D, Radue E-W, McGuire P, Riecher-Rössler A, Borgwardt SJ: Different duration of at-risk mental state associated with neurofunctional abnormalities. A multimodal imaging study. Hum Brain Mapp 2011;33:2281–2294.

61 Allen P, Chaddock CA, Howes OD, Egerton A, Seal ML, Fusar-Poli P, Valli I, Day F, McGuire PK: Abnormal relationship between medial temporal lobe and subcortical dopamine function in people with an ultra high risk for psychosis. Schizophr Bull 2012;38:1040–1049.

62 Allen P, Seal ML, Valli I, Fusar-Poli P, Perlini C, Day F, Wood SJ, Williams SC, McGuire PK: Altered prefrontal and hippocampal function during verbal encoding and recognition in people with prodromal symptoms of psychosis. Schizophr Bull 2011;37:746–756.

63 Allen P, Stephan KE, Mechelli A, Day F, Ward N, Dalton J, Williams SC, McGuire P: Cingulate activity and fronto-temporal connectivity in people with prodromal signs of psychosis. Neuroimage 2010;49:947–955.

64 Natsubori T, Hashimoto R, Yahata N, Inoue H, Takano Y, Iwashiro N, Koike S, Gonoi W, Sasaki H, Takao H, Abe O, Kasai K, Yamasue H: An fMRI study of visual lexical decision in patients with schizophrenia and clinical high-risk individuals. Schizophr Res 2014;157:218–224.

65 Sabb FW, van Erp TG, Hardt ME, Dapretto M, Caplan R, Cannon TD, Bearden CE: Language network dysfunction as a predictor of outcome in youth at clinical high risk for psychosis. Schizophr Res 2010;116:173–183.

66 Egerton A, Borgwardt SJ, Tognin S, Howes OD, McGuire P, Allen P: An overview of functional, structural and neurochemical imaging studies in individuals with a clinical high risk for psychosis. Neuropsychiatry 2011;1:477–493.

67 Fusar-Poli P, Broome MR, Woolley JB, Johns LC, Tabraham P, Bramon E, Valmaggia L, Williams SC, McGuire P: Altered brain function directly related to structural abnormalities in people at ultra high risk of psychosis: longitudinal VBM-fMRI study. J Psych Res 2011;45:190–198.

68 Roiser JP, Howes OD, Chaddock CA, Joyce EM, McGuire P: Neural and behavioral correlates of aberrant salience in individuals at risk for psychosis. Schizophr Bull 2013;39:1328–1336.

69 Valli I, Stone J, Mechelli A, Bhattacharyya S, Raffin M, Allen P, Fusar-Poli P, Lythgoe D, O'Gorman R, Seal M, McGuire P: Altered medial temporal activation related to local glutamate levels in subjects with prodromal signs of psychosis. Biol Psychiatry 2011;69:97–99.

70 Schmidt A, Smieskova R, Aston J, Simon A, Allen P, Fusar-Poli P, McGuire PK, Riecher-Rössler A, Stephan KE, Borgwardt S: Brain connectivity abnormalities predating the onset of psychosis. JAMA Psychiatry 2013;70:903.

71 Benetti S, Mechelli A, Picchioni M, Broome M, Williams S, McGuire P: Functional integration between the posterior hippocampus and prefrontal cortex is impaired in both first episode schizophrenia and the at risk mental state. Brain 2009;132:2426–2436.

72 Dandash O, Fornito A, Lee J, Keefe RSE, Chee MWL, Adcock RA, Pantelis C, Wood SJ, Harrison BJ: Altered striatal functional connectivity in subjects with an at-risk mental state for psychosis. Schizophr Bull 2014;40:904–913.

73 Lord LD, Allen P, Expert P, Howes O, Broome M, Lambiotte R, Fusar-Poli P, Valli I, McGuire P, Turkheimer FE: Functional brain networks before the onset of psychosis: a prospective fMRI study with graph theoretical analysis. Neuroimage Clin 2012;1: 91–98.

74 Orr JM, Turner JA, Mittal VA: Widespread brain dysconnectivity associated with psychotic-like experiences in the general population. Neuroimage Clin 2014;4:343–351.

75 Shim G, Oh JS, Jung W, Jang J, Choi C-H, Kim E, Park H-Y, Choi J-S, Jung M, Kwon J: Altered resting-state connectivity in subjects at ultra-high risk for psychosis: an fMRI study. Behav Brain Funct 2010;6: 58.

76 Fornito A, Bullmore ET: Connectomics: a new paradigm for understanding brain disease. Eur Neuropsychopharmacol 2015;25:733–748.

77 Agartz I, Momenan R, Rawlings RR, Kerich MJ, Hommer DW: Hippocampal volume in patients with alcohol dependence. Arch Gen Psychiatry 1999; 56:356–363.

78 Bremner JD, Narayan M, Anderson ER, Staib LH, Miller HL, Charney DS: Hippocampal volume reduction in major depression. Am J Psychiatry 2000; 157:115–118.

79 Driessen M, Herrmann J, Stahl K, Zwaan M, Meier S, Hill A, Osterheider M, Petersen D: Magnetic resonance imaging volumes of the hippocampus and the amygdala in women with borderline personality disorder and early traumatization. Arch Gen Psychiatry 2000;57:1115–1122.

80 Gurvits TV, Shenton ME, Hokama H, Ohta H, Lasko NB, Gilbertson MW, Orr SP, Kikinis R, Jolesz FA, McCarley RW, Pitman RK: Magnetic resonance imaging study of hippocampal volume in chronic, combat-related posttraumatic stress disorder. Biol Psychiatry 1996;40:1091–1099.

81 Koob GF, Volkow ND: Neurocircuitry of addiction. Neuropsychopharmacology 2010;35:217–238.

82 Mechelli A, Riecher-Rössler A, Meisenzahl EM, Tognin S, Wood SJ, Borgwardt SJ, Koutsouleris N, Yung AR, Stone JM, Phillips LJ, McGorry PD, Valli I, Velakoulis D, Woolley J, Pantelis C, McGuire P: Neuroanatomical abnormalities that predate the onset of psychosis. Arch Gen Psychiatry 2011;68:1–7.

Prof. Philip McGuire
Institute of Psychiatry, Psychology, and Neuroscience, Department of Psychosis Studies
King's College London, 16 De Crespigny Park
London SE5 8AF (UK)
E-Mail Philip.mcguire@kcl.ac.uk

Riecher-Rössler A, McGorry PD (eds): Early Detection and Intervention in Psychosis: State of the Art and Future Perspectives. Key Issues Ment Health. Basel, Karger, 2016, vol 181, pp 95–102 (DOI: 10.1159/000440917)

Pattern Recognition Methods in the Prediction of Psychosis

Nikolaos Koutsouleris · Joseph Kambeitz

Department of Psychiatry and Psychotherapy, Ludwig Maximilian University, Munich, Germany

Abstract

The analysis of large-scale multidomain databases has become a key avenue in the quest for identifying predictors of psychosis. However, despite large scientific efforts, until today no clinically viable predictive models have been derived from these databases. This might to some extent result from methodological shortcomings of classical statistical approaches that are typically applied to these data. New methods such as multivariate pattern analysis (MVPA) hold the promise to overcome these drawbacks and have therefore been successfully applied in multiple areas of predictive medicine. Most importantly, MVPA facilitates predictions at the single-subject level which is a prerequisite of early recognition findings becoming part of routine diagnostic algorithms. One potential application area of MVPA is the automated classification of clinically relevant disease outcomes. In this regard, the 'first generation' of MVPA studies provided evidence that these methods can differentiate healthy individuals from different psychiatric populations such as patients with depressive, bipolar or schizophrenic disorders. Recently, MVPA methods have been successfully employed in the more challenging classification of different patient populations. However, in terms of early recognition, the most interesting area of application of these methods is the individualized stratification of patients into high-risk and established disease stages as well as the prediction of treatment response. Along this path, predictive modelling could potentially evolve into a clinical tool enabling clinicians to personalize preventive therapy, thus avoiding unnecessary interventions and making the most efficient use of limited clinical resources. The present chapter gives an overview of the methodology of MVPA and current results obtained using this methodology in the emerging field of predictive psychiatry. Clinical implications and further potential applications are discussed.   © 2016 S. Karger AG, Basel

Over the last 20 years the early recognition field has developed operationalized inventories of subtle clinical symptoms which have been shown to mark an elevated clinical risk for the development of a psychotic disorder [1]. Furthermore, research conducted in these clinical high-risk (CHR) populations as well as genetic high-risk individuals and subjects with different degrees of schizotypal personality features has identified a host of abnormalities spanning (1) profiles of neurocognitive deficits in mnemonic and executive tasks [2], (2) neuroanatomical alterations in prefrontal, limbic and temporal brain networks [3, 4], and (3) functional and neurochemical brain abnormalities as measured by functional MRI, EEG and F-DOPA [5]. Both at the clinical and the brain phenotype levels, these abnormalities seem to represent attenuated patterns of the alterations seen in overt psychosis, suggesting that the CHR states evolve at the cross-section of *temporal continua* between full mental health and full-blown illness [6] and *epidemiological continua*, where the disease-related brain patterns intensify with increasing proximity to the cross-sectional and longitudinal dimensions of the psychosis phenotype [7].

These findings have opened a window of possibilities to augment the so far purely clinical early recognition strategies with more 'objective' measurements, thus paving the way for an effective early intervention in the *psychosis prodrome* [8]. So far, however, the vast majority of these studies have used univariate methodological concepts to describe highly complex patterns of abnormalities in the CHR states. Two major methodological properties account for the limitations of these 'classical' statistical methods in generating *clinically applicable* markers for individualized disease prediction [9]. First, instead of holistically modelling patterns of group differences in potentially disease-affected brain systems, they break down these differences into overlapping and unrelated single features, such as voxel-by-voxel MRI measures. Second, the main outcome measure of the classical statistical approach – single-feature significance values corrected for multiple comparisons – has proven useless in terms of individualized inference and personalized medicine, which benchmarks diagnostic and prognostic tests in terms of sensitivity and specificity as well as positive and negative likelihood ratios. Beyond these methodological problems, in a recent meta-analysis Fusar-Poli et al. [10] reported a considerable heterogeneity of disease transition rates across different CHR populations, with the average transition risk measuring ~30% over 3 years. Furthermore, this seminal work and further studies [11, 12] indicated that the transition rates in recently recruited CHR populations significantly declined, thus challenging the validity of the existing CHR criteria in separating individuals in these states both from healthy subjects as well as from patients with other psychiatric diagnoses. Due to this drop of predictive validity in the established CHR inventories, novel analysis methods are urgently required to condense the extensive clinical and neuropsychological batteries to the most parsimonious and predictive canons of clinical items (aim 1), identify neurobiological signatures in the rich sets of multimodal imaging and electrophysiological information (aim 2), and delineate subgroups within the heterogeneous CHR population that share distinct disease pathologies and phenotypes (aim 3).

Such methods recently entered the wider field of predictive psychiatry in the form of multivariate pattern analysis (MVPA) techniques, with promising initial findings in neuroimaging-based disease classification [13, 14], prediction of transition from prodromal to established stages of psychosis [15–17] and prediction of treatment response in depression and dyslexia [18, 19]. These studies demonstrated the superiority of MVPA [20] in 'learning' classification rules in complex, high-dimensional training samples and generalizing these rules to unseen individuals. Hence, MPVA may provide the tools needed to realize the aforementioned major aims. In turn, the successful generalization of MVPA-derived predictive models would have the potential to clear the obstacles toward a risk-stratified and individualized intervention in the early psychosis field. In this regard, other areas of predictive medicine, such as cancer prognosis, have already successfully applied multivariate pattern recognition methods for individualized outcome prediction [21] and achieved scalability of these tools to large and diverse patient populations [22].

Multivariate Pattern Analysis Methods

Machine Learning Strategies
The 'classical' methodology employed in the analysis of multivariate databases such as neurocognitive test batteries, neuroimaging datasets and genome-wide association study repositories is typically based on a univariate approach. As for the case of MRI and genetic data, this means computing a large amount of individual statistical tests for each analysis unit (e.g. voxels in neuroimaging and SNPs in genomic analyses). In consequence, this mass univariate testing strategy requires a post hoc correction procedure to adjust the resulting p values for multiple comparisons, such as Bonferroni, family-wise error or false discovery rate. It is important to note that this approach is based on the assumption that the units of analysis are statistically independent. However, this assumption is at odds with the inherent, highly connected nature of the brain which typically causes disease-specific effects of interest to be organized in relatively low-dimensional manifold structures. Similarly, clinical and neuropsychological variables can be frequently projected on some latent factor structure consisting of few orthogonal variance components in the data. The univariate approach is 'blind' to such hidden structures in the data and hence even in case of statistically significant results at the group level, a substantial overlap is usually observed between the effect distributions of the groups compared. Thus, on the individual level, univariate analysis does not generate meaningful predictions unless the effect size is very large [23]. This limits the sensitivity and specificity of neurobiological findings as the measurement unit effects in the univariate analysis typically do not reach a magnitude of Cohen's d >1.0–1.2. Thus, this methodological approach precludes these data domains from developing into clinically applicable tools meeting the diagnostic and predictive requirements of early recognition.

A promising way to overcome these methodological drawbacks is the use of more recently developed MVPA methods. As an example, MVPA has recently been successfully introduced to the analysis of neuroimaging data [for a summary, see 24]. Instead of focusing on a restricted set of variables (e.g. a 'regions-of-interest' approach in the neuroimaging field) or computing individual statistical tests on all variables in isolation, MVPA takes a holistic approach by considering the whole space of available variables. Even in the absence of any statistical significance, variables can carry predictive information for the current research question. An important feature of MVPA is that it is able to detect these informative patterns in high-dimensional data. One example of a frequently applied classification algorithm for MVPA is the support vector machine (SVM) [20]. The algorithm was originally created for the case of classification problems, but was later modified to also be applicable to regression problems [25]. Most importantly, the SVM can also generate statistical models when nonlinear relationships need to be accounted for. In this case the SVM makes use of the 'kernel trick' and projects the data into a higher-dimensional space where the nonlinear data becomes linearly separable [26]. Besides the SVM, there are multiple alternative classification algorithms that also have generated promising results in high-dimensional classification problems (e.g. with neuroimaging data) such as Gaussian process models, random forests or Fisher's discriminant analysis.

Validation of Predictive Models

As the algorithms applied in MVPA can account for the high dimensionality of the data and are extremely flexible with respect to the relationships they can model, there is the high risk of overfitting to the data when conducting MVPA. The problem with overfitting is that these models will only show poor generalization performance when applied to new data. However, for MVPA to become a tool used in the clinical context for classification and prediction, generalizability is a prerequisite. The ultimate aim is to generate models that allow reliable claims when applied to data of new, previously unseen individuals (e.g. a new patient admitted the hospital). Thus, a substantial part of MVPA is the validation of the generated models.

In order to avoid overfitting and to generate models with good generalizability in MVPA, typically a nested cross-validation framework is employed [27]. Cross-validation describes a technique in which the available data is split. Then one part of the data is used for model generation and the other part is used for testing the generalizability. If parameter optimization is involved, a nested cross-validation setup is *mandatory* as otherwise the analysis will produce generalization estimates that are too optimistic [28]. At the outer cross-validation level, subjects are separated into a training and a test data set (e.g. at a ratio of 10:1). The training data set is used to generate the models within the inner cross-validation. The test data set is used to estimate the accuracy of the model when applied to previously unseen individuals. In the inner cross-validation, subjects are again separated into training and test data sets for model optimization. Here the training data is used to generate multiple predictive models with different parameter settings. The test data set is used to select the parameter set associated with the best model performance. Both cross-validation cycles (inner and outer) can be repeated while permuting subjects into different test and training data sets. This permutation is typically employed to decrease variability in the predictions of predictive models and increase variability in the training populations, thus enhancing generalizability of the trained prediction models.

Visualization of Prediction Rules

The main advantage of MVPA methods – their capacity to model complex structure in the data – may turn into a drawback when it comes to visualizing the extracted predictive patterns. In contrast to parametric or nonparametric univariate approaches, it is in principle invalid to infer statistical significance to a specific unit (feature) of the identified hyperplane. Furthermore, in case of nonlinear models employing the 'kernel trick', a back-projection of the feature weights into the original data space is not straightforward [29]. Moreover, the localization power of the multivariate analysis method depends on the regularization functions built into the respective algorithm – the space of possibilities ranges from highly distributed patterns in L2-regularized algorithms to a highly localized (sparse) solution in case of L1 norm regularization.

Nevertheless, recent methodological developments have allowed the field to analytically derive statistical significance from the arbitrary feature weighting generated by, for example, the SVM [30]. The obtained 'multivariate' p values seem to be much less affected by the multiple comparison problems than their univariate counterparts and may provide a more intuitive and comparable measure of feature relevance compared to the metrics used until now, such as mean feature weight, cross-validation ratio and feature selection frequency. However, further research is needed to identify a correction method that will allow extending the SVM to a statistical inference framework.

Pattern Recognition Applications in the Early Recognition of Psychosis

The following study overview exclusively focuses on early recognition studies that wrapped MVPA methods into rigorous cross-validation or independent test validation strategies to benchmark the feasibility of predicting psychosis in individual CHR persons using neuroimaging data.

In a seminal paper, Pantelis et al. [31] reported on subtle and distributed gray matter reductions in CHR individuals with versus without a subsequent disease transition which were identified by means of voxel-based morphometry [32] in the right medial temporal, lateral temporal and inferior frontal cortex, as well as the cingulate cortex, bilaterally. Findings reported in subsequent voxel-based morphometry studies corroborated the evidence for accumulating prefrontal temporolimbic abnormalities prior to the onset of frank psychosis [33]. However, due to the aforementioned limitations of the univariate methods classically employed for MRI analysis, it remained unclear whether these subtle structural brain differences could provide added value in terms of improved risk stratification in CHR persons.

The first evidence for the predictive value of structural brain imaging on the level of individuals was reported by Koutsouleris et al. [16]. The authors extracted a pattern of distributed gray matter volume abnormalities distinguishing converters from nonconverters with an accuracy of 88% by training nonlinear SVMs on neuroanatomical features obtained through principal component analysis. Again, the main foci of predictive brain structures lay in prefrontal, temporal and cerebellar areas, suggesting that a disruption of cortico-subcortical systems spanning these regions may not only characterize the established disease, but may also predate psychosis several years prior to the onset of the disease. These initial findings were first replicated with a prediction accuracy of 84% in a second, completely independent population of at-risk individuals [15] and then further substantiated (balanced accuracy: 80%) in a third SVM analysis performed in the pooled Basel and Munich CHR cohort [17]. The latter analysis could demonstrate that (1) it may be possible to identify predictive neuroanatomical disease signatures across heterogeneous CHR populations examined by means of different MRI scanner hardware and data acquisition protocols, and (2) that the individual expression of these brain signatures may be strongly linked with different 'survival' curves in terms of disease transition risk. Finally, another MVPA-based imaging analysis in the FePsy cohort [34] assessed the feasibility of distinguishing between CHR subjects with a subsequent disease transition from first-episode psychosis patients with an accuracy of 80%, suggesting that the transition from the prodromal to the first-episode stage is subserved by a dynamic pathophysiological process that leads to accumulating structural brain abnormalities in prefrontal, perisylvian and subcortical brain structures. Given the recent data from Koutsouleris et al. [35] who found that neuroanatomical schizophrenia likeness did not differ between CHR subjects with attenuated psychosis and first-episode patients, it remains to be answered whether these dynamic brain changes result from transition-specific brain processes or alternatively whether neuroanatomical resilience processes are present in CHR subjects without a subsequent disease transition. Finally, MVPA methods have been recently applied to functional neuroimaging data of persons with psychosis proneness in order to identify abnormalities in the mesolimbic and salience networks induced by aversive visual stimuli [36]. These findings suggest that MVPA-based analysis of fMRI data may potentially enhance candidate biomarkers of the psychosis prodrome.

Challenges Ahead

Based on these data, several large-scale CHR projects have commenced to probe the predictive value of MVPA-based neuroanatomical and neurofunctional risk stratification models in the multicenter study settings across the US and Europe (see e.g.

PRONIA, http://pronia.eu, and PsyScan, http://ec.europa.eu/research/health/medical-research/brain-research/projects/psyscan_en.html). These projects will generate the comprehensive and heterogeneous multidomain databases needed to thoroughly test the real-world generalization capacity of MVPA-based predictive models and identify parsimonious data combinations which can be realistically translated into a future biomarker-based early recognition of psychosis.

References

1 Fusar-Poli P, Borgwardt S, Bechdolf A, Addington J, Riecher-Rössler A, Schultze-Lutter F, Keshavan M, Wood S, Ruhrmann S, Seidman LJ, et al: The psychosis high-risk state: a comprehensive state-of-the-art review. JAMA Psychiatry 2013;70:107–120.

2 Fusar-Poli P, Deste G, Smieskova R, Barlati S, Yung AR, Howes O, Stieglitz R-D, Vita A, McGuire P, Borgwardt S: Cognitive functioning in prodromal psychosis: a meta-analysis. Arch Gen Psychiatry 2012;69:562–571.

3 Fusar-Poli P, Borgwardt S, Crescini A, Deste G, Kempton MJ, Lawrie S, McGuire PM, Sacchetti E: Neuroanatomy of vulnerability to psychosis: a voxel-based meta-analysis. Neurosci Biobehav Rev 2011; 35:1175–1185.

4 Fusar-Poli P, Radua J, McGuire P, Borgwardt S: Neuroanatomical maps of psychosis onset: voxel-wise meta-analysis of antipsychotic-naive VBM studies. Schizophr Bull 2012;38:1297–1307.

5 Fusar-Poli P, Perez J, Broome M, Borgwardt S, Placentino A, Caverzasi E, Cortesi M, Veggiotti P, Politi P, Barale F, et al: Neurofunctional correlates of vulnerability to psychosis: a systematic review and meta-analysis. Neurosci Biobehav Rev 2007;31:465–484.

6 Wood SJ, Pantelis C, Velakoulis D, Yücel M, Fornito A, McGorry PD: Progressive changes in the development toward schizophrenia: studies in subjects at increased symptomatic risk. Schizophr Bull 2008;34: 322–329.

7 Ettinger U, Meyhöfer I, Steffens M, Wagner M, Koutsouleris N: Genetics, cognition, and neurobiology of schizotypal personality: a review of the overlap with schizophrenia. Front Psychiatry 2014;5:18.

8 Koutsouleris N, Ruhrmann S, Falkai P, Maier W: Personalised medicine in psychiatry and psychotherapy. A review of the current state-of-the-art in the biomarker-based early recognition of psychoses (in German). Bundesgesundheitsblatt Gesundheitsforschung Gesundheitsschutz 2013;56:1522–1530.

9 Davatzikos C: Why voxel-based morphometric analysis should be used with great caution when characterizing group differences. Neuroimage 2004;23:17–20.

10 Fusar-Poli P, Bonoldi I, Yung AR, Borgwardt S, Kempton MJ, Valmaggia L, Barale F, Caverzasi E, McGuire P: Predicting psychosis: meta-analysis of transition outcomes in individuals at high clinical risk. Arch Gen Psychiatry 2012;69:220–229.

11 Wiltink S, Velthorst E, Nelson B, McGorry PM, Yung AR: Declining transition rates to psychosis: the contribution of potential changes in referral pathways to an ultra-high-risk service. Early Interv Psychiatry 2015;9:200–206.

12 Yung AR, Yuen HP, Berger G, Francey S, Hung T-C, Nelson B, Phillips L, McGorry P: Declining transition rate in ultra high risk (prodromal) services: dilution or reduction of risk? Schizophr Bull 2007;33: 673–681.

13 Kambeitz J, Kambeitz-Ilankovic L, Leucht S, Wood S, Davatzikos C, Malchow B, Falkai P, Koutsouleris N: Detecting neuroimaging biomarkers for schizophrenia: a meta-analysis of multivariate pattern recognition studies. Neuropsychopharmacology 2015; 40:1742–1751.

14 Orrù G, Pettersson-Yeo W, Marquand AF, Sartori G, Mechelli A: Using support vector machine to identify imaging biomarkers of neurological and psychiatric disease: a critical review. Neurosci Biobehav Rev 2012;36:1140–1152.

15 Koutsouleris N, Borgwardt S, Meisenzahl EM, Bottlender R, Möller H-J, Riecher-Rössler A: Disease prediction in the at-risk mental state for psychosis using neuroanatomical biomarkers: results from the FePsy study. Schizophr Bull 2012;38:1234–1246.

16 Koutsouleris N, Meisenzahl E, Davatzikos C, Bottlender R, Frodl T, Scheuerecker J, Schmitt GJE, Zetzsche T, Decker P, Reiser M, et al: Use of neuroanatomical pattern classification to identify subjects in at-risk mental states of psychosis and predict disease transition. Arch Gen Psychiatry 2009;66:700–712.

17 Koutsouleris N, Riecher-Rössler A, Meisenzahl EM, Smieskova R, Studerus E, Kambeitz-Ilankovic L, Saldern S, von Cabral C, Reiser M, Falkai P, et al: Detecting the psychosis prodrome across high-risk populations using neuroanatomical biomarkers. Schizophr Bull 2015;41:471–482.

18 Costafreda SG, Chu C, Ashburner J, Fu CH: Prognostic and diagnostic potential of the structural neuroanatomy of depression. PLoS One 2009;4:e6353.

19 Hoeft F, McCandliss BD, Black JM, Gantman A, Zakerani N, Hulme C, Lyytinen H, Whitfield-Gabrieli S, Glover GH, Reiss AL, et al: Neural systems predicting long-term outcome in dyslexia. Proc Natl Acad Sci USA 2011;108:361–366.

20 Noble WS: What is a support vector machine? Nat Biotechnol 2006;24:1565–1567.

21 Krishnan M, Temel JS, Wright AA, Bernacki R, Selvaggi K, Balboni T: Predicting life expectancy in patients with advanced incurable cancer: a review. J Support Oncol 2013;11:68–74.

22 Karamouzis MV, Fotiadis DI: Machine learning applications in cancer prognosis and prediction. Comput Struct Biotechnol J 2014;13:8–17.

23 Sullivan GM, Feinn R: Using effect size – or why the p value is not enough. J Grad Med Educ 2012;4:279–282.

24 Kambeitz J, Koutsouleris N: Neuroimaging in psychiatry: multivariate analysis techniques for diagnosis and prognosis (in German). Nervenarzt 2014;85:714–719.

25 Smola A, Schölkopf B: A tutorial on support vector regression. Stat Comput 2004;14:199–222.

26 Schölkopf B, Smola A: Learning with Kernels. Support Vector Machines, Regularization, Optimization and Beyond. Cambridge, MIT Press, 2002.

27 Filzmoser P, Liebmann B, Varmuza K: Repeated double cross validation. J Chemometrics 2009;23:160–171.

28 Varma S, Simon R: Bias in error estimation when using cross-validation for model selection. BMC Bioinformatics 2006;7:91.

29 Lao Z, Shen D, Xue Z, Karacali B, Resnick SM, Davatzikos C: Morphological classification of brains via high-dimensional shape transformations and machine learning methods. Neuroimage 2004;21:46–57.

30 Gaonkar B, Davatzikos C: Deriving statistical significance maps for SVM based image classification and group comparisons. Med Image Comput Comput Assist Interv 2012;15:723–730.

31 Pantelis C, Velakoulis D, McGorry PD, Wood SJ, Suckling J, Phillips LJ, Yung AR, Bullmore ET, Brewer W, Soulsby B, et al: Neuroanatomical abnormalities before and after onset of psychosis: a cross-sectional and longitudinal MRI comparison. Lancet 2003;361:281–288.

32 Good CD, Johnsrude IS, Ashburner J, Henson RN, Friston KJ, Frackowiak RS: A voxel-based morphometric study of ageing in 465 normal adult human brains. Neuroimage 2001;14:21–36.

33 Borgwardt SJ, Riecher-Rössler A, Dazzan P, Chitnis X, Aston J, Drewe M, Gschwandtner U, Haller S, Pflüger M, Rechsteiner E, et al: Regional gray matter volume abnormalities in the at risk mental state. Biol Psychiatry 2007;61:1148–1156.

34 Borgwardt S, Koutsouleris N, Aston J, Studerus E, Smieskova R, Riecher-Rössler A, Meisenzahl EM: Distinguishing prodromal from first-episode psychosis using neuroanatomical single-subject pattern recognition. Schizophr Bull 2013;39:1105–1114.

35 Koutsouleris N, Meisenzahl EM, Borgwardt S, Riecher-Rössler A, Frodl T, Kambeitz J, Köhler Y, Falkai P, Möller H-J, Reiser M, et al: Individualized differential diagnosis of schizophrenia and mood disorders using neuroanatomical biomarkers. Brain 2015;138:2059–2073.

36 Modinos G, Pettersson-Yeo W, Allen P, McGuire PK, Aleman A, Mechelli A: Multivariate pattern classification reveals differential brain activation during emotional processing in individuals with psychosis proneness. Neuroimage 2012;59:3033–3041.

Priv.-Doz. Dr. med. Nikolaos Koutsouleris
Department of Psychiatry and Psychotherapy
Ludwig Maximilian University, Nussbaumstrasse 7
DE–80336 Munich (Germany)
E-Mail Nikolaos.Koutsouleris@med.uni-muenchen.de

Riecher-Rössler A, McGorry PD (eds): Early Detection and Intervention in Psychosis: State of the Art and Future Perspectives. Key Issues Ment Health. Basel, Karger, 2016, vol 181, pp 103–115 (DOI: 10.1159/000440918)

Connectivity Abnormalities in Emerging Psychosis

André Schmidt[a] · Stefan Borgwardt[b]

[a]Department of Psychiatry (UPK), University of Basel, Basel, Switzerland; [b]Department of Psychosis Studies, Institute of Psychiatry, Psychology and Neuroscience, King's College London, London, UK

Abstract

With the advent of modern neuroimaging techniques it was possible to improve our understanding of the potential pathogenetic mechanisms of psychosis. Using functional magnetic resonance imaging and diffusion tensor imaging, numerous studies have elucidated that the core hallmark of psychosis may be abnormal connectivity, although it still remains unclear which regions are most affected. A critical point is that brain connectivity abnormalities, whether structural or functional, are already evident in the psychosis high-risk state and further develop along the psychosis continuum. This suggests that the assessment of the brain connectivity pattern with neuroimaging approaches may permit the detection of the early phases of the illness and may also allow predictions of the course of the disease. In the present chapter, we present an overview of neuroimaging findings of abnormal structural and functional connectivity in subjects at high risk for psychosis. We first report structural connectivity findings derived from diffusion tensor imaging studies, which may serve as a base for the later presented changes in functional and effective connectivity findings obtained from functional magnetic resonance imaging during tasks and resting state. In the last part of this chapter, we also discuss some potential avenues in this field to get one step closer towards a network connectivity-driven classification of the psychosis high-risk state, which may also predict the onset of psychosis. © 2016 S. Karger AG, Basel

Brain imaging has emerged as a powerful tool to improve the specificity and validity of an early diagnosis and to sustain preventive intervention prior the onset of illness [1]. Although no imaging marker for clinics has been established so far, experimental evidence derived from magnetic resonance imaging (MRI) has repeatedly indicated that psychosis is characterized by abnormal structural and functional connectivity [2]. These studies support the dysconnectivity hypothesis of schizophrenia [3, 4] and its refinements [5, 6], proposing that the disorder results from abnormal integration across brain regions rather than from changes in local brain properties. Importantly, brain connectivity changes in psychosis evolve along a continuum, emerging before disease onset and proceeding with ongoing illness [7]. This suggests that the assessment of brain connectivity abnormalities may help to detect the transition from the high-risk state to established psychosis [8].

Brain connectivity can be measured according to structural, functional and effective connectivity [9]. Structural connectivity can be inferred from diffusion MRI [10] and reflects how brain regions are interconnected by white matter fiber bundles. The most commonly studied metrics in clinical diffusion tensor imaging (DTI) studies are fractional anisotropy (FA) and mean diffusivity. FA measures the diffusion directionality of water molecules along white matter tracts, which allows the estimation of the orientation of axon bundles, whereas mean diffusivity describes the magnitude of water diffusion within the tracts in all directions [for a review on these parameters, see 11, 12]. Previous DTI investigations have reported that microstructural changes in white matter may reflect a critical pathophysiological marker for psychosis [13] and that they are already evident before the onset of psychosis [2, 14–16]. Functional connectivity generally describes a correlation (undirected) between brain regions inferred either from blood oxygenation level-dependent functional MRI (fMRI) or coherence in electro- or magnetoencephalogram signals acquired during task performance or resting state [9]. Numerous fMRI studies have consistently provided evidence of abnormal functional connectivity during different tasks and rest in different phases of psychosis [2]. Finally, effective connectivity measures how neural activity in one region is caused by activity in another. This approach constitutes model-based formulations of context-specific directed connectivity that are based on the biophysics of neuronal interactions, such as dynamic causal modeling [9]. Abnormalities in effective connectivity have been reported in early stages of psychosis, with most of them being detected during working memory paradigms [17].

In the present chapter, we present an overview of neuroimaging findings of abnormal structural and functional connectivity in subjects at high risk for psychosis. We first report structural connectivity findings in order to provide a better understanding of the later presented changes in functional and effective connectivity findings obtained from fMRI during tasks and resting state. Finally, we provide further directions in this field to approach a connectivity-driven classification of the psychosis high-risk state which may also predict the onset of psychosis.

Structural Connectivity Abnormalities

Compared to healthy controls, clinical high-risk subjects for psychosis show decreased FA values along several long association fibers such as the inferior longitudinal fasciculus, inferior fronto-occipital fasciculus, superior longitudinal fasciculus, body and splenium of the corpus callosum, stria terminalis, right internal and external capsules, superior and posterior corona radiata, and cerebral peduncles [18–21]. Reduced FA in the superior longitudinal fasciculus, inferior longitudinal fasciculus and inferior fronto-occipital fasciculus has also been reported in subjects with a genetic high-risk state who showed intermediate values between healthy controls and chronic patients [22, 23]. Furthermore, genetic high-risk subjects also showed reduced FA in the right genu of the corpus callosum [24] and the anterior limb of internal capsule [25].

Although most cross-sectional studies have reported reduced FA in widespread brain regions including the superior longitudinal fasciculus, there is also evidence reporting increased FA in the genu of the corpus callosom [26], acuate fasciculus [23], anterior cingulum, bilateral pontine tegmental white matter and right and superior frontal white matter in high-risk populations [27, 28] [for a review, see 7]. Other studies found no FA difference relative to controls [29, 30]. Inconsistencies in studies with high-risk samples may result from different software packages applied or adjusting or not for different covariates. Another important point that complicates comparisons across studies is the high clinical heterogeneity in high-risk populations [31].

Comparing subjects with a subsequent transition to psychosis with those without transition, FA values in the superior longitudinal fasciculus seem to be reduced in clinical high-risk subjects with a subsequent transition to psychosis [21]. Longitudinal comparison of data in individuals who developed psychosis revealed a reduction in white matter volume in the region of the left fronto-occipital fasciculus, whereas participants who had not developed psychosis showed no reductions in white matter volume but increases in a region subjacent to the right inferior parietal lobule [32]. In line with these FA reductions, another longitudinal study showed that high-risk subjects with a later transition to psychosis also revealed decreased FA in the anterior limb of the left internal capsule, body of the corpus callosum, left superior corona radiata and left superior fronto-occipital fasciculus. In contrast, nonconverters showed a slight increase in these regions, although these within-group changes were not themselves significant [33]. The authors suggest that the onset of schizophrenia may be associated with a progressive reduction in the integrity of the frontal white matter [18]. In contrast, applying fiber tracking of the uncinate and arcuate fasciculi, dorsal and anterior cingulate, and subdivisions of the corpus callosum, no differences were found between high-risk subjects with transition to psychosis at follow-up and subjects without transition [14]. At baseline, FA was significantly reduced in a subregion of the corpus callosum in the clinical high-risk group as a whole compared to controls. This reduction was also found in the 34 individuals who did not transition during the 1-year follow-up. In contrast, nonconverters showed a significant improvement in subthreshold positive symptoms at follow-up, which was correlated with an increase in FA in the same corpus callosum region [34]. Furthermore, while there were no group differences in the integrity of the left/right superior cerebellar peduncles at baseline, controls showed a normative increase while the high-risk group showed a decrease in FA over 12 months. Moreover, neurological soft signs predicted a longitudinal decrease in cerebellar-thalamic FA and elevations in negative but not positive symptoms 12 months later [35].

Although there is a large body of evidence for FA development in emerging psychosis, less is clear regarding how mean diffusivity is altered in high-risk populations. Only one study so far has investigated mean diffusivity in clinical high-risk subjects and reported increased values in several clusters in the right hemisphere, most notably in the superior longitudinal fasciculus, posterior corona radiata and corpus callosum (splenium and body) [29].

In summary, the main trends that have emerged are that the psychosis high-risk state is associated with FA reductions in widespread white matter tract, with the most consistent finding in the superior longitudinal fasciculus. However, there is also evidence of increased FA. Differences among studies may be due to methodological differences, heterogeneity of samples and effects of medication. It is therefore important to adjust DTI findings for age, gender and antidepressant medication, all of which are known to significantly affect DTI metrics [19, 36–39]. Longitudinal designs with large samples are further needed to draw robust conclusions as to whether FA and mean diffusivity assessments are useful for detecting the onset of psychosis.

Functional Connectivity Abnormalities

Studies during Resting State

Studies on resting state functional connectivity in high-risk populations is ongoing and evidence is therefore limited in the literature. However, a recent study reported increased amygdala connectivity with a brainstem region around noradrenergic arousal nuclei in high-risk subjects relative to healthy controls [40]. Using a seed-based correlation approach, high-risk patients showed reduced functional connectivity of Broca's area to the right dorsolateral prefrontal cortex and left medial superior frontal cortex. Conversely, they also showed increased functional connectivity of Broca's area to the left dorsolateral prefrontal cortex and right anterior insula [41]. Fornito et al. [42] recently found that individuals with early psychosis and their unaffected relatives showed corticostriatal dysregulation, with dorsal striatal hypoconnectivity and ventral striatal hyperconnectivity with cortical targets. Furthermore, the default mode network in genetic high-risk individuals showed reduced functional connectivity in the prefrontal areas, posterior cingulate cortex and precuneus. Notably, this reduced connectivity in the prefrontal cortices correlated with total and general scores on the Positive and Negative Syndrome Scale [43]. In contrast, another study found that high-risk subjects had significantly greater positive connectivity than did controls between the posterior cingulate cortex seed region and other areas in the bilateral anterior cingulate cortex, medial prefrontal cortex, precuneus and lateral parietal cortex [44].

Schmidt · Borgwardt

Several investigations have been conducted to examine inter-network connectivity. This is important as, for example, interactions between brain systems such as the default mode and the frontoparietal cognitive system are critical for the flexibility of normal cognitive control and its disruption in pathological conditions [45]. In particular, hyperconnectivity in the default network of high-risk individuals was associated with reduced connectivity in the task-related network comprising frontoparietal brain regions [44], and may indicate deficient capacity for appropriate cognitive processing. Indeed, activity in the default mode is inversely correlated with cognitive control [46, 47]. Such a reduced negative correlation between the default mode network and the task-positive network has been observed in other studies with clinical high-risk patients [48, 49]. In accordance with studies in clinical high-risk subjects, the inverse correlation between the default mode network and the task-positive network is also diminished in genetic high-risk individuals [50]. Thus, a resting state fMRI study found reduced inter-network connectivity between the frontoparietal network and the cingulo-opercular network and a cerebellar network in individuals with psychosis and their unaffected siblings, and that these reductions were associated with both cognitive impairments and clinical symptoms [51]. This is important evidence, as it suggests that antagonism between the default mode and frontoparietal activity is mediated by the cingulo-opercular system [52].

Task-Induced fMRI Studies
Using dynamic causal modeling with a focus on endogenous connections (i.e. not modulated by a specific task condition), studies have reported reduced connectivity from the right posterior hippocampus to the right inferior frontal gyrus [53] and from the superior temporal gyrus to the middle frontal gyrus in clinical high-risk subjects during a working memory task [54]. In contrast, another study found increased endogenous connectivity between the left middle temporal gyrus and anterior cingulate gyrus during the Hayling Sentence Completion Task [55]. This study also explored task-induced modulation of connectivity, but found no difference between healthy controls and high-risk individuals. By focusing on task-induced modulation of connectivity, a more recent study found that working memory-induced connectivity from the middle frontal gyrus to the superior parietal lobule was significantly reduced in high-risk subjects [56]. In this study, the extent of connectivity from the right middle frontal gyrus to the superior parietal lobule was negatively related to the Brief Psychiatric Rating Scale total score, suggesting a mechanistic relation between the degree of functional network integrity and the clinical expression of schizophrenia. It is interesting to note that the expression of frontoparietal connectivity during working memory processing in high-risk subjects was intermediate between healthy controls and first-episode psychosis patients. Furthermore, the abnormal modulation of connectivity in first-episode psychosis patients was normalized by treatment with antipsychotics [57] (fig. 1).

Using functional connectivity approaches (undirected correlations) in genetic high-risk populations, reductions in connectivity between the right dlPFC and multiple

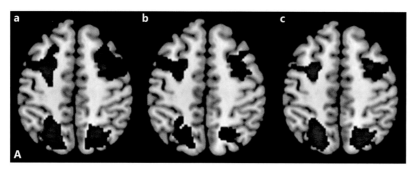

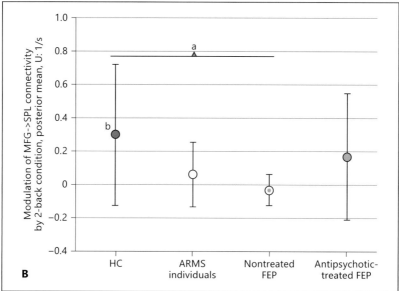

Fig. 1. A Healthy controls (a). individuals with an at-risk mental state (b) and patients experiencing a first-episode psychosis (c). Activations are reported at a whole-brain-corrected cluster threshold of p < 0.001 and a voxel size threshold of 1,400. **B** Data are shown for healthy controls (HC; n = 19), individuals with an at-risk mental state (ARMS; n = 15) and individuals with a first-episode psychosis (FEP) who were treated with antipsychotics (n = 8) or nontreated (n = 12) during scanning. The y-axis denotes the mean for all study participants and all 12 dynamic causal models (using Bayesian model averaging) with regard to the posterior mean of the modulatory effect; this encodes changes in connection strength induced by the 2-back working memory condition. [a] Significant differences among groups at p < 0.05. [b] Significant t test within each group (relative to zero) at p < 0.05. Error bars indicate SD derived from Bayesian parameter averages. With permission from Schmidt et al. [57].

brain regions in unaffected siblings were found during a 4-choice reaction time task [58]. In contrast to these reductions in connectivity, genetic high-risk subjects showed increased activation in frontoparietal regions during the working encoding phase relative to the healthy control group [59]. This result corresponds with previous evidence showing increased frontoparietal connectivity in genetic high-risk subjects [60, 61], which has been interpreted as a compensatory mechanism [62], probably for

       Schmidt · Borgwardt

prefrontal cortex dysfunction during working memory processing [63]. Using dynamic causal modeling to assess directed connectivity, a previous study found that the connection strength with the nonlinear modulation between the thalamus and the inferior frontal gyrus was significantly reduced in high-risk subjects with psychotic symptoms and 4 ill subjects who subsequently developed schizophrenia in contrast to the healthy controls. Furthermore, there was a significant correlation between the individual connection strength and the presence of delusions in high-risk subjects with psychotic symptoms. Another dynamic causal modeling study showed that genetic high-risk subjects revealed significant reductions in coupling across both frontostriatal and frontoarietal pathways during sustained attention task [64]. Using psychophysiological interaction to explore effective connectivity, it was shown that high-risk subjects who subsequently developed psychosis showed greater midbrain-PFC connectivity during verbal fluency task compared with those who did not become psychotic [65].

In summary, these studies reveal a broad spectrum of abnormalities in functional brain connectivity in high-risk subjects for psychosis, suggesting that the assessment of functional brain connectivity pattern may permit an early detection of the disease. One of the most consistent findings is alteration in frontoparietal connectivity [2], which may indicate that abnormalities in this pathway particularly reflect a vulnerability marker for emerging psychosis. However, more longitudinal studies in high-risk subjects are needed with larger samples, including a meaningful number of converters in relation to nonconverters.

Potential Developments for Future Research

A potential limitation of most of the abovementioned studies is that they have often analyzed connectivity strengths among a restricted number of brain regions. Although this can be an advantage if the included regions comprise highly sensitive clinical data, which are not confounded by unimportant and noisy data from other regions, such approaches neglect the comprehensive network organization of the brain. Thus, we need to understand how the entire architecture of the brain is altered in the psychosis high-risk state. Network studies in humans are motivated by the idea that brain function is not solely attributable to local regions and connections, but rather emerges from the topology of the network as a whole, the connectome of the brain [66, 67]. Methodological advances allow us to quantify topological properties of complex systems such as modularity [68], hierarchy [69], centrality [70] and the distribution of networks hubs [71]. 'Brain hubs' represent specific regions that play a central role in the overall network organization, as indexed by a high degree, low clustering, short path length, high centrality and participation in multiple communities across the network [72]. Graph theory analysis has emerged as a very helpful approach to infer complex network properties of the brain, and will play an increasingly important part in the effort to comprehend the physics of the brain's connectome [67] and how it is altered in psychosis [73]. One achievement of graph theory is the detection of the so-called 'rich club' [74]. The rich club phenomenon in networks is said to be present when the hubs of a network tend to be more densely connected among themselves than nodes of a lower degree [75]. Rich club organization can provide important information on the higher-order structure of a network, particularly on the level of resilience, hierarchal ordering and specialization [75]. Interestingly, a previous study revealed that rich club organization is significantly affected in schizophrenia patients, together with a reduced density of rich club connections predominantly comprising the white matter pathways that link the midline frontal, parietal and insular hub regions. This reduction in rich club density was found to be further associated with lower levels of global communication capacity [76]. This study provides novel biological evidence that schizophrenia is characterized by a selective disruption of structural brain connectivity among central hub regions of the brain, potentially leading to reduced communication capacity and altered functional brain dynamics [76]. Moreover, this study also found an increased coupling between structural connectivity strength and functional connectivity during resting-state fMRI in patients with schizophrenia. Along this line, another study found that psychotic patients showed decreased functional connectivity and impaired white matter integrity in a distributed network encompassing frontal, temporal, thalamic and striatal regions [77], suggesting that graph theory is useful to study the structure-function relationship (fig. 2). Furthermore and perhaps most relevant, a very recent DTI study showed that abnormal rich club organization is already evident in unaffected siblings of schizophrenia patients when compared with healthy subjects, but less affected than in schizophrenia patients, which suggests that impaired rich club connectivity is related to familial vulnerability for schizophrenia and may therefore reflect genetic vulnerability [78]. More global data-driven correlation approaches across the whole brain with graph theory are thus promising approaches to detect robust network connectivity abnormalities in the psychosis high-risk state.

Fig. 2. A (i) Confirming previous findings, rich club members included the bilateral precuneus, superior frontal cortex, superior parietal cortex, and the insula in both the healthy and patient populations. This figure is based on the group-averaged cortical network in controls (at a rich club level of k >15) [79]. (ii) Edges across individual brain networks (both controls and patients) were divided into 3 distinct classes: rich club connections linking rich club members (red), feeder connections linking rich club members to non-rich club members (orange) and local connections connecting non-rich club members (yellow edges). (iii) Examining the density of rich club, feeder and local connections between the populations of controls and patients revealed a significant reduction in rich club density in patients but no significant effect in density of feeder and local connections. The figure shows mean (SD) density values for each of the 3 classes, scaled to the mean density values of the control group. ROI = Region of interest. **B** Rich club, feeder and local connectivity. Bar graphs indicate connectivity strength (i.e. sum of reconstructed fibers) for rich club, feeder and local connections. A significant ordered difference, such that controls > siblings > patients, was found for rich club connectivity (p = 0.014). * Significantly ordered difference across groups. With permission from Collin et al. [78].

(For figure see next page.)

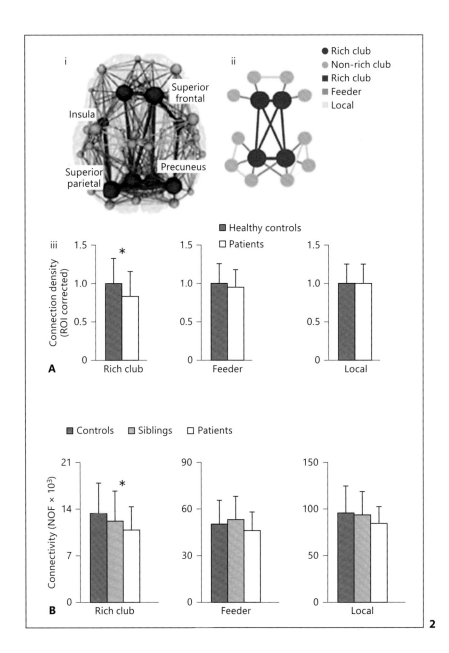

Conclusions

Although further extensive work is needed, the assessment of network connectivity endophenotypes is promising to detect a subsequent transition from the high-risk of psychosis to the onset of the frank disease [7]. The two concepts, graph theoretical approaches to infer complex network properties of the brain from a more global perspective and model-based formulations of context-specific effective (directed) connectivity should be used in conjunction. For instance, whole-brain network topology measures based on graph theory can first be used to detect dysconnected brain regions, which may also show a relation to clinical endophenotypes. This sensitive clinical information could then serve as a base to construct later model-based assays of effective connectivity. Finally, effective connectivity estimates might further be fed into classification procedures. Such approaches, as recently demonstrated in chronic patients [80], provide a mechanistic understanding of brain signal and thus may increase the accuracy of machine learning engines [81].

References

1 Fusar-Poli P, McGuire P, Borgwardt S: Mapping prodromal psychosis: a critical review of neuroimaging studies. Eur Psychiatry 2012;27:181–191.

2 Pettersson-Yeo W, Allen P, Benetti S, McGuire P, Mechelli A: Dysconnectivity in schizophrenia: where are we now? Neurosci Biobehav Rev 2011;35:1110–1124.

3 Friston KJ, Frith CD: Schizophrenia: a disconnection syndrome? Clin Neurosci 1995;3:89–97.

4 Friston KJ: The disconnection hypothesis. Schizophr Res 1998;30:115–125.

5 Stephan K, Baldeweg T, Friston K: Synaptic plasticity and dysconnection in schizophrenia. Biol Psychiatry 2006;59:929–939.

6 Stephan KE, Friston KJ, Frith CD: Dysconnection in schizophrenia: from abnormal synaptic plasticity to failures of self-monitoring. Schizophr Bull 2009;35:509–527.

7 Schmidt A, Diwadkar VA, Smieskova R, Harrisberger F, Lang UE, McGuire P, Fusar-Poli P, Borgwardt S: Approaching a network connectivity-driven classification of the psychosis continuum: a selective review and suggestions for future research. Front Hum Neurosci 2014;8:1047.

8 Schmidt A, Borgwardt S: Abnormal effective connectivity in the psychosis high-risk state. Neuroimage 2013;81:119–120.

9 Park HJ, Friston K: Structural and functional brain networks: from connections to cognition. Science 2013;342:1238411.

10 Basser PJ, Pierpaoli C: Microstructural and physiological features of tissues elucidated by quantitative-diffusion-tensor MRI. J Magn Reson B 1996;111:209–219.

11 Jellison BJ, Field AS, Medow J, Lazar M, Salamat MS, Alexander AL: Diffusion tensor imaging of cerebral white matter: a pictorial review of physics, fiber tract anatomy, and tumor imaging patterns. AJNR Am J Neuroradiol 2004;25:356–369.

12 Le Bihan D, Mangin JF, Poupon C, Clark CA, Pappata S, Molko N, Chabriat H: Diffusion tensor imaging: concepts and applications. J Magn Reson Imaging 2001;13:534–546.

13 Kubicki M, McCarley R, Westin CF, Park HJ, Maier S, Kikinis R, Jolesz FA, Shenton ME: A review of diffusion tensor imaging studies in schizophrenia. J Psychiatr Res 2007;41:15–30.

14 Peters BD, Blaas J, de Haan L: Diffusion tensor imaging in the early phase of schizophrenia: what have we learned? J Psychiatr Res 2010;44:993–1004.

15 Canu E, Agosta F, Filippi M: A selective review of structural connectivity abnormalities of schizophrenic patients at different stages of the disease. Schizophr Res 2015;161:19–28.

16 Samartzis L, Dima D, Fusar-Poli P, Kyriakopoulos M: White matter alterations in early stages of schizophrenia: a systematic review of diffusion tensor imaging studies. J Neuroimaging 2014;24:101–110.

17 Dauvermann MR, Whalley HC, Schmidt A, Lee GL, Romaniuk L, Roberts N, Johnstone EC, Lawrie SM, Moorhead TW: Computational neuropsychiatry – schizophrenia as a cognitive brain network disorder. Front Psychiatry 2014;5:30.

18 Carletti F, Woolley JB, Bhattacharyya S, Perez-Iglesias R, Fusar Poli P, Valmaggia L, Broome MR, Bramon E, Johns L, Giampietro V, Williams SC, Barker GJ, McGuire PK: Alterations in white matter evident before the onset of psychosis. Schizophr Bull 2012;38:1170–1179.

19 Karlsgodt KH, Niendam TA, Bearden CE, Cannon TD: White matter integrity and prediction of social and role functioning in subjects at ultra-high risk for psychosis. Biol Psychiatry 2009;66:562–569.

20 Peters BD, Schmitz N, Dingemans PM, van Amelsvoort TA, Linszen DH, de Haan L, Majoie CB, den Heeten GJ: Preliminary evidence for reduced frontal white matter integrity in subjects at ultra-high-risk for psychosis. Schizophr Res 2009;111:192–193.

21 Bloemen OJ, de Koning MB, Schmitz N, Nieman DH, Becker HE, de Haan L, Dingemans P, Linszen DH, van Amelsvoort TA: White-matter markers for psychosis in a prospective ultra-high-risk cohort. Psychol Med 2010;40:1297–1304.

22 Clark KA, Nuechterlein KH, Asarnow RF, Hamilton LS, Phillips OR, Hageman NS, Woods RP, Alger JR, Toga AW, Narr KL: Mean diffusivity and fractional anisotropy as indicators of disease and genetic liability to schizophrenia. J Psychiatr Res 2011;45:980–988.

23 Knöchel C, O'Dwyer L, Alves G, Reinke B, Magerkurth J, Rotarska-Jagiela A, Prvulovic D, Hampel H, Linden DE, Oertel-Knöchel V: Association between white matter fiber integrity and subclinical psychotic symptoms in schizophrenia patients and unaffected relatives. Schizophr Res 2012;140:129–135.

24 Camchong J, Lim KO, Sponheim SR, Macdonald AW: Frontal white matter integrity as an endophenotype for schizophrenia: diffusion tensor imaging in monozygotic twins and patients' nonpsychotic relatives. Front Hum Neurosci 2009;3:35.

25 Muñoz Maniega S, Lymer GK, Bastin ME, Marjoram D, Job DE, Moorhead TW, Owens DG, Johnstone EC, McIntosh AM, Lawrie SM: A diffusion tensor MRI study of white matter integrity in subjects at high genetic risk of schizophrenia. Schizophr Res 2008;106:132–139.

26 Kim SN, Park JS, Jang JH, Jung WH, Shim G, Park HY, Hwang JY, Choi CH, Kang DH, Lee JM, Kwon JS: Increased white matter integrity in the corpus callosum in subjects with high genetic loading for schizophrenia. Prog Neuropsychopharmacol Biol Psychiatry 2012;37:50–55.

27 Hoptman MJ, Nierenberg J, Bertisch HC, Catalano D, Ardekani BA, Branch CA, Delisi LE: A DTI study of white matter microstructure in individuals at high genetic risk for schizophrenia. Schizophr Res 2008; 106:115–124.

28 Bora E, Fornito A, Radua J, Walterfang M, Seal M, Wood SJ, Yücel M, Velakoulis D, Pantelis C: Neuroanatomical abnormalities in schizophrenia: a multimodal voxelwise meta-analysis and meta-regression analysis. Schizophr Res 2011;127:46–57.

29 Clemm von Hohenberg C, Pasternak O, Kubicki M, Ballinger T, Vu MA, Swisher T, Green K, Giwerc M, Dahlben B, Goldstein JM, Woo TU, Petryshen TL, Mesholam-Gately RI, Woodberry KA, Thermenos HW, Mulert C, McCarley RW, Seidman LJ, Shenton ME: White matter microstructure in individuals at clinical high risk of psychosis: a whole-brain diffusion tensor imaging study. Schizophr Bull 2014;40: 895–903.

30 Peters BD, de Haan L, Dekker N, Blaas J, Becker HE, Dingemans PM, Akkerman EM, Majoie CB, van Amelsvoort T, den Heeten GJ, Linszen DH: White matter fibertracking in first-episode schizophrenia, schizoaffective patients and subjects at ultra-high risk of psychosis. Neuropsychobiology 2008;58:19–28.

31 Simon AE, Umbricht D, Lang UE, Borgwardt S: Declining transition rates to psychosis: the role of diagnostic spectra and symptom overlaps in individuals with attenuated psychosis syndrome. Schizophr Res 2014;159:292–298.

32 Walterfang M, McGuire PK, Yung AR, Phillips LJ, Velakoulis D, Wood SJ, Suckling J, Bullmore ET, Brewer W, Soulsby B, Desmond P, McGorry PD, Pantelis C: White matter volume changes in people who develop psychosis. Br J Psychiatry 2008;193: 210–215.

33 Carletti F, Woolley JB, Bhattacharyya S, Perez-Iglesias R, Fusar Poli P, Valmaggia L, Broome MR, Bramon E, Johns L, Giampietro V, Williams SC, Barker GJ, McGuire PK: Alterations in white matter evident before the onset of psychosis. Schizophr Bull 2012; 38:1170–1179.

34 Katagiri N, Pantelis C, Nemoto T, Zalesky A, Hori M, Shimoji K, Saito J, Ito S, Dwyer DB, Fukunaga I, Morita K, Tsujino N, Yamaguchi T, Shiraga N, Aoki S, Mizuno M: A longitudinal study investigating subthreshold symptoms and white matter changes in individuals with an 'at risk mental state' (ARMS). Schizophr Res 2015;162:7–13.

35 Mittal VA, Dean DJ, Bernard JA, Orr JM, Pelletier-Baldelli A, Carol EE, Gupta T, Turner J, Leopold DR, Robustelli BL, Millman ZB: Neurological soft signs predict abnormal cerebellar-thalamic tract development and negative symptoms in adolescents at high risk for psychosis: a longitudinal perspective. Schizophr Bull 2014;40:1204–1215.

36 Lebel C, Caverhill-Godkewitsch S, Beaulieu C: Age-related regional variations of the corpus callosum identified by diffusion tensor tractography. Neuroimage 2010;52:20–31.

37 Abe O, Yamasue H, Yamada H, Masutani Y, Kabasawa H, Sasaki H, Takei K, Suga M, Kasai K, Aoki S, Ohtomo K: Sex dimorphism in gray/white matter volume and diffusion tensor during normal aging. NMR Biomed 2010;23:446–458.

38 Hsu JL, Leemans A, Bai CH, Lee CH, Tsai YF, Chiu HC, Chen WH: Gender differences and age-related white matter changes of the human brain: a diffusion tensor imaging study. Neuroimage 2008;39:566–577.

39 Korgaonkar MS, Williams LM, Song YJ, Usherwood T, Grieve SM: Diffusion tensor imaging predictors of treatment outcomes in major depressive disorder. Br J Psychiatry 2014;205:321–328.

40 Anticevic A, Tang Y, Cho YT, Repovs G, Cole MW, Savic A, Wang F, Krystal JH, Xu K: Amygdala connectivity differs among chronic, early course, and individuals at risk for developing schizophrenia. Schizophr Bull 2014;40:1105–1116.

41 Jung WH, Jang JH, Shin NY, Kim SN, Choi CH, An SK, Kwon JS: Regional brain atrophy and functional disconnection in Broca's area in individuals at ultra-high risk for psychosis and schizophrenia. PLoS One 2012;7:e51975.

42 Fornito A, Harrison BJ, Goodby E, Dean A, Ooi C, Nathan PJ, Lennox BR, Jones PB, Suckling J, Bullmore ET: Functional dysconnectivity of corticostriatal circuitry as a risk phenotype for psychosis. JAMA Psychiatry 2013;70:1143–1151.

43 Jang JH, Jung WH, Choi JS, Choi CH, Kang DH, Shin NY, Hong KS, Kwon JS: Reduced prefrontal functional connectivity in the default mode network is related to greater psychopathology in subjects with high genetic loading for schizophrenia. Schizophr Res 2011;127:58–65.

44 Shim G, Oh JS, Jung WH, Jang JH, Choi CH, Kim E, Park HY, Choi JS, Jung MH, Kwon JS: Altered resting-state connectivity in subjects at ultra-high risk for psychosis: an fMRI study. Behav Brain Funct 2010;6:58.

45 Cocchi L, Zalesky A, Fornito A, Mattingley JB: Dynamic cooperation and competition between brain systems during cognitive control. Trends Cogn Sci 2013;17:493–501.

46 Lawrence NS, Ross TJ, Hoffmann R, Garavan H, Stein EA: Multiple neuronal networks mediate sustained attention. J Cogn Neurosci 2003;15:1028–1038.

47 McKiernan KA, Kaufman JN, Kucera-Thompson J, Binder JR: A parametric manipulation of factors affecting task-induced deactivation in functional neuroimaging. J Cogn Neurosci 2003;15:394–408.

48 Wotruba D, Michels L, Buechler R, Metzler S, Theodoridou A, Gerstenberg M, Walitza S, Kollias S, Rössler W, Heekeren K: Aberrant coupling within and across the default mode, task-positive, and salience network in subjects at risk for psychosis. Schizophr Bull 2014;40:1095–1104.

49 Fryer SL, Woods SW, Kiehl KA, Calhoun VD, Pearlson GD, Roach BJ, Ford JM, Srihari VH, McGlashan TH, Mathalon DH: Deficient suppression of default mode regions during working memory in individuals with early psychosis and at clinical high-risk for psychosis. Front Psychiatry 2013;4:92.

50 Whitfield-Gabrieli S, Thermenos HW, Milanovic S, Tsuang MT, Faraone SV, McCarley RW, Shenton ME, Green AI, Nieto-Castanon A, LaViolette P, Wojcik J, Gabrieli JD, Seidman LJ: Hyperactivity and hyperconnectivity of the default network in schizophrenia and in first degree relatives of persons with schizophrenia. Proc Natl Acad Sci U S A 2009;106:1279–1284.

51 Repovs G, Csernansky JG, Barch DM: Brain network connectivity in individuals with schizophrenia and their siblings. Biol Psychiatry 2011;69:967–973.

52 Bressler SL, Menon V: Large-scale brain networks in cognition: emerging methods and principles. Trends Cogn Sci 2010;14:277–290.

53 Benetti S, Mechelli A, Picchioni M, Broome M, Williams S, McGuire P: Functional integration between the posterior hippocampus and prefrontal cortex is impaired in both first episode schizophrenia and the at risk mental state. Brain 2009;132:2426–2436.

54 Crossley NA, Mechelli A, Fusar-Poli P, Broome MR, Matthiasson P, Johns LC, Bramon E, Valmaggia L, Williams SC, McGuire PK: Superior temporal lobe dysfunction and frontotemporal dysconnectivity in subjects at risk of psychosis and in first-episode psychosis. Hum Brain Mapp 2009;30:4129–4137.

55 Allen P, Stephan KE, Mechelli A, Day F, Ward N, Dalton J, Williams SC, McGuire P: Cingulate activity and fronto-temporal connectivity in people with prodromal signs of psychosis. Neuroimage 2010;49:947–955.

56 Schmidt A, Smieskova R, Simon A, Allen P, Fusar-Poli P, McGuire PK, Bendfeldt K, Aston J, Lang UE, Walter M, Radue EW, Riecher-Rössler A, Borgwardt SJ: Abnormal effective connectivity and psychopathological symptoms in the psychosis high-risk state. J Psychiatry Neurosci 2014;39:239–248.

57 Schmidt A, Smieskova R, Aston J, Simon A, Allen P, Fusar-Poli P, McGuire PK, Riecher-Rössler A, Stephan KE, Borgwardt S: Brain connectivity abnormalities predating the onset of psychosis: correlation with the effect of medication. JAMA Psychiatry 2013;70:903–912.

58 Woodward ND, Waldie B, Rogers B, Tibbo P, Seres P, Purdon SE: Abnormal prefrontal cortical activity and connectivity during response selection in first episode psychosis, chronic schizophrenia, and unaffected siblings of individuals with schizophrenia. Schizophr Res 2009;109:182–190.

59 Choi JS, Park JY, Jung MH, Jang JH, Kang DH, Jung WH, Han JY, Choi CH, Hong KS, Kwon JS: Phase-specific brain change of spatial working memory processing in genetic and ultra-high risk groups of schizophrenia. Schizophr Bull 2012;38:1189–1199.

60 Delawalla Z, Csernansky JG, Barch DM: Prefrontal cortex function in nonpsychotic siblings of individuals with schizophrenia. Biol Psychiatry 2008;63:490–497.

61 Whalley HC, Simonotto E, Flett S, Marshall I, Ebmeier KP, Owens DG, Goddard NH, Johnstone EC, Lawrie SM: fMRI correlates of state and trait effects in subjects at genetically enhanced risk of schizophrenia. Brain 2004;127:478–490.

62 Whalley HC, Simonotto E, Marshall I, Owens DG, Goddard NH, Johnstone EC, Lawrie SM: Functional disconnectivity in subjects at high genetic risk of schizophrenia. Brain 2005;128:2097–2108.

63 Anticevic A, Repovs G, Barch DM: Working memory encoding and maintenance deficits in schizophrenia: neural evidence for activation and deactivation abnormalities. Schizophr Bull 2013;39:168–178.

64 Diwadkar VA, Bakshi N, Gupta G, Pruitt P, White R, Eickhoff SB: Dysfunction and dysconnection in cortical-striatal networks during sustained attention: genetic risk for schizophrenia or bipolar disorder and its impact on brain network function. Front Psychiatry 2014;5:50.

65 Allen P, Luigjes J, Howes OD, Egerton A, Hirao K, Valli I, Kambeitz J, Fusar-Poli P, Broome M, McGuire P: Transition to psychosis associated with prefrontal and subcortical dysfunction in ultra high-risk individuals. Schizophr Bull 2012;38:1268–1276.

66 Sporns O, Tononi G, Kötter R: The human connectome: a structural description of the human brain. PLoS Comput Biol 2005;1:e42.

67 Bullmore E, Sporns O: Complex brain networks: graph theoretical analysis of structural and functional systems. Nat Rev Neurosci 2009;10:186–198.

68 Girvan M, Newman ME: Community structure in social and biological networks. Proc Natl Acad Sci U S A 2002;99:7821–7826.

69 Ravasz E, Barabási AL: Hierarchical organization in complex networks. Phys Rev E Stat Nonlin Soft Matter Phys 2003;67:026112.

70 Barthelemy M: Betweenness centrality in large complex networks. Eur Phys J B 2004;38:163–168.

71 Guimerà R, Nunes Amaral LA: Functional cartography of complex metabolic networks. Nature 2005;433:895–900.

72 Sporns O, Honey CJ, Kötter R: Identification and classification of hubs in brain networks. PLoS One 2007;2:e1049.

73 van den Heuvel MP, Fornito A: Brain networks in schizophrenia. Neuropsychol Rev 2014;24:32–48.

74 van den Heuvel MP, Sporns O: Rich-club organization of the human connectome. J Neurosci 2011;31:15775–15786.

75 Colizza V, Flammini A, Serrano MA, Vespignani A: Detecting rich-club ordering in complex networks. Nat Phys 2006;2:110–115.

76 van den Heuvel MP, Sporns O, Collin G, Scheewe T, Mandl RC, Cahn W, Goñi J, Hulshoff Pol HE, Kahn RS: Abnormal rich club organization and functional brain dynamics in schizophrenia. JAMA Psychiatry 2013;70:783–792.

77 Cocchi L, Harding IH, Lord A, Pantelis C, Yucel M, Zalesky A: Disruption of structure-function coupling in the schizophrenia connectome. Neuroimage Clin 2014;4:779–787.

78 Collin G, Kahn RS, de Reus MA, Cahn W, van den Heuvel MP: Impaired rich club connectivity in unaffected siblings of schizophrenia patients. Schizophr Bull 2014;40:438–448.

79 de Reus MA, van den Heuvel MP: Estimating false positives and negatives in brain networks. Neuroimage 2013;70:402–409.

80 Brodersen KH, Deserno L, Schlagenhauf F, Lin Z, Penny WD, Buhmann JM, Stephan KE: Dissecting psychiatric spectrum disorders by generative embedding. Neuroimage Clin 2013;4:98–111.

81 Varoquaux G, Thirion B: How machine learning is shaping cognitive neuroimaging. Gigascience 2014;3:28.

Dr. André Schmidt
Department of Psychiatry (UPK), University of Basel
Wilhelm Klein-Strasse 27
CH–4012 Basel (Switzerland)
E-Mail andre.schmidt@unibas.ch

Riecher-Rössler A, McGorry PD (eds): Early Detection and Intervention in Psychosis: State of the Art and Future Perspectives. Key Issues Ment Health. Basel, Karger, 2016, vol 181, pp 116–132 (DOI: 10.1159/000440919)

Neurocognition and Motor Functioning in the Prediction of Psychosis

Erich Studerus[a] · Martina Papmeyer[a, b] · Anita Riecher-Rössler[a]

[a]Center for Gender Research and Early Detection, University of Basel Psychiatric Clinics, Basel, and [b]Division of Systems Neuroscience of Psychopathology, Translational Research Center, University Hospital of Psychiatry, University of Bern, Bern, Switzerland

Abstract

Meta-analyses suggest that – among help-seeking individuals – only about one third of those meeting internationally established criteria for an at-risk mental state (ARMS) for psychosis will later develop psychosis, and about one third will have a clinical remission within two years. Hence, further risk stratification among ARMS individuals is urgently needed to improve the cost-benefit ratio of preventive interventions. Cognitive and motor functioning deficits are promising candidates for improving the prediction of psychosis in ARMS individuals because they are hallmark features of schizophrenic psychoses, they precede the onset of frank psychosis by many years, and they can be assessed at relatively low costs. In this chapter, we critically evaluate the potential of cognitive and motor functioning parameters for improving the prediction of psychosis in ARMS individuals. We first summarize current evidence on cognitive and motor functioning differences between ARMS individuals who later developed psychosis and those who did not, and then address the question of whether cognitive and motor functioning variables are independently associated with transition to psychosis. Specifically, we review all available studies that included cognitive and/or motor functioning variables into prediction models integrating variables from multiple domains and thereby evaluate their added predictive value. Finally, we provide a detailed discussion of methodological issues in the current research and give recommendations for improvements.   © 2016 S. Karger AG, Basel

The early detection and treatment of schizophrenic psychoses already in their prodromal stage have become major aims in psychiatric research during the last two decades [1]. Consequently, a number of operational criteria have been established internationally that aim at identifying the schizophrenia prodrome. The criteria most widely employed are the so-called 'ultra-high-risk' criteria [2], which require the fulfillment of at least one out of three clinical symptom presentations: 'attenuated' psychotic symptoms, brief limited intermittent psychotic symptoms, or a significant decrease in functioning in the context of a genetic risk for schizophrenia. Further frequently used criteria include the basic symptoms criteria [3], which require the presence of subjective disturbances of cognitive processing or the perception of the self and the world. Both criteria sets have been demonstrated to have predictive validities when applied to help-seeking individuals. That is, among those who meet at least one of these criteria, about 36% develop frank psychosis within a three-year time period [4]. Furthermore, among those who develop psychosis, about 73% are diagnosed with schizophrenic psychoses [5]. However, since only about one third of those identified by current risk criteria develop psychosis and about one third go into remission from their clinical high-risk state within two years [6], further risk stratification is urgently needed to identify subgroups with specific needs and response patterns and thus improve the cost-benefit ratio of preventive interventions [7]. Hence, it has been suggested to develop prediction models that integrate information from various assessment domains, including psychopathology, sociodemographic characteristics, neurocognition, blood parameters, neuroimaging, and neurophysiology [8].

Neurocognitive and motor functioning variables likely play an important role in such multidomain prediction models for several reasons. First, cognitive deficits are considered core features of schizophrenic psychoses which may be even more defining for these disorders than positive psychotic symptoms [cf. 9]. Although they also frequently occur in other psychiatric disorders, such as major depression, bipolar disorder, or attention deficit hyperactivity disorder [for a review, see 10], in schizophrenia patients cognitive underperformance seems to be more prevalent [11], more severe [12, 13], more stable over the course of the illness, and more independent of clinical symptoms [14]. Meta-analyses suggest that, at psychosis onset, cognitive performance is on average about one standard deviation (SD) below that of age-matched healthy control subjects [15–17]. Furthermore, deficits have been consistently demonstrated in all cognitive domains with medium to large effect sizes and cannot be attributed to the effects of antipsychotics because unmedicated and medicated patients are similarly affected [17]. The greatest impairments appear to be present in the domains of verbal memory, speed of processing, and working memory, whereas motor functioning and dexterity seem to be least affected [15–17]. However, effect sizes are quite similar across domains and factor analyses indicate that one underlying factor explains most of the variance in each domain, suggesting that cognitive dysfunction in schizophrenia is broad and generalized [18, 19].

Second, cognitive and motor functioning deficits are already present almost a decade before the onset of frank psychosis [9] and can also be observed – albeit to a lesser extent – in first-degree relatives of schizophrenia patients [20], suggesting a potential role as endophenotypic markers. A recent meta-analysis of prospective investigations of birth or genetic high-risk cohorts and follow-back investigations of population samples indicated that, by age 16, individuals who subsequently developed schizophrenia spectrum disorders displayed significant deficits in IQ (Cohen's $d = 0.51$) and motor function ($d = 0.56$), but not in general academic ($d = 0.25$) or mathematical achievement ($d = 0.21$) [21]. Likewise, a meta-analysis of population-based cohorts and nested case-control studies indicated that low IQ increased the risk of developing schizophrenia in a dose-dependent fashion [22]. Early cognitive deficits seem to be relatively specific for schizophrenic psychoses as these have been observed in children and adolescents who later developed schizophrenia, but not in those who later developed depression or bipolar disorder [9, 23, 24]. Current evidence therefore suggests that cognitive and motor functioning deficits observed in schizophrenic psychoses are mostly the result of aberrant neurodevelopment continuing throughout the first two decades of life and not of neurodegenerative processes [25]. That is, individuals who later develop schizophrenia often show continuous problems in skills acquisition during childhood and adolescence, and thus increasingly fall behind their peers in terms of cognitive and intellectual performance. In line with the neurodevelopmental theory [26], studies that have assessed cognitive functioning in clinical high-risk subjects indicate that cognitive deficits are already present in almost all domains before transition to psychosis [27–29] and do not decline from before to after transition [30].

Third, cognitive and motor functioning can usually be assessed at lower costs and in less time than variables from other domains, such as neuroimaging. Furthermore, as instructions and procedures can be highly standardized, cognitive assessments might be more objective than clinical assessments of psychopathology. Finally, most early detection clinics already routinely perform neuropsychological testing for clinical purposes. Thus, the inclusion of neurocognitive variables into risk prediction models would not prolong existing examinations of patients at risk for psychosis.

In the following, we critically evaluate the potential of cognitive and motor functioning variables for improving the prediction of psychosis and risk stratification in individuals with an at-risk mental state (ARMS) for psychosis. By using the term 'ARMS individuals', we refer to individuals meeting the internationally established criteria described above for a clinical risk for psychosis (i.e., ultra-high-risk or basic symptoms criteria). We review all available studies that have investigated baseline cognitive and motor performance differences between ARMS individuals who later made a transition to psychosis (ARMS-T) and those who did not (ARMS-NT). Two types of studies will be discussed separately: (1) studies that have analyzed mean group differences in cognitive and motor functioning between ARMS-T and ARMS-NT individuals, and (2) studies that have included cognitive and/or motor functioning variables in multivariate prediction models and thus evaluated their added predictive values. Finally, we will discuss methodological problems and limitations of previous studies and give an outlook on future research in this area.

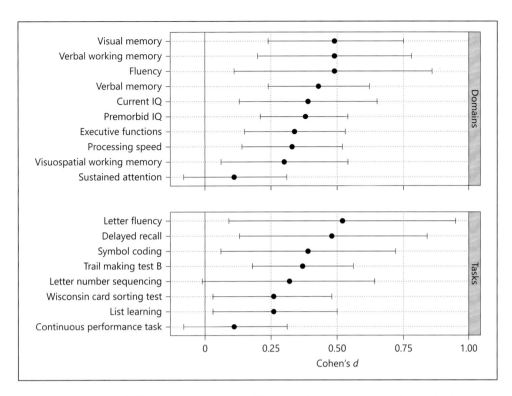

Fig. 1. Mean weighted effect sizes for cognitive differences between at-risk patients with later transition to psychosis and those without later transition according to Bora et al. [27].

Cognitive and Motor Dysfunction in the Prediction of Psychosis

Difference between ARMS-T and ARMS-NT

To date, associations between cognitive performance and later transition to psychosis have been investigated in at least four systematic reviews [31–34] and three meta-analyses [27–29], all of them concluding that ARMS-T individuals have more severe deficits than ARMS-NT individuals. The most recent and hence most up-to-date meta-analysis by Bora et al. [27], which was based on data from nine samples (263 ARMS-T and 586 ARMS-NT), reported that ARMS-T individuals performed significantly worse than ARMS-NT individuals in nine out of ten studied cognitive domains and in seven out of eight studied individual tasks (fig. 1). The only nonsignificant differences were found in the domain of sustained attention and the continuous performance and letter/number sequencing tasks. The effect sizes (Cohen's d) were mostly modest and ranged between 0.11 and 0.49 for the cognitive domains studied and between 0.26 and 0.52 for the individual tasks. The largest cognitive performance differences were detected in the domains of verbal fluency ($d = 0.49$), visual memory ($d = 0.49$), working memory ($d = 0.49$), and verbal memory ($d = 0.43$). Among the individual tasks, letter fluency ($d = 0.52$), delayed recall ($d = 0.48$), and digit symbol coding ($d = 0.39$) showed the best discrimination. The latter finding is in line with meta-analyses on schizophrenia patients which showed that digit symbol coding is the single best cognitive task for discriminating schizophrenia patients from healthy controls [35].

Since the completion of the meta-analysis of Bora et al. [27], at least four more studies have investigated associations between cognitive performance and later transition to psychosis in ARMS samples that did not overlap with Bora et al. [27]. Ziermans et al. [36] compared 10 ARMS-T and 33 ARMS-NT individuals using a neuropsychological test battery covering the domains of general intelligence, verbal memory, psychomotor functioning, and executive functioning, and found that ARMS-T performed worse than ARMS-NT individuals only in the full-scale ($d = 0.99$) and performance IQ ($d = 0.96$). Healey et al. [37] compared social cognition in 25 ARMS-T and 122 ARMS-NT individuals using theory of mind and social adjustment tasks. They found a statistical trend for a higher trustworthiness score in the social adjustment task in ARMS-T compared to ARMS-NT individuals. Gill et al. [38] measured smell identification using the University of Pennsylvania Smell Identification Test (UPSIT) and the Brief Smell Identification Test (BSIT) in 19 ARMS-T and 52 ARMS-NT individuals, and found no significant differences between the two groups (Cohen's $d = 0.20$ and 0.17 for the UPSIT and BSIT, respectively). Lin et al. [39] also applied the UPSIT in 31 ARMS-T and 50 ARMS-NT individuals, and found no significant difference between the two groups ($d = 0.20$). An earlier study of the same group [40] using a smaller and partially overlapping sample had found a significantly worse smell identification in ARMS-T compared to ARMS-NT individuals. There is one further study [41] that had previously investigated associations between olfaction and transition to psychosis, but it was not included in the meta-analysis by Bora et al. [27] due to the small number of studies in this domain. It measured smell identification using the BSIT in 13 ARMS-T and 55 ARMS-NT individuals, and found no significant differences between the two groups ($d = 0.19$). To sum up, there are now three nonoverlapping studies comparing olfactory performance between ARMS-T and ARMS-NT individuals. None of them found significant group differences, but all of them showed that ARMS-T individuals tended to have worse smell identification abilities with very similarly small effect sizes ($d = 0.19–0.20$). Hence, these studies might not have found significant results due to a lack of power. On the other hand, a random effects meta-analysis of these three group differences revealed that the overall group difference is still not significant ($p = 0.193$).

The domain of motor functioning was also not covered in the meta-analysis by Bora et al. [27] because only few studies have investigated associations between motor functioning and later transition to psychosis in ARMS patients. Hence, in the following, we summarize the results in this domain on a per study basis.

The predictive potential of movement abnormalities such as nondrug-induced choreoathetoid and ballistic, dystonic, and stereotypic movements, which are collectively referred to as 'spontaneous dyskinesias', was investigated in three studies [42–44], although two studies [43, 44] had partially overlapping samples. In the first study

Studerus · Papmeyer · Riecher-Rössler

[44], movement abnormalities were coded from videotapes made during the baseline clinical interview of 40 ARMS individuals of whom 10 later developed psychosis. Coding was conducted using the Dyskinesia Identification System: Condensed User Scale (DISCUS) [45]. It was found that movement abnormalities in the face (p = 0.01, d = 1.13) and upper body region (p < 0.01, d = 1.24), but not the lower limb region (p = 0.77, d = 0.11), significantly predicted later transition to psychosis. The second study [43] applied the same assessment method to 80 ARMS individuals of whom 24 later developed psychosis, and found that abnormalities in the upper body region (p = 0.01, d = 0.69), but not facial region (p = 0.22, d = 0.3), predicted psychosis. The third study [42] assessed movement abnormalities using the Abnormal Involuntary Movement Scale (AIMS) [46] in 148 ARMS individuals of whom 28 later developed psychosis. ARMS-T individuals demonstrated significantly more severe ratings than ARMS-NT individuals on AIMS total, nonglobal, severity of abnormal movements and awareness of movement scales and on specific indices of dyskinetic movements of the facial muscles, jaw, upper extremity, and trunk, but not lower extremities.

A further study of our own group [47] assessed neurological soft signs using the shortened version of the Neurological Evaluation Scale (NES) [48] in a sample of 53 ARMS individuals of whom 16 later developed psychosis. Neither of the two NES scales related to motor functioning (i.e., motor coordination and sequencing of complex motor acts) was predictive for later transition to psychosis.

The predictive potential of motor speed was investigated in at least six studies [49–53]. Keefe et al. [50] assessed motor speed using the Finger Oscillation Test in 28 ARMS individuals of whom 11 later developed psychosis, and did not find it to be associated with later transition to psychosis. Lencz et al. [49] measured motor speed with the Trail Making Test A (TMT-A) [54], the Finger Tapping Test [55], and the Grooved Pegboard Test [56] in 33 ARMS patients of whom 12 later converted to psychosis. They reported that a composite score of these three measures was not predictive of later transition to psychosis. Although the TMT-A has been categorized as a measure of speed of processing in previous meta-analyses [27–29], it can also serve as an index of motor speed due to its low cognitive load [cf. 31]. At least three further studies [51–53] have investigated whether baseline TMT-A performance predicts later transition to psychosis in clinical high-risk samples. All of them found that TMT-A performance was not predictive of later transition to psychosis, although in one study [52] this might have been due to insufficient power as ARMS-T individuals showed moderately worse motor speed than ARMS-NT individuals (d = 0.40).

Taken together, current evidence suggests ARMS-T individuals show worse cognitive performances than ARMS-NT individuals across all cognitive domains except for sustained attention and olfaction. In the domain of motor functioning, previous studies indicate that movement abnormalities or spontaneous dyskinesias, particularly in the upper body region, are more severe in ARMS-T compared to ARMS-NT individuals. Motor speed and neurological soft signs of motor functions on the other hand do not seem to be worse in ARMS-T as compared to ARMS-NT individuals.

However, it should be noted that effect sizes for cognitive performance differences between ARMS-T and ARMS-NT individuals tend to be rather small. Even in the domains with the largest differences (i.e., verbal fluency, verbal and visual memory, and working memory), Cohen's d was only 0.5, indicating a performance overlap of 67% between the two groups. Therefore, it does not appear feasible to predict psychosis with high accuracy on the basis of neuropsychological measures only.

Although the most recent meta-analysis [27] suggests somewhat higher performance differences in verbal fluency, visual working memory, and visual memory than in other domains, it remains unclear whether this is due to particularly severe deficits in these domains or merely the result of different measurement properties of assessment instruments. For example, it is possible that frequently used measures of verbal fluency, visual working memory, and visual memory are more reliable (i.e., are assessed with less measurement error) or simultaneously sensitive to a greater number of somewhat differentially impaired abilities than measures of other cognitive domains, and thereby give rise to larger effect size estimates [for a more detailed discussion of these issues, see 19, 57].

However, even if we take cognitive performance differences between ARMS-T and ARMS-NT individuals at their face values, they do not seem to vary substantially across most domains, suggesting that cognitive impairments of ARMS-T individuals are rather unspecific and generalized. One possible reason for this is that the traditional neurocognitive measures used in most studies are multidimensional and not easily classified into single cognitive domains [29]. Thus, they might tap many different cognitive processes simultaneously and not be pure enough to reveal deficits that are specific for the prodrome of schizophrenic psychoses. Future studies should therefore use measures of discrete cognitive processes, allowing for the interpretation of specific deficits that could be linked to specific neural systems. Such measures have recently been developed and validated by the Cognitive Neuroscience Test Reliability and Clinical Applications for Schizophrenia (CNTRACS) Consortium [58]. Nevertheless, it may even be feasible to considerably improve predictive accuracy when using traditional neuropsychological measures by discovering specific discriminative patterns of cognitive deficits. In support of this, Koutsouleris et al. [52] could predict transition to psychosis with a relatively high accuracy of 77.5% by performing automated pattern classification with variables of a conventional neuropsychological test battery.

The meta-analysis by Bora et al. [27] also revealed that a lower transition rate was significantly associated with larger IQ differences between ARMS-T and ARMS-NT individuals. In other words, in samples with high transition rates, ARMS-T and ARMS-NT groups tended to have more similar cognitive abilities than in samples with low transition rates. Bora et al. [27] speculated that this might be because samples with a high transition rate are more 'risk enriched' and thus contain more severely ill ARMS-NT individuals than samples with a low transition rate. As transition rates have been declining in recent years [for a review, see 59], newer studies might therefore be more successful in finding group differences. Furthermore, cognition-based prediction models developed in samples with high transition rates might show substantially reduced predictive accuracy when applied to samples with low transition rates and vice versa.

Added Predictive Value of Cognitive and Motor Functioning Measures

Although a large body of evidence from group comparisons between ARMS-T and ARMS-NT individuals indicates that cognitive and motor functioning measures do have at least some potential to improve the prediction of psychosis, few studies have rigorously tested whether these variables are independent predictors of psychosis. This is unfortunate because studies in both ARMS individuals and schizophrenia patients suggest that cognitive performance and psychopathological symptoms might not be orthogonal. In individuals with a lifetime history of nonaffective psychosis and schizophrenia patients, there is meta-analytic evidence that cognitive performance is modestly negatively correlated with disorganization and negative symptoms, but not with positive and depressive symptoms [60, 61]. Similar associations are likely present in ARMS individuals as two studies [62, 63] found that neurocognitive performance was correlated predominantly with psychopathology in the negative symptom dimension. However, other studies [64, 65] could not confirm statistically significant relationships in ARMS individuals, possibly due to insufficient power. In addition to negative symptoms, cognitive performance in ARMS individuals is also likely associated at least to some degree with social and role functioning [64, 66], structural MRI [67], mismatch negativity [68], and neural oscillations [69]. As most of these variables are also associated with later transition to psychosis themselves, it is likely that the relationship between cognitive performance and transition to psychosis is partially confounded by them.

At least six studies [36, 49, 70–72] have included neurocognitive measures in prediction models containing variables from multiple domains and thus evaluated their added predictive values. The first study [49] was based on 33 ARMS individuals recruited by the Recognition and Prevention clinic in New York, of whom 12 developed nonaffective psychotic disorders. Neurocognitive performance and clinical symptoms were assessed at baseline using a comprehensive neuropsychological test battery and the Scale of Prodromal Symptoms (SOPS) [73], respectively. Univariate tests of sociodemographic, clinical, and neurocognitive variables identified only two significant predictors of transition to psychosis, namely SOPS positive symptoms and verbal memory. When these two variables were entered into one Cox regression model, they both remained significant, suggesting that they were both independently associated with the outcome.

The second study [70] was conducted in the framework of the Früherkennung von Psychosen (FePsy) project [74] in Basel, Switzerland, and included 53 ARMS individuals, of whom 21 developed psychosis. A multivariate prediction model was developed using variables from three domains: positive symptoms from the Brief

Psychiatric Rating Scale (BPRS) [75], negative symptoms from the Scale for the Assessment of Negative Symptoms (SANS) [76], and neurocognitive measures from a comprehensive neuropsychological test battery [77]. Using domain-wise backward variable elimination, BPRS suspiciousness was selected from positive symptoms, SANS alogia and anhedonia/asociality were selected from negative symptoms, and verbal IQ and speed of processing variables were selected from neurocognitive measures as the most important predictors. When these five predictor variables were entered into a single model and subjected to stepwise backward elimination, three variables remained in the model: BPRS suspiciousness, SANS alogia/asociality, and speed of information processing. The predictive performance of the final integrated model was better than each of the three models developed from single domains. Since at least one variable of each domain remained significant in the integrated model, the results of this study suggest that each of the three domains contains nonredundant predictive information. However, it was also shown that there is partial overlap between clinical and neurocognitive variables as verbal IQ and SANS alogia were eliminated in the final model.

The third study [71] was based on data of the North American Prodrome Longitudinal Study (NAPLS), a multicenter study of eight research centers. It investigated the predictive potential of eight cognitive domains in a sample of 167 ARMS individuals, of whom 54 later developed psychosis. Univariate tests revealed that only verbal memory was associated with transition to psychosis. However, when the neurocognitive variables were added separately to a multivariate prediction algorithm developed in an earlier study [78], none of them were significant, indicating that none added unique variance to prediction beyond the earlier selected clinical variables (i.e., genetic risk for schizophrenia with recent functional deterioration, unusual thought content, suspicion/paranoia, social impairment, and history of any drug abuse).

The fourth study [53] was based on 325 ARMS individuals recruited by the Personal Assessment and Crisis Evaluation (PACE) Clinic in Melbourne, of whom 81 developed psychosis. Since participants recruited between 1994 and 2000 had completed a different test battery than those recruited between 2000 and 2006, these time periods were analyzed separately. To identify the most predictive variables, the authors applied stepwise backward elimination first to neurocognitive and clinical variables separately and then to the variables that were selected during the first step. In the first time period, General Assessment of Functioning (GAF) [79] was selected from clinical variables and visual reproduction and arithmetic were selected from neurocognitive variables. However, only GAF and visual reproduction remained in the final model. In the second time period, GAF and thought content from the Comprehensive Assessment of At-Risk Mental States (CAARMS) [80] were selected from clinical variables. Furthermore, matrix reasoning, which assesses visual abstract manipulation, was selected from neurocognitive variables. However, only thought content and matrix reasoning remained in the final model. Since the preselected neurocognitive variables – except for arithmetic in the first time period – remained significant after adjusting for psychopathology, the results of this study suggest that neurocognitive performance uniquely contributes to the prediction of psychosis. However, given that only few neurocognitive variables were identified to be predictive, and given that these predictors had relatively small hazard rates, the authors concluded that the predictive validity of neurocognitive performance (as assessed using traditional neuropsychological tasks) is likely to be very weak.

The fifth study [72] was based on data collected at the Cologne Early Recognition and Intervention Center (FETZ). The sample consisted of 97 ARMS individuals, of whom 44 developed psychosis. Predictive variables were selected from dichotomized neurocognitive performance measures and at-risk criteria according to the ultra-high-risk and basic symptom approach. By using univariate variable screening followed by domain-wise stepwise variable selection, a predictive model was derived that consisted of the two binary predictors: deficit in speed of processing (i.e., 1 SD below the normative mean in the Digit Symbol Test) and fulfillment of both 'attenuated' psychotic symptoms and subjective cognitive disturbances (COGDIS) criteria. Since speed of processing remained significant in the final model, the results of this study indicate that it improves the prediction of psychosis beyond what can be achieved by commonly applied at-risk criteria.

The sixth study [36] included 43 adolescent ARMS patients recruited at University Medical Center Utrecht, of whom 10 transitioned to psychosis. Stepwise backward variable elimination was separately applied to variables of the Structured Interview for Prodromal Syndromes (SIPS) [73], the Bonn Scale for the Assessment of Basic Symptoms-Prediction List (BSABS-P) [81], and a comprehensive neuropsychological test battery. The positive symptom scale was selected from the SIPS, cognitive disturbances from the BSAPS-P, and full-scale IQ from neurocognitive variables as significant predictors. However, when these variables were integrated into one model and subjected to stepwise backward elimination, only SIPS-positive symptoms and full-scale IQ remained in the model and only SIPS positive symptoms was statistically significant. The authors therefore concluded that the predictive value of neurocognitive measures is limited when clinical measures are added to the equation.

In summary, the majority of existing studies support the notion that neurocognitive measures uniquely contribute to the prediction of psychosis. However, neurocognitive measures in general seem to be weaker predictors than clinical measures, and it seems that their strength of association with transition to psychosis is attenuated when clinical measures are taken into account. Furthermore, no clear picture has yet emerged about which cognitive tasks and domains are most important to include into multivariate prediction models, as some studies selected speed of processing [70, 72], while others selected IQ [36, 53], verbal memory [49], or visual memory [53] measures. These inconsistent results might be due to relatively small sample sizes and/or poor modeling strategies in previous studies. Hence, in the next section, we will discuss the most important methodological problems and offer recommendations for improvement.

Methodological Problems

Since the number of participants in the smaller group (i.e., ARMS-T) determines the effective sample size [82], previous multivariate prediction of psychosis studies using neurocognitive measures only had effective sample sizes between 10 and 85 (mean = 37). In fact, the effective sample sizes in several studies were even lower due to incomplete data or because not all participants were assessed by the same test battery [e.g. 53]. Low sample sizes are common in the field of early detection of psychosis because ARMS individuals are difficult to recruit and follow-up durations of many years are needed to detect later transitions to psychosis. Furthermore, due to their symptomatology (e.g. suspiciousness), ARMS individuals are often noncompliant, which can lead to high dropout rates and incomplete data. The low sample size problem becomes more obvious when we compare the average sample size of prediction of psychosis studies to those of other disease outcomes. For example, systematic reviews on the methodological quality of studies predicting cancer [83], type 2 diabetes [84], and chronic kidney disease [85] found average sample sizes of at least several hundred patients.

For developing clinical prediction models, current textbooks recommend event per variable (EPV) ratios of at least 10 [82, 86]. That is, the effective sample size should be at least 10 times as high as the number of considered predictors. However, this is only a reasonable lower bound for prespecified models. For reliable selection among candidate predictors, an EPV ratio of 50 might be required [87]. Unfortunately, all of the six prediction of psychosis studies described above had an EPV ratio lower than 10. Consequently, the prediction models developed in these studies are likely overfitted and not performing well in independent data sets. Moreover, the problem of overfitting has likely been aggravated in these studies as they all used data-driven variable selection methods (e.g. univariate tests and/or stepwise variable selection). Stepwise variable selection methods, which unfortunately were used in all six studies, have been criticized by methodologists because – due to multiple testing – they frequently select variables that are significantly associated with the outcome by chance [88]. Likewise, they frequently fail to include all variables that actually have an influence on the response. Moreover, due to the so-called 'testimation bias', regression coefficients and statistical significances of selected predictors are systematically overestimated [cf. 82].

Since univariate screening and stepwise procedures induce more bias with decreasing EPV ratio [82], their use in prediction of psychosis research is particularly problematic. A more sensible approach in this field would be to rely more on external knowledge for selecting candidate predictors [82]. Furthermore, to reduce overfitting, regression coefficients of prediction models should be estimated by modern shrinkage methods, such as the least absolute shrinkage and selection operator (LASSO). The LASSO has the advantage that it not only performs shrinkage of regression coefficients but also a variable selection that is often more accurate than the one achieved

Studerus · Papmeyer · Riecher-Rössler

by stepwise methods [89]. Moreover, to assess the degree of overfitting and to adjust for overoptimism in predictive performance evaluation, models should be internally validated by using resampling methods, such as bootstrapping or repeated k-fold cross validation. Although two [70, 72] of the prediction studies described above performed internal cross-validation by applying resampling procedures, they both only cross-validated the final model or models nested within the final model, and thus did not take into account the uncertainty introduced by the variable selection. Future studies should perform internal cross-validation in line with current recommendations [82, 88], that is, they should repeat automated variable selection at each iteration of the resampling procedure. This would not only lead to more realistic predictive performance estimates, but would also allow to more rigorously test whether neurocognitive measures improve the prediction of psychosis beyond clinical measures. Since previous studies only showed that neurocognitive measures improve the non-cross-validated or the so-called 'apparent' predictive performance, we cannot rule out the possibility that they fail to do so in more rigorous testing situations, such as internal and external cross-validation.

Successful external validation, that is the demonstration that the predictive model performs well in data sets collected at different centers, is even more difficult to achieve than internal validation, and – to our knowledge – has not been performed in any prediction of psychosis studies using neuropsychological or motor functioning variables. Given that external validation is an essential requirement for the clinical use of these models [90], it is not surprising that none of these models has yet been adopted in clinical practice. Unfortunately, it is unlikely that many of the published prediction of psychosis models will be externally validated in the near future because inclusion and transition criteria, clinical interviews, and neuropsychological test batteries between two centers are rarely identical. In general, the more variables and domains a prediction model includes, the more difficult it is to find an external validation data set for it. Clearly, progress in this area can only be made if criteria and assessment instruments are better harmonized across centers. Luckily, several multicenter studies are now under way that will facilitate external validation studies in the future (e.g. NAPLS 2 [91], EU-GEI [92], PSYSCAN, and PRONIA).

A further limitation is that most studies had relatively short follow-up durations, typically ranging between one and two years with only few exceptions [e.g. 36, 53, 70]. Although meta-analytic evidence indicates that most transitions occur within the first year of follow-up [4], a minimum follow-up duration of several years is needed to reliably detect all transitions to psychosis [93]. Thus, studies with short follow-up durations likely had misclassified some ARMS-T individuals as ARMS-NT individuals. This in turn might have attenuated cognitive performance differences between the two groups. On the other hand, follow-up duration was not significantly associated with between-group differences in the meta-analysis of Bora et al. [27], indicating that short follow-up durations did not substantially bias results. Furthermore, many studies applied Cox regression, which avoided the problem of misclassifying ARMS individuals by using time to transition as the outcome measure and by considering the outcome as right-censored in individuals who did not develop psychosis during the follow-up [82].

Conclusions

Current evidence suggests that ARMS-T individuals perform moderately worse than ARMS-NT individuals across a wide range cognitive and motor functioning domains. Differences seem to be most pronounced in the domains of verbal fluency, visual memory, working memory, and verbal memory, and not or only mildly present in the domains of sustained attention, olfaction, motor speed, movement abnormalities in the lower extremities, and neurological soft signs related to motor functioning. Nevertheless, most cognitive domains show similar effect sizes, suggesting that ARMS-T individuals demonstrate cognitive impairments that are mostly quantitatively but not qualitatively different from those seen in ARMS-NT individuals. However, this might also be due to the relatively low specificity of traditional neurocognitive tasks. Studies using measures of discrete cognitive processes are needed to further clarify whether the prodrome of schizophrenic psychoses is associated with specific patterns of cognitive and motor functioning deficits.

Regarding the added predictive value of cognitive and motor performance measures, the majority of studies reported that an integrated model of neurocognitive and clinical variables achieved better predictive performance than a model based on clinical variables alone, suggesting that cognitive variables contain nonredundant predictive information that can be exploited to improve the prediction of psychosis. However, available evidence also suggests that cognitive measures are less predictive than clinical measures and that their association with transition to psychosis is attenuated when clinical measures are taken into account. Furthermore, the results of existing studies must be interpreted with great caution because they relied on relatively small sample sizes, have not been correctly validated internally and externally, and applied modeling strategies that are prone to overfitting and overoptimistic predictive performance estimation. As a consequence of this, neurocognitive variables selected for multivariate prediction models are quite inconsistent across studies and no multivariate prediction model containing neurocognitive measures has been adopted in clinical practice. Since large sample sizes are needed for developing and validating clinical prediction models [82] and since ARMS individuals are difficult to recruit and follow up, future research efforts should be directed towards large multicenter studies to fully evaluate the role of neurocognition and motor functioning in the prediction of psychosis. Furthermore, strictly independent external validation studies must be performed to honestly estimate the clinical utility of these measures for risk stratification and targeted intervention.

References

1 Fusar-Poli P, Borgwardt S, Bechdolf A, Addington J, Riecher-Rössler A, Schultze-Lutter F, et al: The psychosis high-risk state a comprehensive state-of-the-art review. JAMA Psychiatry 2013;70:107–120.

2 Yung AR, Phillips LJ, McGorry PD, McFarlane CA, Francey S, Harrigan S, et al: Prediction of psychosis. A step towards indicated prevention of schizophrenia. Br J Psychiatry Suppl 1998;172:14–20.

3 Schultze-Lutter F: Subjective symptoms of schizophrenia in research and the clinic: the basic symptom concept. Schizophr Bull 2009;35:5–8.

4 Fusar-Poli P, Bonoldi I, Yung AR, Borgwardt S, Kempton MJ, Valmaggia L, et al: Predicting psychosis: meta-analysis of transition outcomes in individuals at high clinical risk. Arch Gen Psychiatry 2012; 69:220–229.

5 Fusar-Poli P, Bechdolf A, Taylor MJ, Bonoldi I, Carpenter WT, Yung AR, et al: At risk for schizophrenic or affective psychoses? A meta-analysis of DSM/ICD diagnostic outcomes in individuals at high clinical risk. Schizophr Bull 2013;39:923–932.

6 Simon AE, Borgwardt S, Riecher-Rössler A, Velthorst E, de Haan L, Fusar-Poli P: Moving beyond transition outcomes: meta-analysis of remission rates in individuals at high clinical risk for psychosis. Psychiatry Res 2013;209:266–272.

7 Ruhrmann S, Schultze-Lutter F, Schmidt SJ, Kaiser N, Klosterkötter J: Prediction and prevention of psychosis: current progress and future tasks. Eur Arch Psychiatry Clin Neurosci 2014;264(suppl 1):9–16.

8 Riecher-Rössler A, Gschwandtner U, Borgwardt S, Aston J, Pfluger M, Rössler W: Early detection and treatment of schizophrenia: how early? Acta Psychiatr Scand Suppl, 2006, pp 73–80.

9 Kahn RS, Keefe RS: Schizophrenia is a cognitive illness: time for a change in focus. JAMA Psychiatry 2013;70:1107–1112.

10 Millan MJ, Agid Y, Brune M, Bullmore ET, Carter CS, Clayton NS, et al: Cognitive dysfunction in psychiatric disorders: characteristics, causes and the quest for improved therapy. Nat Rev Drug Discov 2012;11:141–168.

11 Reichenberg A, Harvey PD, Bowie CR, Mojtabai R, Rabinowitz J, Heaton RK, et al: Neuropsychological function and dysfunction in schizophrenia and psychotic affective disorders. Schizophr Bull 2009;35: 1022–1029.

12 Bora E, Yucel M, Pantelis C: Cognitive functioning in schizophrenia, schizoaffective disorder and affective psychoses: meta-analytic study. Br J Psychiatry 2009;195:475–482.

13 Krabbendam L, Arts B, van Os J, Aleman A: Cognitive functioning in patients with schizophrenia and bipolar disorder: a quantitative review. Schizophr Res 2005;80:137–149.

14 Keefe RSE: Should cognitive impairment be included in the diagnostic criteria for schizophrenia? World Psychiatry 2008;7:22–28.

15 Mesholam-Gately RI, Giuliano AJ, Goff KP, Faraone SV, Seidman LJ: Neurocognition in first-episode schizophrenia: a meta-analytic review. Neuropsychology 2009;23:315–336.

16 Schaefer J, Giangrande E, Weinberger DR, Dickinson D: The global cognitive impairment in schizophrenia: consistent over decades and around the world. Schizophr Res 2013;150:42–50.

17 Fatouros-Bergman H, Cervenka S, Flyckt L, Edman G, Farde L: Meta-analysis of cognitive performance in drug-naive patients with schizophrenia. Schizophr Res 2014;158:156–162.

18 Dickinson D, Goldberg TE, Gold JM, Elvevag B, Weinberger DR: Cognitive factor structure and invariance in people with schizophrenia, their unaffected siblings, and controls. Schizophr Bull 2011;37: 1157–1167.

19 Dickinson D, Harvey PD: Systemic hypotheses for generalized cognitive deficits in schizophrenia: a new take on an old problem. Schizophr Bull 2009;35: 403–414.

20 Snitz BE, Macdonald AW 3rd, Carter CS: Cognitive deficits in unaffected first-degree relatives of schizophrenia patients: a meta-analytic review of putative endophenotypes. Schizophr Bull 2006;32:179–194.

21 Dickson H, Laurens KR, Cullen AE, Hodgins S: Meta-analyses of cognitive and motor function in youth aged 16 years and younger who subsequently develop schizophrenia. Psychol Med 2012;42:743–755.

22 Khandaker GM, Barnett JH, White IR, Jones PB: A quantitative meta-analysis of population-based studies of premorbid intelligence and schizophrenia. Schizophr Res 2011;132:220–227.

23 Meier MH, Caspi A, Reichenberg A, Keefe RS, Fisher HL, Harrington H, et al: Neuropsychological decline in schizophrenia from the premorbid to the postonset period: evidence from a population-representative longitudinal study. Am J Psychiatry 2014; 171:91–101.

24 Lewandowski KE, Cohen BM, Ongur D: Evolution of neuropsychological dysfunction during the course of schizophrenia and bipolar disorder. Psychol Med 2011;41:225–241.

25 Bora E: Neurodevelopmental origin of cognitive impairment in schizophrenia. Psychol Med 2015;45: 1–9.

26 Pino O, Guilera G, Gomez-Benito J, Najas-Garcia A, Rufian S, Rojo E: Neurodevelopment or neurodegeneration: review of theories of schizophrenia. Actas Esp Psiquiatr 2014;42:185–195.

27 Bora E, Lin A, Wood SJ, Yung AR, McGorry PD, Pantelis C: Cognitive deficits in youth with familial and clinical high risk to psychosis: a systematic review and meta-analysis. Acta Psychiatr Scand 2014; 130:1–15.

28 Fusar-Poli P, Deste G, Smieskova R, Barlati S, Yung AR, Howes O, et al: Cognitive functioning in prodromal psychosis: a meta-analysis. Arch Gen Psychiatry 2012;69:562–571.

29 Giuliano AJ, Li H, Mesholam-Gately RI, Sorenson SM, Woodberry KA, Seidman LJ: Neurocognition in the psychosis risk syndrome: a quantitative and qualitative review. Curr Pharm Des 2012;18:399–415.

30 Bora E, Murray RM: Meta-analysis of cognitive deficits in ultra-high risk to psychosis and first-episode psychosis: do the cognitive deficits progress over, or after, the onset of psychosis? Schizophr Bull 2014;40: 744–755.

31 Pukrop R, Klosterkötter J: Neurocognitive indicators of clinical high-risk states for psychosis: a critical review of the evidence. Neurotox Res 2010;18:272–286.

32 Brewer WJ, Wood SJ, Phillips LJ, Francey SM, Pantelis C, Yung AR, et al: Generalized and specific cognitive performance in clinical high-risk cohorts: a review highlighting potential vulnerability markers for psychosis. Schizophr Bull 2006;32:538–555.

33 Addington J, Barbato M: The role of cognitive functioning in the outcome of those at clinical high risk for developing psychosis. Epidemiol Psychiatr Sci 2012;21:335–342.

34 Valli I, Tognin S, Fusar-Poli P, Mechelli A: Episodic memory dysfunction in individuals at high-risk of psychosis: a systematic review of neuropsychological and neurofunctional studies. Curr Pharm Des 2012; 18:443–458.

35 Dickinson D, Ramsey ME, Gold JM: Overlooking the obvious: a meta-analytic comparison of digit symbol coding tasks and other cognitive measures in schizophrenia. Arch Gen Psychiatry 2007;64:532–542.

36 Ziermans T, de Wit S, Schothorst P, Sprong M, van Engeland H, Kahn R, et al: Neurocognitive and clinical predictors of long-term outcome in adolescents at ultra-high risk for psychosis: a 6-year follow-up. PLoS One 2014;9:e93994.

37 Healey KM, Penn DL, Perkins D, Woods SW, Addington J: Theory of mind and social judgments in people at clinical high risk of psychosis. Schizophr Res 2013;150:498–504.

38 Gill KE, Evans E, Kayser J, Ben-David S, Messinger J, Bruder G, et al: Smell identification in individuals at clinical high risk for schizophrenia. Psychiatry Res 2014;220:201–204.

39 Lin A, Brewer WJ, Yung AR, Nelson B, Pantelis C, Wood SJ: Olfactory identification deficits at identification as ultra-high risk for psychosis are associated with poor functional outcome. Schizophr Res 2015; 161:156–162.

40 Brewer WJ, Wood SJ, McGorry PD, Francey SM, Phillips LJ, Yung AR, et al: Impairment of olfactory identification ability in individuals at ultra-high risk for psychosis who later develop schizophrenia. Am J Psychiatry 2003;160:1790–1794.

41 Woodberry KA, Seidman LJ, Giuliano AJ, Verdi MB, Cook WL, McFarlane WR: Neuropsychological profiles in individuals at clinical high risk for psychosis: relationship to psychosis and intelligence. Schizophr Res 2010;123:188–198.

42 Callaway DA, Perkins DO, Woods SW, Liu L, Addington J: Movement abnormalities predict transitioning to psychosis in individuals at clinical high risk for psychosis. Schizophr Res 2014;159:263–266.

43 Mittal VA, Walker EF, Bearden CE, Walder D, Trottman H, Daley M, et al: Markers of basal ganglia dysfunction and conversion to psychosis: neurocognitive deficits and dyskinesias in the prodromal period. Biol Psychiatry 2010;68:93–99.

44 Mittal VA, Walker EF: Movement abnormalities predict conversion to axis I psychosis among prodromal adolescents. J Abnorm Psychol 2007;116: 796–803.

45 Kalachnik JE, Young RC, Offerman D: A tardive dyskinesia evaluation and diagnosis form for applied facilities. Psychopharmacol Bull 1984;20:303–307.

46 Guy W: ECDEU assessment manual for psychopharmacology. Rockville, US Department of Health, Education, and Welfare, Public Health Service, Alcohol, Drug Abuse, and Mental Health Administration, National Institute of Mental Health, Psychopharmacology Research Branch, Division of Extramural Research Programs, 1976.

47 Tamagni C, Studerus E, Gschwandtner U, Aston J, Borgwardt S, Riecher-Rössler A: Are neurological soft signs pre-existing markers in individuals with an at-risk mental state for psychosis? Psychiatry Res 2013;210:427–431.

48 Buchanan RW, Heinrichs DW: The Neurological Evaluation Scale (NES): a structured instrument for the assessment of neurological signs in schizophrenia. Psychiatry Res 1989;27:335–350.

49 Lencz T, Smith CW, McLaughlin D, Auther A, Nakayama E, Hovey L, et al: Generalized and specific neurocognitive deficits in prodromal schizophrenia. Biol Psychiatry 2006;59:863–871.

50 Keefe RS, Perkins DO, Gu H, Zipursky RB, Christensen BK, Lieberman JA: A longitudinal study of neurocognitive function in individuals at-risk for psychosis. Schizophr Res 2006;88:26–35.

51 Kim HS, Shin NY, Jang JH, Kim E, Shim G, Park HY, et al: Social cognition and neurocognition as predictors of conversion to psychosis in individuals at ultra-high risk. Schizophr Res 2011;130:170–175.

52 Koutsouleris N, Davatzikos C, Bottlender R, Patschurek-Kliche K, Scheuerecker J, Decker P, et al: Early recognition and disease prediction in the at-risk mental states for psychosis using neurocognitive pattern classification. Schizophr Bull 2012;38:1200–1215.

53 Lin A, Yung AR, Nelson B, Brewer WJ, Riley R, Simmons M, et al: Neurocognitive predictors of transition to psychosis: medium- to long-term findings from a sample at ultra-high risk for psychosis. Psychol Med 2013;43:2349–2360.

54 Reitan RM: Manual for Administration of Neuropsychological Test Batteries for Adults and Children. Indianapolis, Neuropsychology Laboratory, Indiana University Medical Center, 1979.

55 Reitan RM, Wolfson D: The Halstead-Reitan Neuropsychological Test Battery: Theory and Clinical Interpretation. Tucson, Neuropsychology Press, 1985.

56 Matthews C, Klove H: Instruction Manual for the Adult Neuropsychology Test Battery. Madison, University of Wisconsin Medical School, 1964.

57 Macdonald AW 3rd, Kang SS: Misinterpreting schizophrenia relatives' impairments. Am J Med Genet B Neuropsychiatr Genet 2009;150B:443–444.

58 Gold JM, Barch DM, Carter CS, Dakin S, Luck SJ, MacDonald AW 3rd, et al: Clinical, functional, and intertask correlations of measures developed by the cognitive neuroscience test reliability and clinical applications for schizophrenia consortium. Schizophr Bull 2012;38:144–152.

59 Simon AE, Umbricht D, Lang UE, Borgwardt S: Declining transition rates to psychosis: the role of diagnostic spectra and symptom overlaps in individuals with attenuated psychosis syndrome. Schizophr Res 2014;159:292–298.

60 Dominguez MD, Viechtbauer W, Simons CJP, van Os J, Krabbendam L: Are psychotic psychopathology and neurocognition orthogonal? A systematic review of their associations. Psychol Bull 2009;135:157–171.

61 Nieuwenstein MR, Aleman A, de Haan EHF: Relationship between symptom dimensions and neurocognitive functioning in schizophrenia: a meta-analysis of WCST and CPT studies. Wisconsin Card Sorting Test. Continuous Performance Test. J Psychiatr Res 2001;35:119–125.

62 Lindgren M, Manninen M, Laajasalo T, Mustonen U, Kalska H, Suvisaari J, et al: The relationship between psychotic-like symptoms and neurocognitive performance in a general adolescent psychiatric sample. Schizophr Res 2010;123:77–85.

63 Becker HE, Nieman DH, Dingemans PM, van de Fliert JR, De Haan L, Linszen DH: Verbal fluency as a possible predictor for psychosis. Eur Psychiatry 2010;25:105–110.

64 Niendam TA, Bearden CE, Johnson JK, McKinley M, Loewy R, O'Brien M, et al: Neurocognitive performance and functional disability in the psychosis prodrome. Schizophr Res 2006;84:100–111.

65 Pukrop R, Ruhrmann S, Schultze-Lutter F, Bechdolf A, Brockhaus-Dumke A, Klosterkötter J: Neurocognitive indicators for a conversion to psychosis: comparison of patients in a potentially initial prodromal state who did or did not convert to a psychosis. Schizophr Res 2007;92:116–125.

66 Carrion RE, Goldberg TE, McLaughlin D, Auther AM, Correll CU, Cornblatt BA: Impact of neurocognition on social and role functioning in individuals at clinical high risk for psychosis. Am J Psychiatry 2011;168:806–813.

67 Koutsouleris N, Gaser C, Patschurek-Kliche K, Scheuerecker J, Bottlender R, Decker P, et al: Multivariate patterns of brain-cognition associations relating to vulnerability and clinical outcome in the at-risk mental states for psychosis. Hum Brain Mapp 2012;33:2104–2124.

68 Higuchi Y, Sumiyoshi T, Seo T, Miyanishi T, Kawasaki Y, Suzuki M: Mismatch negativity and cognitive performance for the prediction of psychosis in subjects with at-risk mental state. PLoS One 2013;8:e54080.

69 Ramyead A, Kometer M, Studerus E, Koranyi S, Ittig S, Gschwandtner U, et al: Aberrant current source-density and lagged phase synchronization of neural oscillations as markers for emerging psychosis. Schizophr Bull 2015;41:919–929.

70 Riecher-Rössler A, Pflueger MO, Aston J, Borgwardt SJ, Brewer WJ, Gschwandtner U, et al: Efficacy of using cognitive status in predicting psychosis: a 7-year follow-up. Biol Psychiatry 2009;66:1023–1030.

71 Seidman LJ, Giuliano AJ, Meyer EC, Addington J, Cadenhead KS, Cannon TD, et al: Neuropsychology of the prodrome to psychosis in the NAPLS consortium: relationship to family history and conversion to psychosis. Arch Gen Psychiatry 2010;67:578–588.

72 Michel C, Ruhrmann S, Schimmelmann BG, Klosterkötter J, Schultze-Lutter F: A stratified model for psychosis prediction in clinical practice. Schizophr Bull 2014;40:1533–1542.

73 Miller TJ, McGlashan TH, Rosen JL, Cadenhead K, Cannon T, Ventura J, et al: Prodromal assessment with the structured interview for prodromal syndromes and the scale of prodromal symptoms: predictive validity, interrater reliability, and training to reliability. Schizophr Bull 2003;29:703–715.

74 Riecher-Rössler A, Gschwandtner U, Aston J, Borgwardt S, Drewe M, Fuhr P, et al: The Basel early-detection-of-psychosis (FEPSY)-study – design and preliminary results. Acta Psychiatr Scand 2007;115: 114–125.

75 Lukoff D, Nuechterlein K, Ventura J: Manual for the expanded brief psychiatric rating scale. Schizophr Bull 1986;12:594–602.

76 Andreasen NC: The Scale for the Assessment of Negative Symptoms (SANS): conceptual and theoretical foundations. Br J Psychiatry Suppl, 1989, pp 49–58.

77 Pflueger MO, Gschwandtner U, Stieglitz RD, Riecher-Rössler A: Neuropsychological deficits in individuals with an at risk mental state for psychosis – working memory as a potential trait marker. Schizophr Res 2007;97:14–24.

78 Cannon TD, Cadenhead K, Cornblatt B, Woods SW, Addington J, Walker E, et al: Prediction of psychosis in youth at high clinical risk: a multisite longitudinal study in North America. Arch Gen Psychiatry 2008; 65:28–37.

79 Diagnostic and Statistical Manual of Mental Disorders: DSM-IV. Washington, American Psychiatric Association, 1994.

80 Yung A, Phillips L, McGorry P, Ward J, Donovan K, Thompson K: Comprehensive Assessment of At-Risk Mental States (CAARMS). Melbourne, University of Melbourne, Department of Psychiatry, Personal Assessment and Crisis Evaluation Clinic, 2002.

81 Schultze-Lutter F, Klosterkötter J: Bonn Scale for the Assessment of Basic Symptoms-Prediction List (BSABS-P). Cologne, University of Cologne, 2002.

82 Steyerberg EW: Clinical prediction models a practical approach to development, validation, and updating. New York, Springer, 2009.

83 Mallett S, Royston P, Waters R, Dutton S, Altman DG: Reporting performance of prognostic models in cancer: a review. BMC Med 2010;8:21.

84 Collins GS, Mallett S, Omar O, Yu LM: Developing risk prediction models for type 2 diabetes: a systematic review of methodology and reporting. BMC Med 2011;9:103.

85 Collins GS, Omar O, Shanyinde M, Yu LM: A systematic review finds prediction models for chronic kidney disease were poorly reported and often developed using inappropriate methods. J Clin Epidemiol 2013;66:268–277.

86 Harrell FE: Regression Modeling Strategies with Applications to Linear Models, Logistic Regression, and Survival Analysis. New York, Springer, 2001.

87 Steyerberg EW, Eijkemans MJ, Harrell FE Jr, Habbema JD: Prognostic modeling with logistic regression analysis: in search of a sensible strategy in small data sets. Med Decis Making 2001;21:45–56.

88 Nunez E, Steyerberg EW, Nunez J: Regression modeling strategies (in Spanish). Rev Esp Cardiol 2011; 64:501–507.

89 Tibshirani R: The LASSO method for variable selection in the Cox model. Stat Med 1997;16:385–395.

90 Royston P, Altman DG: External validation of a Cox prognostic model: principles and methods. BMC Med Res Methodol 2013;13:33.

91 Addington J, Cadenhead KS, Cornblatt BA, Mathalon DH, McGlashan TH, Perkins DO, et al: North American Prodrome Longitudinal Study (NAPLS 2): overview and recruitment. Schizophr Res 2012;142: 77–82.

92 European Network of National Networks Studying Gene-Environment Interactions in Schizophrenia (EU-GEI), van Os J, Rutten BP, Myin-Germeys I, Delespaul P, Viechtbauer W, et al: Identifying gene-environment interactions in schizophrenia: contemporary challenges for integrated, large-scale investigations. Schizophr Bull 2014;40:729–736.

93 Fusar-Poli P, Yung AR, McGorry P, van Os J: Lessons learned from the psychosis high-risk state: towards a general staging model of prodromal intervention. Psychol Med 2014;44:17–24.

Prof. Anita Riecher-Rössler
Center for Gender Research and Early Detection, University of Basel Psychiatric Clinics
Kornhausgasse 7
CH–4051 Basel (Switzerland)
E-Mail Anita.Riecher@upkbs.ch

Riecher-Rössler A, McGorry PD (eds): Early Detection and Intervention in Psychosis: State of the Art and Future Perspectives. Key Issues Ment Health. Basel, Karger, 2016, vol 181, pp 133–141 (DOI: 10.1159/000440920)

Electroencephalographic Predictors of Psychosis

Stephan Ruhrmann

Department of Psychiatry and Psychotherapy, University of Cologne, Cologne, Germany

Abstract

Currently, prediction of psychosis is almost exclusively based on clinical criteria. This approach already enables a clinically useful estimation of risk. In combination with algorithms for risk stratification, the first steps towards an individualized risk prediction have been made. However, to achieve the most important goal of a preventive intervention dynamically targeted to the changing individual needs of subjects at risk of psychosis, risk estimation has to be informed by further reliable and valid sources. Neurobiological parameters are among the most promising candidates. Psychopathological as well as neurocognitive studies indicate that disturbances of information processing play a central role already in clinical high-risk (CHR) states. On a neurobiological level, electroencephalographic methods provide a noninvasive, real-time access to such processes. Meanwhile, two studies using quantitative electroencephalographic analysis have reported predictor models. Based on a well-established event-related potential (ERP), the P300, Nieman et al. [Schizophr Bull 2014;40: 1482–1490] proposed a prediction model that also includes an item of the premorbid adjustment scale. The model enabled not only statistically and clinically significant risk stratification with regard to hazard rates (ranging from 0.04 to 1.34), but also with regard to the time to event. However, the best evidence for a biological marker of risk has currently been provided for another ERP, mismatch negativity (MMN). Several studies have reported significant baseline differences between CHR subjects with and without a later transition to psychosis, and two independent studies [Bodatsch et al: Biol Psychiatry 2011;69:959–966; Perez et al: Biol Psychiatry 2014;75:459–469] have demonstrated a convincing predictive value of the MMN.   © 2016 S. Karger AG, Basel

Growing scientific insight into the complex nature of the pathogenesis of diseases like diabetes or heart failure led to the introduction of a new concept of prevention. As part of this concept, indicated prevention was defined by the presence of a marker which identifies persons as 'being at sufficiently high risk to require the preventive intervention' [1, p. 108]. This approach, which was originally restricted to clinically asymptomatic subjects, was later adapted for psychiatry, thereby including the manifestations of early signs and symptoms pointing to a disease process without crossing the diagnostic thresholds [2]. Based on this conceptual framework, several clinical criteria for a clinically increased risk for psychosis were developed and evaluated [3]. The transition rates predicted by these clinical high-risk (CHR) criteria are several times higher than the incidence rates in the general population [4]. However, at least during the next 3 years (the usual follow-up period) following the initial risk estimation, the majority of the CHR subjects do not develop a psychosis [4]. Furthermore, transition rates vary markedly across studies [4–6]. Multilevel algorithms were developed to further individualize the estimation of risk and, thus, the selection of preventive measures [5, 7]. Based on clinical and demographical characteristics, the concept of a prognostic index was introduced into psychiatric prediction as a result of the European Prediction of Psychosis Study (EPOS) [8]. This regression-based stratification approach has been a major step towards an individualization of risk prediction, not only with regard to magnitude of risk, but also with regard to the individual time to transition. However, although the highest risk class in this model showed a markedly shorter time to transition and although a suggested subdivision of the at-risk state into two sequential phases [9] has meanwhile found some clinical support, a sufficient estimation of the individual time to transition by clinical variables alone does not seem expectable. Including measures of neurobiological processes associated with the development of a first manifest psychosis could fill this gap and might enable an improved estimation of the magnitude of risk.

Disturbances of information processing seem to play a central role for the pathogenesis of psychosis. Regarding CHR states, this notion is already supported on the level of psychopathology. Cognitive and perceptive basic symptoms are defined as subtle, subjective disturbances thought to be very closely related to neurobiological aberrations of information processing. Recent results have indicated that the transition rate can become more than twice as high when symptomatic ultra-high-risk criteria occur in combination with cognitive basic symptoms and not only alone [10]. Following this trail, cognitive test batteries were evaluated [11–15], and recent studies found reduced processing speed in combination with psychopathological variables to be predictive for transition [7, 16] as well as social functioning [17, 18]. A further step towards the underlying neurobiology is provided by investigating brain activity real-time with electroencephalographic methods.

Predicting Psychosis by Electroencephalography

Quantitative EEG Parameters
One standard approach for the evaluation of EEG signals is the analysis of the power spectrum. This enables a quantification of resting EEG activity by estimating the power density of different EEG frequency bands.

Zimmerman et al. [19] investigated baseline recordings in a group of adult CHR subjects, 13 with and 15 without a transition to psychosis during a follow-up period of at least 4 years. Considering delta, theta, alpha 1, alpha 2, beta 1–3 bands, as well as the Scale for the Assessment of Negative Symptoms (SANS) total score, a combination of theta absolute power with the SANS total score revealed the best percentage of correct classifications (89%). Interestingly, such associations between negative symptoms and EEG power had also been observed in different stages of schizophrenia [19]. In a more recent study, Ramyead et al. [20] demonstrated an increased medial prefrontal current source density of gamma oscillations in CHR subjects with a later transition to a nonaffective psychosis. In these, but not in subjects without a transition or in healthy controls, this current source density correlated highly and positively with performance in a test of abstract reasoning abilities (explained variance 54%), possibly indicating a compensatory increase of gamma oscillations. Further analyses revealed that subjects with a later transition showed an abnormal interregional synchronization decreasing with longer distance of areas. This was particularly discernible in subjects with higher negative and – most pronounced – higher positive symptom scores.

Van Tricht et al. [21] evaluated the predictive value of resting EEG data of 113 adult and adolescent CHR subjects followed for 18 months within EPOS; 22 developed a first psychotic episode. Delta, theta, lower and upper alpha as well as beta frequency bands and the individual alpha peak frequency were analyzed. The final Cox regression model comprised occipital-parietal alpha peak frequency, frontal delta and frontal theta power. The resulting prognostic score (PS) could be stratified into three risk classes with hazard rates of 0.057, 0.16 and 0.81. Furthermore, the highest risk class showed a shorter time to transition with no overlap of the 95% confidence intervals. Regarding the alpha peak frequency, it seems noteworthy that this parameter has been associated with processing speed in thalamocortical networks and cognitive functions, including working memory [22].

Event-Related Potentials
P300
Another and well-established approach to study information processing by EEG are event-related potentials (ERPs), reflecting the response of the electric activity after administering a defined stimulus [23]. In particular for the P300 component and the mismatch negativity (MMN), aberrations have repeatedly been demonstrated in schizophrenia patients [24, 25]. Thus, these ERPs are the main subjects of the following overview.

The P300 ERP component is usually evoked by an auditory or visual oddball paradigm, comprising an infrequent target appearing on a background of frequent standard stimuli. The P300 amplitude follows the presentation of the target with a latency of about 300 ms. This component is also called P3b; P3a is evoked by the additional presentation of a nontarget distractor. Functionally, the P300 may reflect neural inhibitory activity that occurs with stimulus and task demands and enhances the attentional focus to promote memory storage [26]. Regarding psychosis, decreased P300 amplitudes are a well-established finding in schizophrenia patients and their relatives [25].

Several studies have investigated the P300, comparing CHR samples to healthy controls, and reported lower P3b [27–32] or P3a amplitudes [33–35] in the patient group. As a special feature, Frommann et al. [27] followed the two-stage approach of the German Research Network on Schizophrenia [9]. Compared to healthy controls, they demonstrated smaller P3b amplitudes at midline and left hemispheric electrodes in subjects with a late at-risk state of developing an initial psychotic episode [LRSIP, defined by attenuated positive symptoms and brief limited intermittent psychotic symptoms (BLIPS)], but – except for one temporoparietal electrode site – not in subjects meeting the criteria for an early at-risk state (ERSIP, mainly defined by cognitive-perceptive basic symptoms) [27]. Thereby, the LRSIP group showed significantly reduced amplitudes compared to healthy controls, whereas the comparisons between the ERSIP group and these controls or the LRSIP group did not reveal a significant group interaction. Furthermore, LRSIP subjects reporting BLIPS produced smaller amplitudes at the midline electrode sites Fz and Cz (not at Pz). This is of special interest, as BLIPS are highly predictive of psychosis [4] (although their use as a risk criterion is controversially discussed in the field, as they could also be classified as a very brief or very early variant of a psychotic episode). These results seem to support the notion that the P300 amplitude is not only reduced already before the manifestation of a first psychotic episode, but might also be an indicator of the progression to psychosis. Prospective long-term studies including repeated ERP recordings are required to further investigate this assumption.

Three studies have reported findings in CHR subjects with a transition to psychosis (CHR-T). Atkinson et al. [35] observed a tendency for lower P3a amplitudes in CHR-T subjects than in those without an observable transition (CHR-NT); however, the small number of 6 CHR-T subjects precluded statistical analysis. A power problem can also be assumed for another study that observed no P300 amplitude difference between CHR-NT and CHR-T (n = 7); comparisons of the two groups to healthy controls were not reported [28]. Different to Frommann et al. [27], van Tricht et al. [30] found significantly lower P3b amplitudes at the parietal central (Pz) electrode in 43 CHR-NT as well as in 18 CHR-T than in 28 healthy controls; the follow-up period in the CHR group was 3 years. Furthermore, the CHR-T group showed significantly lower amplitudes than the CHR-NT group. In a subsequently calculated Cox regression analysis, the P3b at Pz turned out to be a predictor of later transition: a 1-μV decrease of the P3b amplitude was associated with a 37% increase of risk. Furthermore, stratification by the mean amplitude revealed a significant difference of survival curves.

Based on this sample, Nieman et al. [36] developed a multifactorial prediction model. Informed by preceding analyses of potential neuropsychological, clinical, environmental, somatic and psychosocial adjustment-related predictor variables, 'semantic verbal fluency', the item 'social anhedonia and withdrawal' from the Scale of Prodromal Symptoms [37], the items 'social-sexual aspects of life during early adolescents (age: 12–15 years)' and 'social-personal adjustment (highest level ever attained)' from the Premorbid Adjustment Scale (PAS) [38], and the parietal P3b amplitude were entered into a stepwise Cox regression analysis. The final model included the P3b amplitude and the PAS 'social-personal adjustment' item. A PS was calculated and stratified into three risk classes. The resulting survival curves differed significantly from each other, hazard rates (lowest to highest risk class) were 0.038, 0.288 and 1.335, and the 95% confidence intervals of the time to transition in the highest risk class did not overlap with the respective intervals of the lower classes. Although indices of diagnostic accuracy are of questionable meaning for predictive models, the PS was entered into a logistic regression (sensitivity optimized PS of –0.57, equaling a probability threshold of 0.4). The resulting sensitivity was 88.9%, specificity 82.5%, positive predictive power 0.70, negative predictive power 0.94, positive likelihood ratio 5.08 and negative likelihood ratio 0.13. These numbers indicate that a low PS markedly decreased the 3-year risk estimation associated with the clinical inclusion criteria. The area under the curve was 0.91 (95% CI: 0.83–0.98) and decreased to 0.86 after bootstrapping of the logistic model, demonstrating an excellent cutoff independent discriminative ability of the PS and validity of the logistic regression model; a cross-validation of the underlying Cox regression model is still pending.

Mismatch Negativity

The MMN is generated 150–250 ms after an auditory stimulus deviating from a regular stimulus sequence with regard to duration or frequency, for example, whereby such differences may lead to different results [39]; it can also be evoked by complex stimuli [40, 41]. Sources have been localized bilaterally supratemporal and predominantly right-frontal [42]. Deficits may reflect disturbances of sensory echoic memory, predictive coding, synaptic plasticity and NMDA receptor function [39, 43–45]. Reductions of both frequency (fMMN) and duration (dMMN) MMN are well established findings in schizophrenia research [24, 39, 46], and some specificity for schizophrenia has been discussed [44].

In the first study of MMN in a CHR population, CHR-related MMN, which was defined by cognitive basic symptoms [47], showed an intermediate position between MMN findings in healthy controls and psychotic patients with no significant differences between the two groups (the group of psychotic patients showed a significantly reduced dMMN compared to the healthy controls). The same result was reported by Bodatsch et al. [48] as long as the complete CHR group was compared to healthy controls and patients with a first psychotic episode. However, when considering CHR-NT and CHR-T separately, differences could be seen: CHR-T exhibited significantly smaller dMMN than CHR-NT and healthy controls. Until now, all following studies except one [34] observed a reduced dMMN in either CHR groups or CHR-T groups compared to healthy controls, and no study found a significant difference between

CHR and psychotic groups [33, 35, 49–52]. Furthermore, a recent meta-analysis of studies comparing MMN of CHR with and without a later transition to psychosis demonstrated a significantly reduced dMMN in CHR-T [53]. No significant result emerged with regard to fMMN. However, only two studies investigated this deviant type, with contradictory results [48, 52]. These two studies also analyzed the predictive value of MMN.

Bodatsch et al. [48] reported a proportional hazards model including dMMN amplitudes at four electrode sites (Fz, F4, C4, C3); the minimum follow-up period was 24 months in CHR-NT, and longer periods were censored. Based on this model, a PS was calculated and stratified by median split into two risk classes which showed significantly different survival curves in a subsequent Kaplan-Meier analysis. The hazard rate was 0.34 in risk class 1 and 0.85 in risk class 2. Furthermore, at 13.3 months, risk class 2 showed a markedly shorter time to transition than risk class 2 with 20.0 months; 95% confidence intervals showed only a marginal overlap. This result was meanwhile partially replicated in an independent sample [52]. Different to the study described above, neither dMMN nor fMMN alone or a model including results from separate trials with these deviants were predictive of psychosis. However, a third paradigm, presenting a stimulus combining both types of deviant information (i.e. differing from the standard stimulus with regard to duration and frequency), was found to be a significant predictor: a unit decrease in MMN (i.e. 1 mV less negative MMN amplitude) was associated with a 1.63-fold increase in the risk for conversion to psychosis. Although different time effects of different amplitude reductions were visible in the reported survival curves, they were unfortunately not further analyzed. The reasons for the stimulus-related differences between both studies requires further research, but it can be concluded that the MMN shows currently the best evidence as a predictor of psychosis.

The overview above zoomed in on the electrophysiological findings of the different studies. It should be noticed that all these findings were made in samples which were preselected by CHR criteria, and thus did not allow a generalization to other samples. Therefore, as a consequence of the presented results, a two- or even multistep approach seems appropriate, combining the currently most sensitive risk detection by CHR criteria with a multiclass stratification of risk. Such an approach should enable a prediction approximating the individual magnitude of risk and time to transition more precisely.

Future Perspective

At present, electroencephalographic paradigms show the best prospects for becoming a neurobiological part of a robust multifactorial prediction model. On a currently still smaller research basis, comparably promising findings are otherwise only reported for structural MRI [54]. Further research will have to investigate whether prediction can be further improved by combining different EEG paradigms and by data about the development of aberrations during repeated recordings, which can be performed at low costs and burden – a major advantage of this approach. Furthermore, the effects of combining different levels of information on predictive accuracy should be further investigated. Two studies following this trail indicate that this could indeed improve prediction [19, 55]. The more facets of risk are included into such models, the more individualized the resulting risk estimation will be – a major precondition for a targeted preventive intervention. Another important step will be the inclusion of course-related measures, including changing patterns of environmental risk and protective factors and their interaction with the dynamic individual state of vulnerability and resilience [56].

References

1 Gordon RS Jr: An operational classification of disease prevention. Public Health Rep 1983;98:107–109.
2 Mrazek PJ, Haggerty HJ: Reducing Risks for Mental Disorders: Frontiers for Preventive Research. Washington, Academy Press, 1994.
3 Fusar-Poli P, Borgwardt S, Bechdolf A, Addington J, Riecher-Rössler A, Schultze-Lutter F, et al: The psychosis high-risk state: a comprehensive state-of-the-art review. JAMA Psychiatry 2013;70:107–120.
4 Schultze-Lutter F, Michel C, Schmidt SJ, Schimmelmann BG, Maric NP, Salokangas RK, et al: EPA guidance on the early detection of clinical high risk states of psychoses. Eur Psychiatry 2015;30:405–416.
5 Ruhrmann S, Schultze-Lutter F, Klosterkötter J: Probably at-risk, but certainly ill – advocating the introduction of a psychosis spectrum disorder in DSM-V. Schizophr Res 2010;120:23–37.
6 Nelson B, Yuen HP, Wood SJ, Lin A, Spiliotacopoulos D, Bruxner A, et al: Long-term follow-up of a group at ultra high risk ('prodromal') for psychosis: the PACE 400 study. JAMA Psychiatry 2013;70:793–802.
7 Riecher-Rössler A, Pflueger MO, Aston J, Borgwardt SJ, Brewer WJ, Gschwandtner U, et al: Efficacy of using cognitive status in predicting psychosis: a 7-year follow-up. Biol Psychiatry 2009;66:1023–1030.
8 Ruhrmann S, Schultze-Lutter F, Salokangas RK, Heinimaa M, Linszen D, Dingemans P, et al: Prediction of psychosis in adolescents and young adults at high risk: results from the prospective European prediction of psychosis study. Arch Gen Psychiatry 2010;67:241–251.
9 Ruhrmann S, Schultze-Lutter F, Klosterkötter J: Early detection and intervention in the initial prodromal phase of schizophrenia. Pharmacopsychiatry 2003; 36(suppl 3):S162–S167.
10 Schultze-Lutter F, Klosterkötter J, Ruhrmann S: Improving the clinical prediction of psychosis by combining ultra-high risk criteria and cognitive basic symptoms. Schizophr Res 2014;154:100–106.
11 Fusar-Poli P, Deste G, Smieskova R, Barlati S, Yung AR, Howes O, et al: Cognitive functioning in prodromal psychosis: a meta-analysis of cognitive functioning in prodromal psychosis. Arch Gen Psychiat 2012; 69:562–571.
12 Pukrop R, Ruhrmann S, Schultze-Lutter F, Bechdolf A, Brockhaus-Dumke A, Klosterkötter J: Neurocognitive indicators for a conversion to psychosis: comparison of patients in a potentially initial prodromal state who did or did not convert to a psychosis. Schizophr Res 2007;92:116–125.
13 Pukrop R, Ruhrmann S: Neurocognitive indicators of high-risk states for psychosis; in Fusar Poli P, Borgwardt S, McGuire P (eds): Vulnerability to Psychosis – From Neuroscience to Psychopathology. Hove, Psychology Press, 2012, pp 73–94.
14 Seidman LJ, Giuliano AJ, Meyer EC, Addington J, Cadenhead KS, Cannon TD, et al: Neuropsychology of the prodrome to psychosis in the NAPLS consortium: relationship to family history and conversion to psychosis. Arch Gen Psychiatry 2010;67:578–588.
15 Frommann I, Pukrop R, Brinkmeyer J, Bechdolf A, Ruhrmann S, Berning J, et al. Neuropsychological profiles in different at-risk states of psychosis: executive control impairment in the early – and additional memory dysfunction in the late – prodromal state. Schizophr Bull 2011;37:861–873.
16 Michel C, Ruhrmann S, Schimmelmann BG, Klosterkötter J, Schultze-Lutter F: A stratified model for psychosis prediction in clinical practice. Schizophr Bull 2014;40:1533–1542.

17 Carrion RE, Goldberg TE, McLaughlin D, Auther AM, Correll CU, Cornblatt BA: Impact of neurocognition on social and role functioning in individuals at clinical high risk for psychosis. Am J Psychiatry 2011;168:806–813.

18 Meyer EC, Carrion RE, Cornblatt BA, Addington J, Cadenhead KS, Cannon TD, et al: The relationship of neurocognition and negative symptoms to social and role functioning over time in individuals at clinical high risk in the first phase of the North American Prodrome Longitudinal Study. Schizophr Bull 2014; 40:1452–1461.

19 Zimmermann R, Gschwandtner U, Wilhelm FH, Pflueger MO, Riecher-Rössler A, Fuhr P: EEG spectral power and negative symptoms in at-risk individuals predict transition to psychosis. Schizophr Res 2010;123:208–216.

20 Ramyead A, Kometer M, Studerus E, Koranyi S, Ittig S, Gschwandtner U, et al: Aberrant current source-density and lagged phase synchronization of neural oscillations as markers for emerging psychosis. Schizophr Bull 2015;41:919–929.

21 Van Tricht MJ, Ruhrmann S, Arns M, Muller R, Bodatsch M, Velthorst E, et al: Can quantitative EEG measures predict clinical outcome in subjects at clinical high risk for psychosis? A prospective multicenter study. Schizophr Res 2014;153:42–47.

22 Richard CC, Veltmeyer MD, Hamilton RJ, Simms E, Paul R, Hermens D, et al: Spontaneous alpha peak frequency predicts working memory performance across the age span. Int J Psychophysiol 2004;53:1–9.

23 Luck SJ, Kappenman ES: The Oxford Handbook of Event-Related Potential Components. Oxford, Oxford University Press, 2013.

24 Umbricht D, Krljes S: Mismatch negativity in schizophrenia: a meta-analysis. Schizophr Res 2005;76:1–23.

25 Bramon E, Rabe-Hesketh S, Sham P, Murray RM, Frangou S: Meta-analysis of the P300 and P50 waveforms in schizophrenia. Schizophr Res 2004;70:315–329.

26 Polich J: Neuropsychology of P300; in Luck SJ, Kappenman ES (eds): The Oxford Handbook of Event-Related Potential Components. Oxford, Oxford University Press, 2013, pp 159–188.

27 Frommann I, Brinkmeyer J, Ruhrmann S, Hack E, Brockhaus-Dumke A, Bechdolf A, et al: Auditory P300 in individuals clinically at risk for psychosis. Int J Psychophysiol 2008;70:192–205.

28 Bramon E, Shaikh M, Broome M, Lappin J, Berge D, Day F, et al: Abnormal P300 in people with high risk of developing psychosis. Neuroimage 2008;41:553–560.

29 Özgürdal S, Gudlowski Y, Witthaus H, Kawohl W, Uhl I, Hauser M, et al: Reduction of auditory event-related P300 amplitude in subjects with at-risk mental state for schizophrenia. Schizophr Res 2008;105:272–278.

30 van Tricht MJ, Nieman DH, Koelman JH, van der Meer JN, Bour LJ, de Haan L, et al: Reduced parietal P300 amplitude is associated with an increased risk for a first psychotic episode. Biol Psychiatry 2010;68:642–648.

31 Oribe N, Hirano Y, Kanba S, del Re EC, Seidman LJ, Mesholam-Gately R, et al: Early and late stages of visual processing in individuals in prodromal state and first episode schizophrenia: an ERP study. Schizophr Res 2013;146:95–102.

32 van der Stelt O, Lieberman JA, Belger A: Auditory P300 in high-risk, recent-onset and chronic schizophrenia. Schizophr Res 2005;77:309–320.

33 Jahshan C, Cadenhead KS, Rissling AJ, Kirihara K, Braff DL, Light GA: Automatic sensory information processing abnormalities across the illness course of schizophrenia. Psychol Med 2012;42:85–97.

34 Mondragon-Maya A, Solis-Vivanco R, Leon-Ortiz P, Rodriguez-Agudelo Y, Yanez-Tellez G, Bernal-Hernandez J, et al: Reduced P3a amplitudes in antipsychotic naive first-episode psychosis patients and individuals at clinical high-risk for psychosis. J Psychiatr Res 2013;47:755–761.

35 Atkinson RJ, Michie PT, Schall U: Duration mismatch negativity and P3a in first-episode psychosis and individuals at ultra-high risk of psychosis. Biol Psychiatry 2012;71:98–104.

36 Nieman DH, Ruhrmann S, Dragt S, Soen F, van Tricht MJ, Koelman JH, et al: Psychosis prediction: stratification of risk estimation with information-processing and premorbid functioning variables. Schizophr Bull 2014;40:1482–1490.

37 McGlashan TH, Miller TJ, Woods SW, Rosen JL, Hoffman RE, Davidson L: Structured Interview for Prodromal Syndromes (Version 3.0). New Haven, PRIME Research Clinic, Yale School of Medicine, 2001.

38 Cannon-Spoor HE, Potkin SG, Wyatt RJ: Measurement of premorbid adjustment in chronic schizophrenia. Schizophr Bull 1982;8:470–484.

39 Näätänen R, Sussman ES, Salisbury D, Shafer VL: Mismatch negativity (MMN) as an index of cognitive dysfunction. Brain Topogr 2014;27:451–466.

40 Pulvermüller F, Kujala T, Shtyrov Y, Simola J, Tiitinen H, Alku P, et al: Memory traces for words as revealed by the mismatch negativity. Neuroimage 2001;14:607–16.

41 Pakarinen S, Teinonen T, Shestakova A, Kwon MS, Kujala T, Hamalainen H, et al: Fast parametric evaluation of central speech-sound processing with mismatch negativity (MMN). Int J Psychophysiol 2013; 87:103–110.

42 Jääskeläinen IP, Pekkonen E, Hirvonen J, Sillanaukee P, Näätänen R: Mismatch negativity subcomponents and ethyl alcohol. Biol Psychol 1996;43:13–25.

43 Näätänen R, Shiga T, Asano S, Yabe H: Mismatch negativity (MMN) deficiency: a break-through biomarker in predicting psychosis onset. Int J Psychophysiol 2015;95:338–344.

44 Baldeweg T, Hirsch SR: Mismatch negativity indexes illness-specific impairments of cortical plasticity in schizophrenia: a comparison with bipolar disorder and Alzheimer's disease. Int J Psychophysiol 2015; 95:145–155.

45 Kompus K, Westerhausen R, Craven AR, Kreegipuu K, Poldver N, Passow S, et al: Resting-state glutamatergic neurotransmission is related to the peak latency of the auditory mismatch negativity (MMN) for duration deviants: an H-MRS-EEG study. Psychophysiology 2015;52:1131–1139.

46 Light GA, Swerdlow NR, Thomas ML, Calkins ME, Green MF, Greenwood TA, et al: Validation of mismatch negativity and P3a for use in multi-site studies of schizophrenia: characterization of demographic, clinical, cognitive, and functional correlates in COGS-2. Schizophr Res 2015;163:63–72.

47 Schultze-Lutter F, Ruhrmann S, Fusar-Poli P, Bechdolf A, Schimmelmann BG, Klosterkötter J: Basic symptoms and the prediction of first-episode psychosis. Curr Pharm Des 2012;18:351–357.

48 Bodatsch M, Ruhrmann S, Wagner M, Müller R, Schultze-Lutter F, Frommann I, et al: Prediction of psychosis by mismatch negativity. Biol Psychiatry 2011;69:959–966.

49 Hsieh MH, Shan JC, Huang WL, Cheng WC, Chiu MJ, Jaw FS, et al: Auditory event-related potential of subjects with suspected pre-psychotic state and first-episode psychosis. Schizophr Res 2012;140:243–249.

50 Shaikh M, Valmaggia L, Broome MR, Dutt A, Lappin J, Day F, et al: Reduced mismatch negativity predates the onset of psychosis. Schizophr Res 2012;134:42–48.

51 Higuchi Y, Sumiyoshi T, Seo T, Miyanishi T, Kawasaki Y, Suzuki M: Mismatch negativity and cognitive performance for the prediction of psychosis in subjects with at-risk mental state. PLoS One 2013;8: e54080.

52 Perez VB, Woods SW, Roach BJ, Ford JM, McGlashan TH, Srihari VH, et al: Automatic auditory processing deficits in schizophrenia and clinical high-risk patients: forecasting psychosis risk with mismatch negativity. Biol Psychiatry 2014;75:459–469.

53 Bodatsch M, Brockhaus-Dumke A, Klosterkötter J, Ruhrmann S: Forecasting psychosis by event-related potentials-systematic review and specific meta-analysis. Biol Psychiatry 2015;77:951–958.

54 Koutsouleris N, Riecher-Rössler A, Meisenzahl EM, Smieskova R, Studerus E, Kambeitz-Ilankovic L, et al: Detecting the psychosis prodrome across high-risk populations using neuroanatomical biomarkers. Schizophr Bull 2015;41:471–482.

55 Nieman DH, Ruhrmann S, Dragt S, Soen F, van Tricht MJ, Koelman JH, et al: Psychosis prediction: stratification of risk estimation with information-processing and premorbid functioning variables. Schizophr Bull 2014;40:1482–1490.

56 Ruhrmann S, Schultze-Lutter F, Schmidt SJ, Kaiser N, Klosterkötter J: Prediction and prevention of psychosis: current progress and future tasks. Eur Arch Psychiatry Clin Neurosci 2014;264(suppl 1):S9–S16.

Prof. Dr. med. habil. Stephan Ruhrmann
Department of Psychiatry and Psychotherapy
University of Cologne , Kerpener Strasse 62
DE–50924 Cologne (Germany)
E-Mail stephan.ruhrmann@uk-koeln.de

Riecher-Rössler A, McGorry PD (eds): Early Detection and Intervention in Psychosis: State of the Art and Future Perspectives. Key Issues Ment Health. Basel, Karger, 2016, vol 181, pp 142–158 (DOI: 10.1159/000440921)

Psychological Methods of Early Intervention in Emerging Psychosis

Hendrik Müller[a] · Andreas Bechdolf[a, b]

[a]Department of Psychiatry and Psychotherapy, University of Cologne, Cologne, and [b]Department of Psychiatry, Psychotherapy and Psychosomatics, Vivantes Klinikum am Urban and Vivantes Klinikum im Friedrichshain, Academic Hospital Charite Medicine Berlin, Berlin, Germany

Abstract

The aim of psychotherapy among individuals at clinical high risk for psychosis (CHR) is to prevent or to delay transition to full-blown psychosis. Remission of attenuated psychotic symptoms and improvements in psychosocial functioning, quality of life and self-esteem are important secondary outcomes. The data on psychoeducation in individuals at CHR is encouraging but still not sufficient. Psychotherapy has been found to be effective in CHR in terms of preventing progression to psychosis. Thereby psychotherapy presents a better benefit/risk ratio than antipsychotic medication and is based on the broadest evidence. We introduce differences in the evaluated approaches and discuss methodological issues. We conclude that the needs of young people at CHR are best met by specially designed, low-threshold outpatient clinical services, where intensive psychotherapy is offered as a part of a stepwise treatment model. Examples for the implementation of such early detection and intervention services are given.   © 2016 S. Karger AG, Basel

Schizophrenia is one of ten main contributing illnesses to the global burden of disease [1]. Not only is this disorder associated with substantial numbers of years lived with disability (WHO, 2001), but its direct health care costs for German society alone are estimated to be EUR 2 billion per year [2]. Post-onset interventions in schizophrenia generally have unfavorable outcomes [3]. Although early detection and intervention strategies have led to substantial improvement in prognosis for a number of nonpsychiatric medical conditions [4–6], these strategies have only started to be applied to schizophrenia over the past 20 years. Nonetheless, enormous progress has been made in this time period in the prevention of first-episode psychosis.

In the following sections we summarize the state of the art of psychological interventions in people at clinical high risk of developing first episode psychosis (CHR).

Rational for Interventions in Emerging Psychosis

There are a number of reasons that provide the rationale for interventions in CHR: (1) schizophrenia often goes untreated for up to 5 years in 75% of the cases with non-psychotic prodromal symptoms (anxiety, depression, cognitive disturbances, negative symptoms) [7], (2) social decline starts prior to the onset of positive symptoms [8], (3) biological changes which are typical for schizophrenia present prior to the onset of frank psychotic symptoms [9], (4) delayed treatment is correlated with an unfavorable outcome [e.g. 10] and (5) psychotic episodes may have neurotoxic effects [11].

An important prerequisite for early intervention in emerging psychosis is to have available and reliable at-risk criteria with sufficient predictive value to predict transition to psychosis. A meta-analysis based on such criteria reported that there is a mean risk of transition to psychosis of 18% after 6 months, 22% after 12 months, 29% after 24 months and 36% after more than 36 months [12] [for details see the chapter by McGorry and Goldstone, this vol., pp. 15–28].

Characteristics of People Meeting Clinical High-Risk Criteria

People who meet criteria for CHR usually present with additional clinical concerns. Many have comorbid diagnoses, in particular anxiety, depression and substance use disorders that are clinically debilitating [13]. High levels of negative symptoms as well as significant impairments in academic performance and occupational functioning are present [8]. Moreover, difficulties with interpersonal relationships and substantially compromised subjective quality of life are often observed [14–17]. Early medium-term studies have indicated that CHR participants continue to present with substantial psychopathological symptoms as well as low social functioning when compared to control group participants (CON) who do not meet CHR criteria [18, 19]. This is true even when CHR participants do not transition to the psychosis threshold. Neurobiological alterations are already present in individuals meeting CHR criteria. When compared to healthy controls and people with schizophrenia, these neurobiological alterations mostly present at an intermediate level. In addition, a broad profile of cognitive deficits is reliably present in CHR individuals [20, 21]. Morphometric studies have shown specific volumetric reductions in regions known to be affected in participants with schizophrenic psychosis, such as the hippocampus [22, 23] or anterior cingulate cortex [24]. Dopamine and glutamate systems are both widely implicated in the pathogenesis of psychosis. Multimodal imaging studies have shown that dysfunction in dopamine and glutamate systems are directly correlated with altered cortical structure [25] and functioning [26–28] in CHR subjects.

Psychological Methods of Early Intervention in Emerging Psychosis

It is important to outline that interventions in CHR exclusively target young people who seek help because they are distressed and impaired by their clinical symptoms or functioning problems but do not yet fulfil the DSM-5 criteria of psychosis. Because of this, interventions in CHR have to work within a rigid ethical framework which has to address several issues (these ethical implications have been extensively discussed in a 2001 special issue of *Schizophrenia Research* [29]). One such issue is that the disclosure of the fact that one is at risk for psychosis may itself put one at risk for depression, anxiety, and demoralization or stigmatization either by oneself or by others [30]. Another important issue is that although the predictive value of the CHR criteria is substantially high, the available evidence suggests that the majority of CHR subjects will not develop a psychotic disorder (at least within 3 years after presentation) [31]. Thus, early intervention has to be particularly well acceptable and tolerable to false-positive young people (i.e. those meeting CHR criteria, who will not move on to develop first-episode psychosis). In this respect, most experts in the field consider psychotherapy as a better treatment alternative, as it presents a better benefit/risk ratio than antipsychotic medication in CHR treatment [e.g. 9, 32]. Their arguments in support of giving priority to evidence-based psychotherapy in favor of antipsychotic treatment in CHR are that (1) psychotherapy is more acceptable, tolerable and less stigmatizing to clients [e.g. 33–35], (2) there is lesser risk of exposing false-positive persons to pharmacological side effects, (3) psychotherapy may be an effective treatment for false-positive persons (depression, anxiety disorders [36]) and (4) psychotherapy is similarly effective in preventing transition to first-episode psychosis as antipsychotics, as well as in improving symptoms and functioning in CHR [32].

Aims of Psychological Early Intervention in Emerging Psychosis

The primary outcome for individuals at CHR is to prevent or delay the onset of full-blown psychosis. Secondary outcomes are to achieve remission of risk symptoms and comorbid axis I or II disorders, as well as to improve psychosocial functioning and quality of life.

Müller · Bechdolf

Psychoeducation in Emerging Psychosis

A possible link between psychotherapeutic approaches and self-help efforts is psychoeducation. Patients with psychotic disorders who receive psychoeducation have lower relapse and rehospitalization rates, higher social and global functioning, and improved quality of life compared to patients who receive standard treatment alone [37].

Therefore, it might be beneficial to use psychoeducation in individuals at CHR. An inherent challenge of early recognition lies in risk assessment. For this reason, psychoeducation should be adjusted to convey a realistic assessment of an individual's risk for psychosis. Other objectives include achieving a better understanding of risk symptoms, as well as improving necessary skills for the management of risk symptoms.

At present, there is pilot data of the beneficial effects of psychoeducation in individuals at CHR from two uncontrolled naturalistic studies and one randomized controlled trial. In these studies, psychoeducation was offered in individual therapy and group formats [38–40]. Hauser et al. [38] investigated the effect of psychoeducation over seven sessions. The before/after comparison showed a significant increase in knowledge, higher quality of life, a reduction of the feeling of being entrapped by the risk symptoms and an improvement in the global clinical impression. On a qualitative level, psychoeducation was assessed to be very useful by the patients themselves. The differentiation of risk-symptoms from frank psychotic symptoms, as well as learning how to cope with stress was considered helpful by the patients. It is important to note that overall, psychoeducation has had a positive effect in individuals at CHR.

In a multifamily group by O'Brien et al. [39], initial psychoeducation was followed by up to 18 sessions of communication and problem-solving training, as well as instructions for symptom management. The evaluation of the program showed that both individuals at CHR and their relatives reported that they benefited from the intervention. Furthermore, individuals at CHR had fewer attenuated positive symptoms, as well as improved level of functioning with respect to school and work performance. The efficacy of psychoeducation as an element of psychological intervention was first indicated by Zarafonitis et al. [40] in a randomized controlled trial. In this trial, psychoeducation was offered to CHR clients in individual therapy, as well as across three meetings with their relatives. The authors concluded that psychoeducation is an important element in psychological interventions aimed at preventing transition to psychosis.

To sum up, at present there is no separate scientific evaluation of psychoeducation in individuals at CHR within a randomized controlled trial. However, manualized and well-formulated psychoeducation programs for individuals at CHR are available [41].

Psychotherapy in Emerging Psychosis

Currently, there are nine completed randomized controlled trials in individuals with CHR that evaluate psychotherapeutic interventions. In one trial, the administration of antipsychotics was compared to cognitive behavioral therapy (CBT) plus placebo and supportive therapy plus placebo [42]. Eight trials evaluated psychotherapy alone. Out of these trials, five studies offered CBT alone [43–47], two evaluated a combination of CBT skills training and family intervention [integrated psychotherapy (IPI)] [48, 49], and one evaluated family-focused therapy (FFT) alone [50] (table 1).

The Common Basis of Psychotherapeutic Interventions
Most psychotherapeutic intervention approaches reviewed thus far follow the structure and principles of CBT, and are therefore time limited and have a problem-oriented approach. As a theoretical foundation, all presented concepts are based more or less explicitly on the vulnerability-stress-coping model of schizophrenia [51]. Given these similarities, the theoretical assumptions differ with respect to individually formulated cognitive models and the interventional modules that are used. In the following section we outline these trials in greater detail, and highlight the differences in their psychotherapeutic approaches.

Personal Assessment and Crisis Evaluation
In their ground-breaking interventional trial, McGorry et al. [29] compared CBT plus risperidone (n = 31) with a needs-based intervention program (n = 28) in individuals at CHR. After a 6-month treatment phase, the specific intervention was found to be more superior than the control intervention in preventing transition to psychosis. At 12 months, results were significant provided that only people who were compliant with their antipsychotic medications were included in the analysis. Since both active treatments were combined in one arm of the trial, the design does not allow for separate examination of the effect of psychotherapy. Thus, in the next generation of trials, McGorry and colleagues [42, 52] implemented a design which compared risperidone plus CBT, CBT plus placebo, and supportive therapy plus placebo. In this trial, practitioners and raters were blinded to the pharmacological prescriptions. No statistical differences in transition rates were found at both 6 and 12 months (table 1). The manualized CBT was based on four treatment modules: (1) stress management, (2) reduction of depression or negative symptoms, (3) coping with positive symptoms and (4) treatment of comorbid disorders [53]. A special focus in the Personal Assessment and Crisis Evaluation approach is given to constructive processes. For instance the therapist may try to understand the risk symptoms in attempt to make sense of the unusual perceptions experienced by patients. Or, the therapist may try to foster the critical appraisal of narrative self-representations and self-stigmatization by the patient in order to prevent the client from forming a negative identity of being a psychotic person [53].

Table 1. Results and baseline characteristics of the randomized controlled trials evaluating psychotherapy in individuals at CRH

Author	Results: primary endpoint conversion to psychosis (%)	Results: secondary endpoints	Participants, n (%)	Mean age, years (SD)	Control condition	Duration CBT/CON, months (sessions)
Addington et al. [65], 2010 EDIE Manual	6 months: CBT: 0/27 (0); CON: 3/24 (12.5) 12 months: CBT: 0/27 (0); CON: 3/24 (12.5) 18 months: CBT: 0/27 (0); CON: 3/24 (12.5); NNT = 9; SOPS	CBT reduces attenuated positive symptoms faster than CON; improvements of depression, anxiety and level of functioning in both groups	n = 51 female = 15 (30) male = 36 (70)	20.9 (4.1)	Supportive therapy: therapeutic variables sensu Rogers, psychoeducation, stress-management, problem-solving, crisis-management	6 (20)/–
Bechdolf et al. [47], 2012 IPI Manual	12 months: IPI: 2/63 (3.2); KON: 11/65 (16.9); NNT = 8.7; 24 months: IPI: 4/63 (6.3); KON: 13/65 (20); NNT = 9.3; ERIraos; PANSS	IPI and CON reduce risk-symptoms, level of functioning and social adjustment	n = 128 female = 47 (37) male = 81 (63)	26 (5.8)	Manualized supportive therapy: therapeutic variables sensu Rogers, basic psychoeducation	12 (55)/–
McGorry et al. [41], 2013 Yung et al. [64], 2010 PACE, Manual	6 months: CT + PL: 4/44 (9.1); CON + PL: 2/28 (7.1); NNT = –60 12 months: CT + PL: 7/44 (15.9); CON + PL: 6/28 (21.4); CAARMS	Reduction of psychiatric symptoms, negative-symptoms, depression, level of functioning and quality of life in both groups	n = 72 female = 42 (58) male = 30 (42)	18.4 (3.2)	Supportive therapy: emotional and social support, monitoring, psychoeducation, problem-solving, stress-management	12/–
Miklowitz et al. [49], 2014 FFT-Early-Onset Youth Manual	6 months: FFT: 1/55 (1.8); CON: 5/47 (10.6); SOPS	FFT reduces attenuated positive symptoms as compared to CON; negative symptoms improved irrespectively of group.	n = 129 female = 55 (42,6) male = 74 (57,4)	17.4 (4.1)	Enhanced care: psychoeducation, symptom-management	6 (18)/6 (3)
Morrison et al. [44], 2004 EDIE Manual	12 months: CT: 2/35 (5.7); CON: 5/23 (21.7); 36 months: CT: 7/35 (20); CON: 5/23 (22); PANSS	CT reduces attenuated positive symptoms compared to CON; CT reduces the prescription of antipsychotic drugs	n = 58 female = 18 (31) male = 40 (69)	22 (4.5)	Monitoring: case-management, crisis-management concerning psychological and social problems	6 (26)/6 (13)

Table 1. Continued

Author	Results: primary endpoint conversion to psychosis (%)	Results: secondary endpoints	Participants, n (%)	Mean age, years (SD)	Control condition	Duration CBT/CON, months (sessions)
Morrison et al. [43], 2012 EDIE Manual	6 months: CT: 6/144 (4.1); CON: 6/144 (4.1) 12 months: CT: 7/144 (4.8); CON: 10/144 (6.9) 24 months: CT: 10/144 (6.9); CON: 13/144 (9); CAARMS	CT reduces severity of attenuated positive symptoms compared to CON	n = 288 female = 108 (37) male = 180 (63)	20.7 (4.3)	TAU + monitoring: therapeutic variables sensu Rogers, crisis-management	6 (30)/–
Nordentoft et al. [48], 2006	12 months: IPI: 3/37 (8.1); CON: 10/30 (33.3) 24 months: CBT: 9/37 (24.3); CON: 14/30 (46.6); ICD-10 schizotypal disorder	IPI reduces negative symptoms at 12 months follow up compared to CON	n = 79 female = 26 (32.9) male = 53 (67.1)	24.9 (4.9)	Standard treatment: contact with a physician and social worker; in some cases, the standard social skills training or daily living activities, or supportive counselling with the family	Individual sessions 12 (46)/– family meetings 18 (36)/–
Stain et al. [46], 2014 EDIE Manual	– CAARMS	No group differences are reported	n = 57 female = 34 (60) male = 23 (40)	16.3 (–)	TAU + nondirective *reflective listening*: therapeutic variables sensu Rogers	6 (26)/6 (26)
van der Gaag et al. [45], 2012 EDIE Manual + meta-cognitive Training	6 months: CBT: 5/98 (5.1); CON: 14/103 (13.5) 12 months: CBT: 9/98 (9.1); CON: 20/103 (19.4) 18 months: CBT: 10/98 (10.2); CON: 22/103 (21.3); CAARMS	More remissions in CBT than in CON; CBT reduces feelings of distress and of being entrapped in relation to risk symptoms as compared to CON	n = 201 female = 102 (50) male = 99 (50)	22.7 (5.5)	TAU + monitoring: treatment for comorbid axis I and II disorders according to Dutch and NICE guidelines	6 (26)/–

CT = Cognitive therapy; NNT = number of treatments needed; TAU = treatment as usual.

Early Detection and Intervention Evaluation

Five out of the nine intervention trials presented here are based on the Early Detection and Intervention Evaluation (EDIE) manual by French and Morrison [54]. In the first single-center trial, Morrison et al. [45] found cognitive therapy to be superior to simply monitoring clients in terms of psychosis prevention (p < 0.05). Addington et al. [43], adopted the therapy approach in a single-center trial, and no transitions to psychosis were found in their active treatment arm. Nevertheless, the difference to the control condition was not statistically significant. Morrison et al. [44] tried to replicate the encouraging results from their first trial in a multicenter trial. A twin trial with the same purpose was set by van der Gaag et al. [46]. While Morrison et al. [44] did not find a difference in the transition rates in their large sample (n = 288), this was the opposite for van der Gaag et al. [46]. Their results demonstrated superiority of the experimental condition compared to the control condition with respect to rates of transition to psychosis (p < 0.05).

As a cognitive therapy method, the manual by French and Morrison [54] emphasizes development of alternative cognitions, work on meta-cognition and cognitive schemas. The cognitive model of the EDIE manual assumes that a comparison of the risk symptoms with internalized cultural norms by the patient (e.g. negative prejudices against psychic illnesses among the general public) may result in catastrophic appraisals, such as 'I am crazy and totally different to other people'. Such an appraisal could exacerbate symptoms, as well as feelings of depression and anxiety, which are then maintained by safety behavior and through poor perception of the self and others [54]. Interventions incorporating strategies, such as normalization, and addressing cognitions and cognitive core beliefs with flexibility are therefore important.

Recently, the EDIE manual has been extended by van der Gaag et al. [55] with a special focus on metacognitive processes. Their model states that dopamine hypersensitivity is the basis for cognitive biases which in turn lead to risk symptoms. One example of such biases is the 'jump to conclusion bias' [56]. Individuals at CHR are educated with respect to these biases and learn how to monitor themselves when such biases arise.

Integrated Psychological Interventions

Besides the treatment aproaches for individuals meeting ultra-high-risk criteria, Bechdolf et al. [48] formulated a psychological approach for intervention in individuals at the early initial prodromal states. In a multicenter trial with blinded raters, they demonstrated that IPI was superior to supportive counseling with regard to transition rates to psychosis, both after the interventional period (p < 0.01) and at the 24-month follow-up (p < 0.05).

The IPI includes a total maximum of 55 sessions over a period of 12 months. This is comprised of 25 sessions (maximum) of individual therapy, 15 group sessions, 12 sessions of cognitive remediation and 3 sessions of counselling for relatives. The individual therapy sessions incorporate a number of different modules including psychoeducation, symptom management, stress management and crisis management. The group sessions encompass activity schedules and work on positive affect such as mood and enjoyment, social skills and problem solving. Cognitive remediation involves computer-based training of attention, memory and concentration.

Bechdolf et al. [48] designed a theoretical framework that integrated the vulnerability-stress-coping model, the concept of basic symptoms [57, 58] and cognitive models of psychosis [e.g. 59]. The model predicts that progression from early initial prodromal states to attenuated positive symptoms occurs in a higher risk stage under the influence of cognitive biases [60].

Another multicenter trial based on an IPI protocol by Nordentoft et al. [49] showed that a high-frequency, assertive, community treatment provided by multiprofessional teams was superior to standard care in Danish mental health centers (p < 0.05). The inclusion criteria followed the ICD-10 criteria for schizotypal disorder, and transition was also defined when patients met diagnostic criteria for (F2) psychosis according to ICD-10. The assessment of the symptoms was carried out by independent, nonblinded raters. Interventions were provided on an individual or group level. Modules of the treatment that needed to be adapted included social skills training (role plays), psychoeducation on medication, side effects and drug abuse, problem-solving, and a variety of techniques from CBT and relapse prevention. Depending on the patients' consent, relatives were offered psychoeducational multifamily groups like those of McFarlane et al. [61], including psychoeducation and problem-solving procedures.

Family-Focused Therapy
FFT is a promising strategy in early intervention because it has been found to be highly effective on relapse prevention in schizophrenia [62]. It can therefore, be assumed to be a suitable intervention candidate for the prevention of the disorder as well. In a multicenter trial which evaluated the efficacy of FFT, Miklowitz et al. [50] found FFT to be superior to brief psychoeducation (p < 0.05) in terms of positive attenuated symptoms (primary outcome, assessed by blinded raters).

The first part of the FFT approach is psychoeducation. Here, individual stressors are identified and copings skills (e.g. pleasant event scheduling, relaxation exercises) are provided. The second part of FFT focuses on communication enhancement training. In addition to problem-solving skills training, individuals at CHR and their families are educated on active listening, are taught skills on clear communication, on making positive requests and on how to express positive as well as negative feelings [63].

Methodology of the Trials on Psychotherapy in Emerging Psychosis
Besides a few trials offering multifamily groups either alone [64] or in group settings (in addition to individual settings) [48, 49], the majority of trials have used individual therapy settings [35, 43, 45, 46]. There is some heterogeneity between the

trials in terms of duration of treatment, which varies between a maximum of 18 months [49] to a minimum of 6 months (table 1). There were a couple of trials that did not report the number of sessions received by patients [42, 47]. For the remaining trials, the median number of therapy sessions provided was 11, with a wide range of 9.1–77.

In three trials, treatment fidelity was ensured by regular supervision, but there was no formal measure of therapeutic competence [45, 48, 49]. Subsequent trials measured treatment fidelity and the competence of therapists through both supervision and audio recordings of therapy sessions, which were rated by means of operationalized methods [43, 44, 46, 65].

It has to be noted that in two trials, recruited patients were excluded post hoc from the analysis as it appeared that they were already psychotic at the inclusion of the study, much to their dissimulation. Had these cases remained in the sample, nonsignificant group differences in the transition rates would have been found [45, 46]. With the intention to prevent these post hoc exclusions from their analyses, Morrison et al. [44] did not recruit a number of patients with severe risk symptoms, which probably led to nonsignificant results despite the large sample size of the trial.

In four of the nine presented trials, the primary outcome did not reach significant results at a statistical level [44, 47, 66, 67]. This is probably due to three factors. The first was the difference between the planned sample size and the actual number of patients recruited (30.72% [66], 57.6% [65], 73% [47]), which in turn, may have rendered these trials underpowered. Second, in most of the trials, CON was characterized by a client-centered approach sensu Carl Rogers [68]. Often, additional psychoeducation, problem-solving training and crisis management were provided. Thus, we conclude that in most of the trials, psychotherapy was compared to an active psychosocial treatment (table 1). In light of this, an active control condition may have made it even more difficult to find effects in the aforementioned underpowered trials. Finally, there is substantial heterogeneity in the presented samples in terms of age (range: 16.3–26 years), gender (generally one third female to two thirds male in all but two more recent studies, which had a nearly balanced sex ratio) and transition rate [median: 12 (5.6–18), regardless of group assignment]. This heterogeneity may have affected risk enrichment [69] and therefore may account for some of the variability in the statistical significances.

Unlike the psychosocial control condition, psychotherapy was manual based in almost all trials [44–48, 63, 66, 67]. In three trials, treatment fidelity and competence of the therapists were only ensured by supervision [45, 48]. Subsequent studies ensured treatment fidelity and therapist competence based on ratings of audio-taped therapy sessions using operationalized measures [44, 46, 49, 65, 66].

In sum, earlier single-center trials adopting smaller sample sizes appear to have been superseded by methodologically sound, multicenter trials with larger samples [see also 70].

Conclusions

Currently, 1,063 individuals at CHR were treated in randomized controlled trials focusing on psychotherapy. Thus, psychotherapy in individuals at CHR is the best evaluated individual therapy approach within the area of psychosis prevention.

The EDIE manual was used in five out of the nine studies presented here, and is therefore the best evaluated approach. However, reference is made to the fact that there is also a published manual in German [71].

Psychotherapy is an intervention that can actively address the needs of individuals at CHR, while simultaneously protecting false-positive patients from the side effects of antipsychotic medication. A possibility to reduce the aforementioned heterogeneity in CHR samples could be the stratification of risk into subclasses [72]. However, there is also growing research interest concerning the side effects of psychotherapy [73]. Data on the adverse events and side effects associated with psychotherapy should therefore be systematically collected by future trials involving individuals at CHR.

Six trials have reported outcomes on medium-term follow-ups (≥18 months). Interestingly, two trials focusing on IPI showed lower transition rates in favor of psychotherapy at their 24-month follow-up [48, 49]. In addition, Morrison et al. [74] showed that the probability of being prescribed antipsychotic medication was significantly lower in the cognitive therapy condition at the 36-month follow-up. Thus, it can be concluded that some medium-term effects of psychotherapy are apparent after cessation of the intervention.

Concerning the treatment of attenuated positive symptoms, psychotherapy was found to be superior to, or at least, equally effective as CON in three trials (table 1). In the six trials reporting results on attenuated negative symptoms, one trial showed that psychotherapy was superior to CON [49]. Two trials reported improvements in negative attenuated symptoms, irrespective of treatment group [64, 67]. Data from other secondary outcomes showed that CON was equal to psychotherapy in terms of improving level of psychosocial functioning [42, 43, 48], depression [42, 43] and social anxiety [43].

Especially concerning the level of psychosocial functioning, it is worth emphasizing that social disability occurs way before the onset of the first psychotic symptoms [75]. It is possible that individuals at CHR could therefore additionally benefit from more behaviorally driven goal setting and the accompanying sociotherapeutic support. However, despite promising approaches [76], interventions with individuals at CHR still lack formulated treatments of attenuated negative symptoms.

From the range of therapy sessions reviewed, we are unable to conclude which is the optimal treatment dose. Future analyses have to demonstrate whether there is a relationship between the number of therapy sessions and the primary or secondary outcomes.

Despite these limitations, overall, the advantages of specific treatment (antipsychotics, neuroprotective agents and psychotherapy) in comparison to standard treatment is shown to be more efficacious in terms of preventing psychosis [9, 32, 77–80] by all available meta-analyses. The same applies for psychological treatments in CHR [32, 77, 79]. Furthermore, the median number of treatments needed (min. – max.) in order to prevent one transition is 10.8 (6–14) within 6 months, 9 (7.7–53.8) within 12 months and 11 (9–83.9) for ≥18 months. Thereby, the median number of treatments needed are much better than, for example, the 67 treatments needed for antihypertensive medication in people with hypertension in order to prevent one stroke within 4 years [81].

Clinical Implications

Evidence shows that psychotherapeutic interventions for patients at CHR are safe, effective and well accepted by patients and their families [9, 32, 33, 35, 77]. Given the accuracy with which we can now predict psychosis [see the chapter by McGorry and Goldstone, this vol., pp. 15–28], providing psychosocial preventive interventions to most clinicians and researchers outweighs the risk of not providing it [9, 32]. Thereby, psychotherapy is currently the best evaluated individual therapy approach for the prevention of psychosis, as well as for the reduction of attenuated positive symptoms and improvement of level of functioning [32, 77]. Antipsychotic medication should therefore serve as a second-line treatment only in cases where individuals do not respond to CBT or present with severe deterioration or risk. The data on psychoeducation in individuals at CHR are encouraging but still not sufficient. From the available data, it can be concluded that psychoeducation may be a safe and accepted intervention for both individuals at CHR and their relatives. As it provides one intervention within a staging approach, methodologically sound trials are needed to demonstrate the possible benefits of psychoeducation.

The recent progress in CHR research is best documented by the fact that the attenuated psychosis syndrome – modelled after the UHR category APS – has been included in the research chapter of DSM-5 [82].

Although there is now substantial evidence to promote specialized CHR treatment, these services should work within a rigid ethical framework as pointed out earlier. Therefore, clinical services for individuals at CHR should meet a number of objectives and requirements. First, these services should provide a nonstigmatizing, low-threshold setting for young help-seeking patients and their families. Second, staff should have experience and sufficient training in assessing potential at-risk symptoms. Third, they must also have a detailed conceptual frame-work, and experience in offering patients and families information regarding the risk of psychosis as well as assistance to cope with it. Finally, a variety of specific clinical interventions (e.g. monitoring, motivational interviewing with regards to substance use, supportive therapies, CBT and family therapy) and a wide range of pharmacological interventions (e.g. neuroprotective agents, antidepressants and antipsychotic medication) must be available in order to deliver optimal risk-benefit ratios with regard to the over- and undertreatment of individuals at CHR [83]. These requirements are best met by specially designed, low-threshold outpatient clinical services.

Despite the encouraging results presented here, it should be noted that there is still a need for further research in individuals with CHR, and replications of existing studies with longer observation periods should be undertaken. Such studies could shed valuable insight into how long treatment should be maintained. This information could provide a valuable contribution in the quest of formulating a reasonable treatment algorithm for individual intervention options.

Can Early Detection and Intervention of Psychosis Be Implemented in Routine Care?

The Australian government is in the process of conducting a nationwide USD 600 million mental health reform [84] which promotes the implementation of specialized youth-friendly services focusing on interventions in people with CHR and first-episode psychosis, as well as other severe mental illnesses around Australia. In addition, many westernized English-speaking countries, such as the USA, Canada and New Zealand, have also begun setting up specialized early intervention centers [85]. In Europe, the implementation of early intervention services is most strongly recommended by the British treatment guidelines for schizophrenia (NICE) [86]. Indeed, to date there are 145 specialized early intervention centers in Great Britain [87]. Initial cost-effectiveness analyses have indicated that the extra costs (as compared to standard care) in the first year are compensated for by subsequent savings associated with a better course of the disorder later [88–90].

We conclude that the implementation and early detection/intervention of psychosis offers a unique opportunity to not only make a difference in the course of psychosis in young people at CHR, but to also make a positive impact on the families of those at CHR. On an even wider scale, we believe it also provides the opportunity to positively impact the health care system through reducing the burden, disability and economic consequences of psychosis.

Acknowledgement

The authors would like to thank Emily Li for her support in the preparation of this chapter.

Disclosure Statement

The authors received no funding for this review. A.B. has received speaker fees from Bristol Myers Squibb, Eli Lilly and Janssen Cilag, and has received support for investigator-initiated trials from Bristol Myers Squibb. H.M. declares no conflict of interest.

References

1 Whiteford HA, Degenhardt L, Rehm J, et al: Global burden of disease attributable to mental and substance use disorders: findings from the Global Burden of Disease Study 2010. Lancet 2013;382:1575–1586.

2 Konnopka A, Klingberg S, Wittorf A, et al: The cost of schizophrenia in Germany: a systematic review of the literature (in German). Psychiatr Prax 2009;36:211–218.

3 van Os J, Kapur S. Schizophrenia. Lancet 2009;374:635–645.

4 Adams EK, Breen N, Joski PJ: Impact of the National Breast and Cervical Cancer Early Detection Program on mammography and Pap test utilization among white, Hispanic, and African American women: 1996–2000. Cancer 2007;109:348–358.

5 Peters AL, Davidson MB, Schriger DL, et al: A clinical approach for the diagnosis of diabetes mellitus: an analysis using glycosylated hemoglobin levels. Meta-analysis Research Group on the Diagnosis of Diabetes Using Glycated Hemoglobin Levels. JAMA 1996;276:1246–1252.

6 Psaty BM, Lumley T, Furberg CD, et al: Health outcomes associated with various antihypertensive therapies used as first-line agents: a network meta-analysis. JAMA 2003;289:2534–2544.

7 Häfner H, Riecher-Rossler A, Maurer K, et al: First onset and early symptomatology of schizophrenia. A chapter of epidemiological and neurobiological research into age and sex differences. Eur Arch Psychiatry Clin Neurosci 1992;242:109–118.

8 Häfner H, Maurer K, An der Heiden W: ABC Schizophrenia study: an overview of results since 1996. Soc Psychiatry Psychiatr Epidemiol 2013;48:1021–1031.

9 Fusar-Poli P, Borgwardt S, Bechdolf A, et al: The psychosis high-risk state: a comprehensive state-of-the-art review. JAMA Psychiatry 2013;70:107–120.

10 Marshall M, Lewis S, Lockwood A, et al: Association between duration of untreated psychosis and outcome in cohorts of first-episode patients: a systematic review. Arch Gen Psychiatry 2005;62:975–983.

11 Archer T, Karilampi U, Ricci S, et al: Neurotoxic vulnerability underlying schizophrenia spectrum disorders; in Kostrzewa R (ed): Handbook of Neurotoxicity. Berlin, Springer 2014, pp 2181–2205.

12 Fusar-Poli P, Bonoldi I, Yung AR, et al: Predicting psychosis: a meta-analysis of transition outcomes in individuals at high clinical risk. Arch Gen Psychiatry 2012;69:220–229.

13 Fusar-Poli P, Nelson B, Valmaggia L, et al: Comorbid depressive and anxiety disorders in 509 individuals with an at-risk mental state: impact on psychopathology and transition to psychosis. Schizophr Bull 2014;40:120–131.

14 Addington J, Penn D, Woods SW, et al: Social functioning in individuals at clinical high risk for psychosis. Schizophr Res 2008;99:119–124.

15 Bechdolf A, Pukrop R, Kohn D, et al: Subjective quality of life in subjects at risk for a first episode of psychosis: a comparison with first episode schizophrenia patients and healthy controls. Schizophr Res 2005;79:137–143.

16 Lencz T, Smith CW, Auther A, et al: Nonspecific and attenuated negative symptoms in patients at clinical high-risk for schizophrenia. Schizophr Res 2004;68:37–48.

17 Velthorst E, Nieman DH, Linszen D, et al: Disability in people clinically at high risk of psychosis. Br J Psychiatry 2010;197:278–284.

18 Addington J, Cornblatt BA, Cadenhead KS, et al: At clinical high risk for psychosis: outcome for nonconverters. Am J Psychiatry 2011;168:800.

19 Ziermans TB, Schothorst PF, Sprong M, et al: Transition and remission in adolescents at ultra-high risk for psychosis. Schizophr Res 2011;126:58–64.

20 Fusar-Poli P, Deste G, Smieskova R, et al: Cognitive functioning in prodromal psychosis: a meta-analysis. Arch Gen Psychiatry 2012;69:562–571.

21 Giuliano AJ, Li H, I Mesholam-Gately R, et al: Neurocognition in the psychosis risk syndrome: a quantitative and qualitative review. Curr Pharm Des 2012;18:399–415.

22 Phillips LJ, Velakoulis D, Pantelis C, et al: Non-reduction in hippocampal volume is associated with higher risk of psychosis. Schizophr Res 2002;58:145–158.

23 Velakoulis D, Wood SJ, Wong MT, et al: Hippocampal and amygdala volumes according to psychosis stage and diagnosis: a magnetic resonance imaging study of chronic schizophrenia, first-episode psychosis, and ultra-high-risk individuals. Arch Gen Psychiatry 2006;63:139–149.

24 Yücel M, Wood SJ, Phillips LJ, et al: Morphology of the anterior cingulate cortex in young men at ultra-high risk of developing a psychotic illness. Br J Psychiatry 2003;182:518–524.

25 Stone JM, Day F, Tsagaraki H, et al: Glutamate dysfunction in people with prodromal symptoms of psychosis: relationship to gray matter volume. Biol Psychiatry 2009;66:533–539.

26 Fusar-Poli P, Howes O, Allen P, et al: Abnormal prefrontal activation directly related to pre-synaptic striatal dopamine dysfunction in people at clinical high risk for psychosis. Mol Psychiatry 2009;16:67–75.

27 Fusar-Poli P, Howes OD, Allen P, et al: Abnormal frontostriatal interactions in people with prodromal signs of psychosis: a multimodal imaging study. Arch Gen Psychiatry 2010;67:683–691.

28 Fusar-Poli P, Stone JM, Broome MR, et al: Thalamic glutamate levels as a predictor of cortical response during executive functioning in subjects at high risk for psychosis. Arch Gen Psychiatry 2011;68:881–890.

29 Xu Z, Müller M, Heekeren K, et al: Self-labelling and stigma as predictors of attitudes towards help-seeking among people at risk of psychosis: 1-year follow-up. Eur Arch Psychiatry Clin Neurosci 2015, Epub ahead of print.

30 Simon AE, Velthorst E, Nieman DH, et al: Ultra high-risk state for psychosis and non-transition: a systematic review. Schizophr Res 2011;132:8–17.

31 van der Gaag M, Smit F, Bechdolf A, et al: Preventing a first episode of psychosis: meta-analysis of randomized controlled prevention trials of 12 month and longer-term follow-ups. Schizophr Res 2013; 149:56–62.

32 Angermeyer MC, Matschinger H, Schomerus G: Attitudes towards psychiatric treatment and people with mental illness: changes over two decades. Br J Psychiatry 2013;203:146–151.

33 Lauber C, Nordt C, Falcato L, et al: Lay recommendations on how to treat mental disorders. Soc Psychiatry Psychiatr Epidemiol 2001;36:553–556.

34 Morrison AP, Birchwood M, Pyle M, et al: Impact of cognitive therapy on internalised stigma in people with at-risk mental states. Br J Psychiatry 2013;203: 140–145.

35 American Psychiatric Association Practice Guidelines for the Treatment of Psychiatric Disorders: Compendium 2006. Arlington, APA, 2006.

36 Xia J, Merinder LB, Belgamwar MR: Psychoeducation for schizophrenia. Cochrane Database Syst Rev 2011;6:CD002831.

37 Hauser M, Lautenschlager M, Gudlowski Y, et al: Psychoeducation with patients at-risk for schizophrenia – an exploratory pilot study. Patient Educ Couns 2009;76:138–142.

38 O'Brien MP, Zinberg JL, Bearden CE, et al: Psychoeducational multi-family group treatment with adolescents at high risk for developing psychosis. Early Interv Psychiatry 2007;1:325–332.

39 Zarafonitis SW, Pützfeld V, Berning J: Psychoedukation bei Personen mit erhöhtem Psychoserisiko. Psychotherapeut 2012;57:326–334.

40 Bechdolf A: Psychoedukation bei Personen mit erhöhtem Psychoserisiko. Stuttgart, Schattauer, 2006.

41 McGorry PD, Nelson B, Phillips LJ, et al: Randomized controlled trial of interventions for young people at ultra-high risk of psychosis: twelve-month outcome. J Clin Psychiatry 2013;74:349–356.

42 Addington J, Epstein I, Liu L, et al: A randomized controlled trial of cognitive behavioral therapy for individuals at clinical high risk of psychosis. Schizophr Res 2011;125:54–61.

43 Morrison AP, French P, Stewart SL, et al: Early detection and intervention evaluation for people at risk of psychosis: multisite randomised controlled trial. BMJ 2012;344:e2233.

44 Morrison AP, French P, Walford L, et al: Cognitive therapy for the prevention of psychosis in people at ultra-high risk: randomised controlled trial. Br J Psychiatry 2004;185:291–297.

45 van der Gaag M, Nieman DH, Rietdijk J, et al: Cognitive behavioral therapy for subjects at ultrahigh risk for developing psychosis: a randomized controlled clinical trial. Schizophr Bull 2012;38:1180–1188.

46 Stain H, Bucci S, Halperin S, et al: DEPTh: randomized controlled trial of cognitive behavioral therapy for young people at ultra high risk for psychosis. 9th International Conference on Early Psychosis, Tokyo, 2014.

47 Bechdolf A, Wagner M, Ruhrmann S, et al: Preventing progression to first-episode psychosis in early initial prodromal states. Br J Psychiatry 2012;200: 22–29.

48 Nordentoft M, Thorup A, Petersen L, et al: Transition rates from schizotypal disorder to psychotic disorder for first-contact patients included in the OPUS trial. A randomized clinical trial of integrated treatment and standard treatment. Schizophr Res 2006; 83:29–40.

49 Miklowitz DJ, O'Brien MP, Schlosser DA, et al: Family-focused treatment for adolescents and young adults at high risk for psychosis: results of a randomized trial. J Am Acad Child Adolesc Psychiatry 2014; 53:848–858.

50 Nuechterlein KH, Dawson ME: A heuristic vulnerability/stress model of schizophrenic episodes. Schizophr Bull 1984;10:300–312.

51 McGorry PD, Yung AR, Phillips LJ, et al: Randomized controlled trial of interventions designed to reduce the risk of progression to first-episode psychosis in a clinical sample with subthreshold symptoms. Arch Gen Psychiatry 2002;59:921–928.

52 Yung AR, Phillips LJ, Nelson B, et al: Randomized controlled trial of interventions for young people at ultra high risk for psychosis: 6-month analysis. J Clin Psychiat 2011;72:430–440.

53 Gleeson JFM, McGorry PD: Psychological Interventions in Early Psychosis: A Treatment Handbook. Hoboken, Wiley, 2004.

54 French P, Morrison AP: Early Detection and Cognitive Therapy for People at High Risk of Developing Psychosis: A Treatment Approach: Hoboken, Wiley, 2004.

55 Van der Gaag M, Nieman D, van den Berg D: CBT for Those at Risk of a First Episode Psychosis: evidence-based psychotherapy for people with an 'At Risk Mental State'. Taylor & Francis, 2013.

56 Fine C, Gardner M, Craigie J, et al: Hopping, skipping or jumping to conclusions? Clarifying the role of the JTC bias in delusions. Cogn Neuropsychiatry 2007;12:46–77.

57 Klosterkötter J, Hellmich M, Steinmeyer EM, et al: Diagnosing schizophrenia in the initial prodromal phase. Arch Gen Psychiatry 2001;58:158–164.

58 Süllwold L, Huber G. Schizophrene Basisstörungen. Berlin, Springer, 1986.

59 Kingdon DG, Turkington D. Cognitive Therapy of Schizophrenia. New York, Guilford Press, 2005.

60 Larsen T, K, Bechdolf A, Birchwood M: The concept of schizophrenia and phase-specific treatment: cognitive-behavioral treatment in pre-psychosis and in nonresponders. J Am Acad Psychoanal Dyn Psychiatry 2003;31:209–228.

61 McFarlane WR, Lukens E, Link B, et al: Multiple-family groups and psychoeducation in the treatment of schizophrenia. Arch Gen Psychiatry 1995;52:679–687.

62 Pharoah F, Mari J, Rathbone J, et al: Family intervention for schizophrenia. Cochrane Database Syst Rev 2010;12:CD000088.

63 Miklowitz DJ, O'Brien MP, Schlosser DA, et al: Clinicians' Treatment Manual for Family-Focused Therapy for Early-Onset Youth and Young Adults (FFT-EOY). 2012, http://www.nasmhpd.org/sites/default/files/FFT-EOY_Manual_82812.pdf.

64 Miklowitz DJ, O'Brien MP, Schlosser DA, et al: Family-focused treatment for adolescents and young adults at high risk for psychosis: results of a randomized trial. J Am Acad Child Adolesc Psychiatry 2014; 53:848–858.

65 Yung AR, Phillips LJ, Nelson B, et al: Randomized controlled trial of interventions for young people at ultra high risk for psychosis: 6-month analysis. J Clin Psychiatry 2011;72:430.

66 Addington J, Epstein I, Liu L, et al: A randomized controlled trial of cognitive behavioral therapy for individuals at clinical high risk of psychosis. Schizophr Res 2011;125:54–61.

67 McGorry PD, Nelson B, Phillips LJ, et al: Randomized controlled trial of interventions for young people at ultra-high risk of psychosis: twelve-month outcome. J Clin Psychiatry 2013;74:349–356.

68 Rogers CR: Client-Centered Therapy: Its Current Practice, Implications and Theory. London, Constable & Robinson, 2003.

69 Rietdijk J, Klaassen R, Ising H, et al: Detection of people at risk of developing a first psychosis: comparison of two recruitment strategies. Acta Psychiatr Scand 2012;126:21–30.

70 Bechdolf A, Muller H, Stutzer H, et al: Rationale and baseline characteristics of PREVENT: a second-generation intervention trial in subjects at-risk (prodromal) of developing first-episode psychosis evaluating cognitive behavior therapy, aripiprazole, and placebo for the prevention of psychosis. Schizophr Bull 2011;37(suppl 2):S111–S121.

71 Bechdolf A, Güttgemanns J, Gross S: Kognitive Verhaltenstherapie bei Personen mit erhöhtem Psychoserisiko: ein Behandlungsmanual. Mannheim, Huber, 2010.

72 Ruhrmann S, Schultze-Lutter F, Schmidt SJ, et al: Prediction and prevention of psychosis: current progress and future tasks. Eur Arch Psychiatry Clin Neurosci 2014;264:9–16.

73 Barlow DH: Negative effects from psychological treatments: a perspective. Am Psychol 2010;65:13–20.

74 Morrison AP, French P, Parker S, et al: Three-year follow-up of a randomized controlled trial of cognitive therapy for the prevention of psychosis in people at ultrahigh risk. Schizophr Bull 2007;33:682–687.

75 Häfner H, Wolpert EM: New Research in Psychiatry. Göttingen, Hogrefe & Huber, 1996.

76 Perivoliotis D, Morrison AP, Grant PM, et al: Negative performance beliefs and negative symptoms in individuals at ultra-high risk of psychosis: a preliminary study. Psychopathology 2009;42:375–379.

77 Hutton P, Taylor PJ: Cognitive behavioural therapy for psychosis prevention: a systematic review and meta-analysis. Psychol Med 2014;44:449–468.

78 Marshall M, Rathbone J: Early intervention for psychosis. Cochrane Database Syst Rev 2011;37: CD004718.

79 Stafford MR, Jackson H, Mayo-Wilson E, et al: Early interventions to prevent psychosis: systematic review and meta-analysis. BMJ 2013;346:f185.

80 Preti A, Cella M: Randomized-controlled trials in people at ultra high risk of psychosis: a review of treatment effectiveness. Schizophr Res 2010;123:30–36.

81 Yusuf S, Sleight P, Pogue J, et al: Effects of an angiotensin-converting-enzyme inhibitor, ramipril, on cardiovascular events in high-risk patients. The Heart Outcomes Prevention Evaluation Study Investigators. N Engl J Med 2000;342:145–153.

82 Fusar-Poli P, Yung A: Should attenuated psychosis syndrome be included in DSM-5? The debate. Lancet 2012;379:591–592.

83 Häfner H BA, Klosterkötter J, Maurer K: Psychosen – Früherkennung und Frühintervention. Der Praxisleitfaden. Stuttgart, Schattauer, 2012.

84 Australian Government Department of Health: A Ten Year Roadmap for National Mental Health Reform. 2012, http://www.health.gov.au/internet/main/publishing.nsf/Content/mental-roadmap.

85 Birchwood M, Connor C, Lester H, et al: Reducing duration of untreated psychosis: care pathways to early intervention in psychosis services. Br J Psychiatry 2013;203:58–64.

86 National Institute for Health and Clinical Excellence Schizophrenia. Core Interventions in the Treatment and Management of Schizophrenia in Primary and Secondary Care (Update). London, NICE, 2009.

87 Bird V, Premkumar P, Kendall T, et al: Early intervention services, cognitive–behavioural therapy and family intervention in early psychosis: systematic review. Br J Psychiatry 2010;197:350–356.

88 Phillips LJ, Cotton S, Mihalopoulos C, et al: Cost implications of specific and non-specific treatment for young persons at ultra high risk of developing a first episode of psychosis. Early Interv Psychiatry 2009;3:28–34.

89 Valmaggia LR, McCrone P, Knapp M, et al: Economic impact of early intervention in people at high risk of psychosis. Psychol Med 2009;39:1617–1626.

90 Ising H, Smit F, Veling W, et al: Cost-effectiveness of preventing first-episode psychosis in ultra-high-risk subjects: multi-centre randomized controlled trial. Psychol Med 2015;45:1435–1446.

Prof. Dr. med. Andreas Bechdolf
Department of Psychiatry, Psychotherapy and Psychosomatics
Vivantes Klinikum am Urban and Vivantes Klinikum im Friedrichshain
Academic Hospital Charite Medicine Berlin
Dieffenbachstrasse 1, DE–10967 Berlin (Germany)
E-Mail andreas.bechdolf@vivantes.de

Riecher-Rössler A, McGorry PD (eds): Early Detection and Intervention in Psychosis: State of the Art and Future Perspectives. Key Issues Ment Health. Basel, Karger, 2016, vol 181, pp 159–167 (DOI: 10.1159/000440922)

Nonpharmalogical Substances for Early Intervention

Philippe Conus

Service of General Psychiatry, Department of Psychiatry-CHUV, Lausanne University, Lausanne, Switzerland

Abstract

Treatment of ultra-high-risk (UHR) patients was initially based on atypical antipsychotic medication, combined or not with psychotherapy. Considering antipsychotic prescription in patients without full-blown psychosis is questionable, various alternatives have been explored, three of which are discussed in this chapter. First, based on the hypothesis of excessive apoptosis in emerging psychosis, neuroprotection has emerged as a target for treatment. Among neuroprotective substances, polyunsaturated fatty acids (PUFA) have received considerable attention. After trials in chronic and first-episode psychosis patients, a study in UHR subjects revealed that PUFA induced a significantly greater reduction of symptoms and transition rate to psychosis than placebo maintained over 12 months. Second, based on the N-methyl-D-aspartate receptor hypoactivity model of schizophrenia, two preliminary trials based on the administration of glycine in UHR patients were promising, with an impact on positive, negative and cognitive symptoms. Thirdly, based on the observation of a glutathione deficit (GSH, a potent antioxidant) in chronic schizophrenia, redox dysregulation has been identified as a potential mechanism in the development of psychosis. N-acetyl-cysteine, a precursor of GSH, has been trialed in chronic schizophrenia and has shown a beneficial impact on negative symptoms and extrapyramidal side effects; trials are currently underway in first-episode psychosis and UHR patients. Although these developments are promising, the limited evidence-based knowledge on the mechanisms involved in the early stages of psychosis is a major limiting factor for the development of new treatments; additional efforts in translational research are needed in order to better understand the neurobiological mechanisms underlying the emergence of psychotic disorders.
© 2016 S. Karger AG, Basel

The first treatment strategies proposed to ultra-high-risk (UHR) patients were based on the adaptation of existing treatment concepts applied to full-blown psychosis: low-dose antipsychotic medication, cognitive behavioral therapy or a combination of both. The aims of such treatments were mainly to delay or prevent transition to full-blown psychosis, and they have shown a certain degree of efficacy in the context of three randomized controlled studies conducted in UHR patient samples.

The first trial was conducted by McGorry et al. [1] who compared, in a 6-month study, a combination of risperidone (1–2 mg/day) and cognitive behavioral therapy in 31 UHR subjects to a 'needs-based intervention' offered to 28 other UHR subjects. The second trial [2] compared, over a 12-month period, 31 UHR patients who received 5–15 mg of olanzapine per day with 29 patients who received placebo. In the third study, Ruhrmann et al. [3] compared, in a 12-week trial, needs focus therapy with and without adjunction of amisulpride. Taken globally, these trials showed a significant decrease in the rate of transition to psychosis in the short term, but when intervention was shorter than 6 months, the effect was not maintained in the long term, suggesting that the impact of such treatment is mainly to delay the onset of the illness.

Despite these positive results, the use of antipsychotic medication remains controversial in UHR patient samples where the rate of false-positive diagnosis is high. The main limitations of this strategy are related to the potential stigmatization linked to prescription of such treatment to young patients and the important risk of side effects, among which the development of metabolic syndrome, weight gain, sexual dysfunction and extrapyramidal side effects can occur. In addition, long-term follow-up of medication trials have revealed their failure to durably influence the rate of transition to psychosis. More importantly, using antipsychotic medication in UHR patients may not be the best approach at a conceptual level. Indeed, the neurobiological mechanisms occurring in this phase of the illness may be different from those occurring at later stages. Rather than receptor blockade, treatment in the prodromal phase may need to aim at another level, targeting for example certain types of changes in the brain structure and functioning which may be occurring during this phase.

The best choice at this illness stage may, for example, be to develop 'neuroprotective' treatments, a domain which has captured a lot of attention in recent years and which relies on two main concepts. The first is the concept of apoptosis, the mechanism of natural cell death. It has been suggested [4] that this mechanism may become uncontrolled or pathological in certain contexts, leading to the development of brain dysfunction and hence to the emergence of disorders such as psychosis. Apoptosis is based on a set of complex mechanisms, but various compounds may inhibit or regulate excessive apoptosis and therefore result in 'neuroprotection'. Various substances with putative neuroprotective properties have been identified and are currently under study [5]. The second concept is linked to the hypothesis that the illness process may in this phase involve the development of micro- and macrocircuit disturbances in the brain, based on dysregulation of receptor function, lesions of synapses or neurons, and disruption of myelination. Various novel treatment strategies have been developed on the basis of these two concepts, three of which will be discussed here below in more detail.

Polyunsaturated Fatty Acids

Polyunsaturated fatty acids (PUFAs) or omega-3 and omega-6 fatty acids are essential to normal brain development, synaptic plasticity and functioning. Considering they cannot be synthesized by humans, they must be ingested in sufficient amounts. Indeed, PUFAs are major constituents of cell membrane phospholipids and play a central role in receptor binding, neurotransmission and signal transduction [4]. It has been shown that PUFA deprivation during pregnancy (in animals as well as humans) is associated with developmental and behavioral abnormalities and that these are improved by PUFA supplementation. In addition, decreased PUFA levels in blood and postmortem brain cell membranes have been observed in various neuropsychiatric conditions such as schizophrenia, bipolar disorders, major depression and ADHD, suggesting they may play a role in these disorders.

PUFAs have captured additional interest considering they may serve as peripheral biomarkers in the context of various illnesses through measurement of their concentration in erythrocyte membranes. For example, Amminger et al. [6] found that PUFA levels are correlated with the rate of conversion to psychosis in UHR patients. In a later study, the same group [7] found that lower levels of PUFAs were related to higher levels of negative symptoms in UHR subjects. Finally, Peters et al. [8] found that erythrocyte membrane PUFA concentrations appear to be related to brain white matter integrity in early psychosis.

Various studies have explored the impact of PUFA supplementation in patients. Seven trials have been conducted in samples of patients with chronic schizophrenia. The design of these studies was generally the addition of PUFA to usual medication and assessment of its potential impact on symptom intensity, quality of life, functional level and side effects. Two studies [9, 10] found no impact and five [11–15] found a limited impact on various symptom dimensions. Globally, the small amplitude of the effect may be linked to the fact that, in chronic patients, the deleterious effect of increased apoptosis is already established, limiting the potential benefit of PUFA supplementation.

One randomized controlled trial has been conducted in a sample of 69 first-episode psychosis patients [16]. In the frame of this double-blind, parallel-group augmentation trial, subjects were randomized either to 2 g/day of purified ethyl-eicosapentaenoic acid (E-EPA, a long-chain PUFA) or to placebo, in addition to a flexible dose of atypical antipsychotic (risperidone, olanzapine or quetiapine), over a period of 12 weeks. Outcome measures were symptoms, functional level and side effects. While there was no significant difference between groups on any dimension at the 12-week endpoint, survival analysis of time to first response revealed that the patient group which received E-EPA had a faster response to treatment. In addition, E-EPA patients needed lower amounts of antipsychotic medication and had fewer side effects. The authors concluded that addition of PUFA to standard treatment may contribute to faster treatment response, decreased need for antipsychotic medication and moderation of side effects, and that the absence of a difference between groups may have been linked to limited sample size, potential influence of PUFA in the diet of the placebo group, type of PUFA used in the trial and ceiling effect due to the high rate of response to antipsychotic medication. Similarly to trials conducted in samples of chronic patients, it may well be that consequences of apoptosis were already established at this stage of illness, limiting the potential influence of the treatment.

More recently, treatment with PUFA has been tried in UHR patients [17]. In this randomized placebo-controlled trial, Amminger et al. [17] aimed at determining whether omega-3 PUFA prescribed to UHR subjects could prevent transition to first-episode psychosis and/or reduce psychiatric symptoms and improve functioning. A sample of 81 participants fulfilling UHR criteria were randomly assigned to 12 weeks of 1.2 g/day of omega-3 PUFA or placebo and assessed again 1 year after study baseline. Outcome measures were the rate of transition to psychosis, the evolution of symptoms and the level of side effects. While 98% of the patients completed the study (suggesting that PUFAs were well accepted by patients), data analysis revealed that the transition rate to psychosis at 12 months was significantly lower in the PUFA group than in the placebo group (4.9 vs. 27.5%, respectively, p = 0.007). In addition, PUFA patients had significantly lower levels of symptoms on PANNS [18] positive (p = 0.01), negative (p = 0.02) and general (p = 0.01) scales, as well as a better functional level as measured by the GAF [19] score (p = 0.002). There was, however, no difference regarding occurrence of side effects. The authors concluded that long-chain omega-3 PUFAs significantly reduce the risk of progression to psychotic disorder in UHR patients and that their prescription may be a preferable strategy to antipsychotic medication in such patients. While it is remarkable that the effect of PUFA treatment was maintained 9 months after its cessation, the study was limited by its sample size and the short duration of outcome assessment, and therefore needs replication, which is underway in the frame of a large multicenter study.

In a post hoc analysis of their data [20], the authors explored the time at which PUFA began to have an impact on symptoms. Through a mixed-model method, they managed to determine at which point the placebo and active treatment group started to significantly differ. The analysis revealed that subtypes of symptoms responded at different time points, starting with general and total PANSS scores at week 4, positive symptoms at week 8, and negative symptoms and GAF score at week 12, in a temporal cascade that is similar to what is observed with antipsychotic treatment. Interestingly, the beneficial effects on psychopathology, some of which were established as early as in the fourth week of treatment, were maintained throughout the entire 12-month follow-up period, well after the administration of PUFA had been interrupted.

Considering the rising interest in omega-3 PUFA supplementation as a preventive treatment strategy in young people at risk of psychosis, the question of their safety needed to be addressed, which was done in a recent review paper [21]. Based on the available data, the most commonly occurring but clinically rarely significant symptoms are mild gastrointestinal symptoms. The sometimes mentioned slight risk of prolonged bleeding time has not been shown to be clinically relevant. Finally, some differential effects on metabolic parameters, most of which appear beneficial, have been mentioned, but do not constitute an obstacle for treatment. The authors concluded on this basis that the available data suggest that PUFAs are safe, even at high doses.

N-Methyl-D-Aspartate Receptor Agonists

The N-methyl-D-aspartate receptor (NMDAR) hypoactivity model is a leading neurobiological hypothesis of schizophrenia [22]. It is based on the observation of an exacerbation of positive and negative symptoms and cognitive impairment in schizophrenia patients by NMDAR agonists such as ketamine as well as the induction of similar effects in healthy humans. Evidence suggests that NMDAR hypoactivity may connect to other prominent models of psychosis, as it contributes to the development of dopamine hyperactivity in the striatum and to deficits in cortical synaptic plasticity.

Two pilot studies, reported in the same paper, have recently been conducted in UHR subjects on the basis of this concept [23] through the administration of glycine, an amino acid neurotransmitter which acts at the glycine/D-serine modulatory site of the NMDAR as a full coagonist with glutamate. The study aims were first to assess whether the size of any beneficial effect of glycine in UHR promised to be clinically meaningful and second to determine which aspect of the UHR state might be the best therapeutic target in future studies. In the first trial, 10 UHR subjects received open-label glycine at doses titrated to 0.8 g/kg/day for 8 weeks, followed by discontinuation and 16 weeks of evaluation for the durability of effects. In the second trial, 8 subjects were randomized to glycine versus placebo for 12 weeks in the frame of a double-blind design, followed by open-label administration of glycine at same dosages for another 12 weeks. Patients were evaluated every 2 weeks with the Scale of Psychosis-Risk Symptoms [24] as well as before and after treatment with a neurocognitive battery. Within-group and between-group effect sizes (ES) were calculated. ES were large for positive (open-label within-group = 1.10; double-blind between-group = –1.11) and total (–1.39 and –1.15 respectively) symptoms and medium to large (–0.74 and –0.79 respectively) for negative symptoms. Medium-to-large ES were also observed for several neurocognitive measures in the open-label study, although data were sparse. No safety concerns were identified. The authors considered that these results were promising, suggesting an association between glycine administration and reduction of symptoms with good ES and signs of a potential impact on cognitive function in UHR subjects. They concluded that further studies of agents facilitating NMDAR function in UHR patients were supported by these preliminary findings and that other approaches to NMDAR hypofunction should also be trialed through administration of other glycine site agonists (e.g. D-serine) or glycine transporter inhibitors (e.g. sarcosine). A recent case report on a 23-year-old schizophrenia patient who suffered from persistent negative and cognitive symptoms whose mental state improved with the administration of sarcosine at 2 g/day (later adapted to 1 g/day due to appearance of a 'manic-like' syndrome under the initial dosage) may be a first positive signal in this direction [25].

Redox Dysregulation

While various risk factors for schizophrenia have been identified, there is a need for the emergence of a theory which would allow the identification of a 'final common pathway' or 'hub' through which these factors converge to lead to the basic pathophysiological mechanisms involved in the emergence of the disorder. Research conducted over the last 20 years by Do et al. [26] led them to conceptualize such a candidate hub related to redox dysregulation resulting from a deficit in glutathione (GSH), a tripeptide known as the major intracellular nonprotein antioxidant. GSH is involved both in protection against cellular damage due to reactive oxygen and nitrogen species, and in maintenance of the thiol redox status that is critical to cell cycle regulation, cell differentiation and receptor activation (including NMDA receptor for example).

While evidence of oxidative stress damage has often been reported in peripheral tissues and postmortem brain of schizophrenia patients, its etiology is unclear. Do et al. [26] proposed that a genetically based deficit of GSH synthesis may be at the root of decreased antioxidant capacities in schizophrenia patients. This group has recently demonstrated an association between schizophrenia and a trinucleotide repeat polymorphism in the gene of a key enzyme involved in GSH synthesis, which suggests a genetic basis for redox dysregulation in at least a subgroup of schizophrenia patients [27]. Such a deficit in GSH has been demonstrated in schizophrenia patients, both in cerebrospinal fluid and in the prefrontal cortex with magnetic resonance spectroscopy [28]. A genetic origin is suggested by data gathered from 2 case-controlled studies where a 'high-risk' polymorphism, associated with low GSH levels, was found in close to 40% of patients, a prevalence 3 times higher than in control subjects [27].

More recently, Steullet et al. [29] have pushed the concept a step further and identified the potential interplay between glutamatergic system NMDAR hypofunction, neuroinflammation and redox dysregulation in constituting a hub towards which most of the genetic and environmental risk factors converge, leading, during neurodevelopment, both to microcircuit and macrocircuit impairments, and to symptoms of the illness as a consequence of altered functional and structural connectivity.

In this context, the idea to increase GSH levels in patients emerged as a potential avenue for treatment. Various characteristics of N-acetyl cysteine (NAC), a drug commercialized as an antidote for paracetamol intoxication and as an add-on treatment for bronchitis, suggest it may be a promising candidate in this aspect. First, NAC induces the in vivo synthesis of GSH through increased availability of cysteine, its metabolite. Second, NAC plays an important modulating role in expression of genes linked to oxidative stress. Third, NAC has a direct antioxidant effect via its free thiol group. Finally, NAC directly protects nervous cells against free radicals.

A recent publication [30] has explored the interaction between GSH deficit and myelin maturation, considering oligodendrocytes are highly vulnerable to altered redox states. In patients, the authors found that white matter integrity, as measured by multimodal brain imaging, was correlated to GSH levels. In an animal model of GSH deficit through the knockout of the genes coding for one of the key enzymes involved in its metabolism (GCLM-KO), a number of mature oligodendrocytes and myelin markers were decreased in the prefrontal cortex. At the molecular level, GSH deficit induced a decrease in the proliferation of oligodendrocyte progenitors that could be reversed by NAC. Taken together, these elements suggest that GSH and redox dysregulation play a critical role in the myelination process and white matter maturation in the prefrontal cortex of rodents and humans, a mechanism which may underlie the development of the schizophrenia syndrome.

These elements suggest that the development of new therapeutic approaches based on this hypothesis may have an impact on schizophrenia patients. The results of the first clinical trial based on NAC administration in schizophrenia patients were published in 2008 [31]. In this double-blind, randomized, placebo controlled trial, 140 patients with chronic schizophrenia received NAC (2 g/day) or placebo as an adjunction to usual medication for a duration of 24 weeks. The results showed that NAC induced a significantly greater decrease in negative symptoms and side effects (akathisia) than placebo. In a post hoc analysis of a subgroup of patients drawn from the same sample, EEG analysis revealed that NAC-treated patients displayed an improvement of mismatch negativity, an auditory-related, NMDA-dependent, evoked potential typically impaired in schizophrenia [32]. These results are encouraging considering mismatch negativity is a preattentional component of auditory perception which may gate some cognitive and functional capacities. The next clinical steps are to conduct trials at an earlier stage of the disorder, considering an earlier intervention may have a more pronounced impact at the various levels described above; a trial in first-episode psychosis patients is currently underway in Switzerland and another multicenter trial in UHR subjects is planned in Germany. Besides the potential clinical impact of an increase in levels, a better knowledge of the basic mechanisms linking redox dysregulation and GSH levels to the successive development phases of schizophrenia may pave the way to the identification of new biomarkers that may be useful not only for earlier diagnosis of UHR patients, but also for the assessment of illness stages and treatment response tools which are essential to the development of a clinically applicable staging model of treatment.

Conclusions

Various alternatives are currently being explored in order to provide new and better adapted treatments for UHR patients. While some promising results have been published, they need replication in larger samples before their results can be generalized. In addition, most mechanisms explaining their impact are still hypothetical, and globally, a better understanding and stronger evidence-based knowledge of neurobiological mechanisms involved in the early phase of psychotic disorders may greatly contribute to the development of new treatment strategies.

References

1 McGorry PD, Yung AR, Phillips LJ, Yuen HP, Francey S, Cosgrave EM, Germano D, Bravin J, McDonald T, Blair A, Adlard S, Jackson H: Randomized controlled trial of interventions designed to reduce the risk of progression to first-episode psychosis in a clinical sample with subthreshold symptoms. Arch Gen Psychiatry 2002;59:921–928.

2 McGlashan TH, Zipursky RB, Perkins D, Addington J, Miller T, Woods SW, Hawkins KA, Hoffman RE, Preda A, Epstein I, Addington D, Lindborg S, Trzaskoma Q, Tohen M, Breier A: Randomized, double-blind trial of olanzapine versus placebo in patients prodromally symptomatic for psychosis. Am J Psychiatry 2006;163:790–799.

3 Ruhrmann S, Bechdolf A, Kühn KU, Wagner M, Schultze-Lutter F, Janssen B, Maurer K, Häfner H, Gaebel W, Möller HJ, Maier W, Klosterkötter J; LIPS Study Group: Acute effects of treatment for prodromal symptoms for people putatively in a late initial prodromal state of psychosis. Br J Psychiatry Suppl 2007;51:s88–s95.

4 Berger GE, Wood S, McGorry PD: Incipient neurovulnerability and neuroprotection in early psychosis. Psychopharmacol Bull 2003;37:79–101.

5 Correll CU, Hauser M, Auther AM, Cornblatt BA: Research in people with the psychosis risk syndrome: a review of current evidence and future directions. J Child Psychol Psychiatry 2010;51:390–431.

6 Amminger GP, Schafer MR, Klier CM, Slavik JM, Holzer I, Goldstone S, Whitford TJ, McGorry PD, Berk M: Decreased nervonic acid levels in erythrocyte membranes predict psychosis in help-seeking ultra-high-risk individuals. Mol Psychiatry 2011;17:1150–1152.

7 Amminger PG, McGorry PD: Update on ω–3 polyunsaturated fatty acids in early stage psychotic disorders. Neuropsychoparmacology 2012;37:309–310.

8 Peters BD, Machielsen MW, Hoen WP, Caan MWA, Malhotra AK, Szeszko PR, Duran M, Olabarriaga SD, de Haan L: Polyunsaturated fatty acid concentration predicts myelin integrity in early-phase psychosis. Schizophr Bull 2013;39:830–838.

9 Fenton WS, Dickerson F, Boronow J, Hibbeln JR, Knable M: A placebo-controlled trial of omega-3 fatty acid (ethyl eicosapentaenoic acid) supplementation for residual symptoms and cognitive impairment in schizophrenia. Am J Psychiatry 2001;158:2071–2074.

10 Peet M, Horrobin DF; E-E Multicentre Study Group: A dose-ranging exploratory study of the effects of ethyl-eicosapentaenoate in patients with persistent schizophrenic symptoms. J Psychiatr Res 2002;36:7–18.

11 Mellor JE, Laugharne JDE, Peet M: Omega-3-fatty acid supplementation in schizophrenic patients. Hum Psychopharmacol 1996;11:39–46.

12 Peet M, Brind J, Ramchand CN, Shah S, Vankar GK: Two double-blind placebo-controlled pilot studies of eicosapentaenoic acid in the treatment of schizophrenia. Schizophr Res 2001;49:243–251.

13 Emsley R, Myburgh C, Oosthuizen P, van Rensburg SJ: Randomized, placebo-controlled study of ethyl-eicosapentaenoic acid as supplemental treatment in schizophrenia. Am J Psychiatry 2002;159:1596–1598.

14 Arvindakshan M, Ghate M, Ranjekar PK, Evans DR, Mahadik SP: Supplementation with a combination of omega-3 fatty acids and antioxidants (vitamins E and C) improves the outcome of schizophrenia. Schizophr Res 2003;62:195–204.

15 Sivrioglu EY, Kirli S, Sipahioglu D, Gursoy B, Sarandöl E: The impact of omega-3 fatty acids, vitamins E and C supplementation on treatment outcome and side effects in schizophrenia patients treated with haloperidol: an open-label pilot study. Prog Neuropsychopharmacol Biol Psychiatry 2007;31:1493–1499.

16 Berger GE, Proffitt TM, McConchie M, Yuen H, Wood SJ, Amminger GP, Brewer W, McGorry PD: Ethyl-eicosapentaenoic acid in first-episode psychosis: a randomized, placebo-controlled trial. J Clin Psychiatry 2007;68:1867–1875.

17 Amminger GP, Schäfer MR, Papageorgiou K, Klier CM, Cotton SM, Harrigan SM, Mackinnon A, McGorry PD, Berger GE: Long-chain omega-3 fatty acids for indicated prevention of psychotic disorders: a randomized, placebo-controlled trial. Arch Gen Psychiatry 2010;67:146–154.

18 Kay SR, Fiszbein A, Opler LA: The positive and negative syndrome scale (PANSS) for schizophrenia. Schizophr Bull 1987;13:261–276.

19 Diagnostic and Statistical Manual of Mental Disorders, ed 4. Washington, American Psychiatric Association, 1994.

20 Mossaheb N, Schäfer MR, Schlögelhofer M, Klier CM, Cotton SM, McGorry PD, Amminger GP: Effect of omega-3 fatty acids for indicated prevention of young patients at risk for psychosis: when do they begin to be effective? Schizophr Res 2013;148:163–167.

21 Schlögelhofer M, Amminger GP, Schaefer MR, Fusar-Poli P, Smesny S, McGorry P, Berger G, Mossaheb N: Polyunsaturated fatty acids in emerging psychosis: a safer alternative? Early Interv Psychiatry 2014;8:199–208.

22 Javitt DC: Twenty-five years of glutamate in schizophrenia: are we there yet? Schizophr Bull 2012;38:911–913.

23 Woods SW, Walsh BC, Hawkins KA, Miller TJ, Saksa JR, D'Souza DC, Pearlson GD, Javitt DC, McGlashan TH, Krystal JH: Glycine treatment of the risk syndrome for psychosis: report of two pilot studies. Eur Neuropsychopharmacol 2013;23:931–940.

24 Hawkins KA, McGlashan TH, Quinlan D, Miller TJ, Perkins DO, Zipursky RB, Addington J, Woods SW: Factorial structure of the Scale of Prodromal Symptoms. Schizophr Res 2004;68:339–347.

25 Strzelecki D, Szyburska J, Rabe-Jabłońska J: Two grams of sarcosine in schizophrenia – is it too much? A potential role of glutamate-serotonin interaction. Neuropsychiatr Dis Treat 2014;10:263–266.

26 Do KQ, Conus P, Cuenod M: Redox dysregulation and oxidative stress in schizophrenia: nutrigenetics as a challenge in psychiatric disease prevention. J Nutrigenet Nutrigenomics 2010;3:267–289.

27 Gysin R, Kraftsik R, Boulat O, Bovet P, Conus P, Comte-Krieger E, Polari A, Steullet P, Preisig M, Teichmann T, Cuénod M, Do KQ: Genetic dysregulation of glutathione synthesis predicts alteration of plasma thiol redox status in schizophrenia. Antioxid Redox Signal 2011;15:2003–2010.

28 Do KQ, Trabesinger AH, Kirsten-Krüger M, Lauer CJ, Dydak U, Hell D, Holsboer F, Boesiger P, Cuénod M : Schizophrenia: glutathione deficit in cerebrospinal fluid and prefrontal cortex in vivo. Eur J Neurosci 2000;12:3721–3728.

29 Steullet P, Cabungcal JH, Monin A, Dwir D, O'Donnell P, Cuenod M, Do KQ: Redox dysregulation, neuroinflammation, and NMDA receptor hypofunction: a 'central hub' in schizophrenia pathophysiology? Schizophr Res 2014;pii:S0920-9964(14)00313-2.

30 Monin A, Baumann PS, Griffa A, Xin L, Mekle R, Fournier M, Butticaz C, Klaey M, Cabungcal JH, Steullet P, Ferrari C, Cuenod M, Gruetter R, Thiran JP, Hagmann P, Conus P, Do KQ: Glutathione deficit impairs myelin maturation: relevance for white matter integrity in schizophrenia patients. Mol Psychiatry 2015;20:827–838.

31 Berk M, Copolov D, Dean O, Lu K, Jeavons S, Schapkaitz I, Hunt MA, Judd F, Katz F, Katz P, Jespersen S, Little J, Do KQ, Conus P, Bush AI: N-acetyl cysteine as a glutathione precursor for schizophrenia: a double blind randomised placebo controlled trial. Biol Psychiatry 2008;64:361–368.

32 Lavoie S, Murray MM, Deppen P, Knyazeva MG, Berk M, Boulat O, Bovet P, Conus P, Copolov D, Cuenod M, Meuli R, Solida A, Buclin T, Do KQ: Glutathione precursor, N-acetyl-cysteine, improves mismatch negativity in schizophrenia patients. Neuropsychopharmacology 2008;33:2187–2199.

Prof. Philippe Conus
PGE/DP-CHUV
Hôpital de Cery
CH–1008 Prilly (Switzerland)
E-Mail philippe.conus@chuv.ch

Riecher-Rössler A, McGorry PD (eds): Early Detection and Intervention in Psychosis: State of the Art and Future Perspectives. Key Issues Ment Health. Basel, Karger, 2016, vol 181, pp 168–178 (DOI: 10.1159/000440923)

Pharmacological Intervention in First-Episode Psychosis

Brian O'Donoghue · Marc Walter · Christian G. Huber · Undine E. Lang

Orygen, The National Centre of Excellence in Youth Mental Health, University of Melbourne, Parkville, Vic., Australia

Abstract

Early psychosis represents a distinct period in which specific guidelines for the use of antipsychotic medications apply. Individuals with a first episode of psychosis are typically drug-naive and while they tend to respond to lower doses, they are also more sensitive to side effects. As a result of this, guidelines for the use of antipsychotic medication in early psychosis have been developed and provide guidance on their appropriate use, such as the concept of 'start low, go slow'. While the introduction of second-generation antipsychotic medications led to a reduction in the side effects traditionally associated with the earlier first-generation antipsychotic medication such as extrapyramidal side effects and tardive dyskinesia, they are associated with different side effects, such as metabolic syndrome and sexual dysfunction. Adherence to antipsychotic medication is low, often below 50%, and the reasons for this are multifactorial and include insight, attitudes towards medication and engagement. There is a lack of clarity as to how long individuals who have remitted from a first episode of psychosis should remain on antipsychotic medication. High relapse rates have been observed following the discontinuation of antipsychotic medication; however, there is emerging evidence that earlier discontinuation could be associated with higher functioning in the longer term. This chapter will first introduce the general underlying mechanism of action associated with antipsychotic medication and will broadly discuss the effectiveness of the different antipsychotic medications. International guidelines specific for the use of antipsychotic medication in early psychosis have been developed and the general principles of these guidelines and recommendations specific to certain guidelines will be outlined. There are a wide range of side effects associated with antipsychotic medications; however, two particular side effects will be discussed, namely metabolic syndrome and sexual dysfunction, as they are highly prevalent with the newer second-generation antipsychotic medications. These side effects, in addition to other factors, contribute to the low adherence rates in early psychosis. The clinical dilemma of how long antipsychotic medication should be continued in individuals who have remitted from a first episode of psychosis will be discussed. Finally, the current controversy of whether antipsychotic medication could be responsible for changes in brain structure will be reviewed.

Mechanism of Action of Antipsychotic Medication

The dopamine hypothesis is a long-standing theory in the aetiology of psychotic disorders and has relevance for the underlying mechanism of action of antipsychotic medication. This theory hypothesizes that the symptoms of psychosis are due to an excess dopaminergic function, either by excess dopamine, increased sensitivity to dopamine or increased density of receptors [1]. It is based on the findings that the potency of antipsychotic medications is correlated with the level of dopamine blockage [2]. Furthermore, it has been found that the activation of the dopamine system, such as by amphetamines, can induce psychotic symptoms [3, 4]. Additionally, when dopamine levels are decreased due to inhibition of dopamine synthesis, a reduction in psychotic symptoms is observed [5].

The dopamine hypothesis has evolved and has undergone two modifications in the last two decades. In 1991, Davis et al. [6] proposed the 'modified dopamine hypothesis of schizophrenia', which incorporated the findings that there are areas (the prefrontal cortex) with reduced dopamine levels. Thus, the major advance of the second version of the dopamine hypothesis was to identify areas of increased dopamine (subcortical area) and reduced dopamine (prefrontal cortex) that are associated with psychotic disorders. In a 'third version' of the dopamine hypothesis published in 2009, Howes and Kapur [7] proposed that dopamine dysregulation is the final common pathway leading to psychosis and there are multiple 'hits' that interact to lead to this dopamine dysregulation.

The dopamine hypothesis is important because the clinical effectiveness of antipsychotic medications is related to the affinity for the dopamine receptor [8], in particular the potency of antipsychotic medication is related to the level of D2 receptor blockage [1].

Treatment Guidelines and Dosing

A number of clinical practice guidelines for the use of antipsychotic medication in people experiencing first-episode psychosis (FEP) have been developed and five guidelines will be focused upon in this chapter, namely the International Clinical Practice Guidelines for Early Psychosis [9], Schizophrenia Patient Outcomes Research Team (PORT) psychopharmacological treatment guidelines [10], The National Institute for Health and Care Excellence (NICE) guidelines [11], the Maudsley Prescribing Guidelines [12] and the Australian Clinical Guidelines for Early Psychosis [13]. These guidelines have some similar recommendations that are applicable to FEP individuals, which will be discussed collectively, in addition to any unique recommendations of specific guidelines. All of the guidelines acknowledge that individuals with an FEP represent a unique group and that the research involving antipsychotic medication on individuals with more enduring psychotic disorders may not necessarily apply to those with an FEP. Importantly, these guidelines highlight the need to introduce antipsychotic medication with great care in individuals who are drug naive, the need for using the minimum effective dose and to avoid the use of typical or first-generation antipsychotic medications if possible. Furthermore, the use of polypharmacy with antipsychotic medications is not advised. Another general principle is the need to distinguish non-affective psychotic disorders from affective psychotic disorders, as psychopharmacological management differs between these broad categories.

The International Clinical Practice Guidelines for Early Psychosis are of significant importance as they were developed by 29 invited international experts and the final guidelines were ratified by the International Early Psychosis Association [9]. These guidelines emphasize the need to 'start low, go slow' by commencing with a low dose and titrating upwards very slowly over a period of several weeks. An example of an initial low target dose of 2 mg of risperidone or 7.5 mg of olanzapine was provided.

The PORT psychopharmacological treatment guidelines have undergone two revisions and the most recent guidelines were published in 2009 [10]. The most recent guidelines incorporated the findings of the European First-Episode Schizophrenia Trial (EUFEST) [14]. The PORT guidelines highlighted that there is little difference in the effectiveness of first-generation antipsychotics (FGAs) and second-generation antipsychotics (SGAs), and that the main difference appears to be in the side-effect profile. A unique aspect of the PORT treatment guidelines is that they did not recommend the use of olanzapine as the first line in FEP due to the propensity for significant weight gain with this SGA.

It is common in FEP individuals to have to switch antipsychotic medications due to either poor tolerability or effectiveness. The Maudsley Prescribing Guidelines are updated every 2–3 years and provide recommendations on switching medications, in addition to providing information on the minimum effective dosages for different antipsychotic medications. NICE has also produced specific guidelines for the treatment of psychosis in children and young people [15]. These guidelines emphasize the need to exercise caution in the prescribing of antipsychotic medication and to consider possible side effects in making this decision, in particular the metabolic side effects. The NICE clinical guidelines for the treatment of psychosis in children and young people also advise that if the young person and their parents or caregivers continually express a wish to try psychological interventions alone without the use of antipsychotic medication that this could be facilitated as a trial for 1 month or less, and during this time symptoms, distress and functioning should be assessed regularly [15].

Effectiveness

The introduction of SGA medications was heralded as a major breakthrough for the treatment of psychotic disorders. Subsequently, however, doubt arose regarding their overall efficacy compared to the FGAs. This debate was addressed by Leucht et al. [16], who conducted a meta-analysis that included 150 double-blind studies with a total of

21,533 participants. The meta-analysis found that four of the SGAs (amisulpride, clozapine, olanzapine, risperidone) were better than FGAs for overall efficacy. The study demonstrated that SGAs were less likely to cause extrapyramidal side effects than FGAs; however, with the exception of aripiprazole and ziprasidone, the SGAs caused more weight gain.

In regard to which antipsychotic medication should be the preferred first-line option for the treatment of psychotic disorders, Leucht et al. [17] undertook a multiple-treatment meta-analysis comparing 15 antipsychotic medications and used data from 212 randomized controlled trials that had a total of 43,049 participants. The study found that clozapine was the most effective antipsychotic medication compared to all of the other antipsychotics. Following clozapine, amisulpride, olanzapine and risperidone were significantly more effective than other antipsychotic medications. It should be considered in interpreting these results that clozapine is a third-line treatment and some guidelines now recommend olanzapine to be used in the second line.

Despite the superior effectiveness that has been demonstrated with clozapine, there is a hesitancy in clinical practice to switch individuals to clozapine after two unsuccessful trials of other antipsychotic medications. This is possibly due to concerns about side effects and the image of clozapine as a 'last resort'. Agid et al. [18] evaluated a treatment algorithm within an early psychosis programme and individuals with an FEP who did not respond to two SGAs had a trial of clozapine as early as 25 weeks into the start of their treatment. While over three quarters of participants responded to the initial antipsychotic, of the remainder, less than one quarter responded to the second antipsychotic trial. Those that agreed to commence clozapine experienced a reduction in the severity of symptoms and improvement in clinical global inventory compared to those who selected not to commence clozapine. Surprisingly, there has been limited research on the effectiveness of switching antipsychotic medications in non-responders and at what stage the use of clozapine should be considered. Leucht et al. [19] conducted a systematic review on this topic and found only ten randomized controlled trials on switching antipsychotic medications, but none of these studies were conclusive and they were not conducted in early psychosis cohorts. This lack of an evidence base formed the rationale for the design and conduct of the Optimization of Treatment and Management of Schizophrenia in Europe (OPTiMiSE) Trial. This study aims to recruit 500 participants with an FEP who will be treated with amisulpride. After 4 weeks, non-responders will be randomized to receive either amisulpride or olanzapine for 6 weeks and non-responders will receive an open trial of clozapine. Results of the OPTiMiSE trial are expected in early 2016.

Side Effects and Management

There are a large number of potential side effects associated with antipsychotic medication including sedation, metabolic (weight gain, glucose intolerance and dyslipidaemia), cardiac (QT prolongation, myocarditis), sexual dysfunction, hyperprolactaemia, tardive dyskinesia and extrapyramidal side effects [12]. Furthermore, individuals taking antipsychotic medication can experience dystonic reactions or the rare but serious side effect of neuroleptic malignant syndrome. A review of all of the potential side effects in detail is beyond the scope of this chapter. However, two common side effects, metabolic side effects and sexual dysfunction, will be discussed in detail.

The weight gain associated with SGAs was initially underestimated and it has been hypothesized that this may have been due to medication trials being conducted with individuals in a later phase of an enduring psychotic disorder. It has been argued that young people with no previous exposure to antipsychotic medication are more susceptible to rapid and pronounced weight gain [20]. Alvarez-Jimenez et al. [21] re-examined trial data from studies involving antipsychotic medication and found that young people with an FEP after 3 months of initiation of antipsychotic medication had higher weight gain, such as 7.1–9.2 kg with olanzapine, 4.0–5.6 kg with risperidone and 2.6–3.8 kg with haloperidol. These findings were replicated by Maayan and Correll [22] who undertook a review of antipsychotic related weight gain in youth (not specific for psychotic disorders) and found weight gain of 3.8–16.2 kg with olanzapine, 0.9–9.5 kg with clozapine and 1.9–7.2 kg with risperidone. The aforementioned review by Leucht et al. [17] on the tolerability of different antipsychotic medications also identified olanzapine as having the highest propensity for weight gain.

Poor diet and a sedentary lifestyle are also factors that contribute to weight gain in young people with an FEP. This weight gain can be attenuated or reduced by both pharmacological and non-pharmacological interventions. Alvarez-Jimenez et al. [23] undertook a meta-analysis and found that nutritional counselling, cognitive-behavioural therapy and individual or group interventions could reduce weight gain. Curtis et al. [24] demonstrated that an individualized lifestyle and life skills intervention that included health coaching, dietetic support and supervised exercise prescription for young people with an FEP could attenuate the weight gain associated with antipsychotic medication. It has been recommended that if lifestyle interventions are not successful in either reducing or preventing weight gain, then metformin, which is a medication for diabetes, could be considered [25].

Sexual dysfunction is common amongst individuals with enduring psychotic disorders, as one study found that 82% of men and 96% of women with schizophrenia had at least one form of sexual dysfunction [26]. However, in the limited studies conducted to date, the prevalence of sexual dysfunction in early psychosis appears lower, but it is still clinically significant. In the European First Episode Schizophrenia Trial (EUFEST), 490 individuals with a first episode of a schizophrenia spectrum disorder were randomized to receive either haloperidol, amisulpride, olanzapine, quetiapine or ziprasidone [27]. 31% of males reported decreased libido and 16 and 18% reported erectile and ejaculatory dysfunction, respectively. There was a similar prevalence of decreased libido in females (28%) and 12% reported amenorrhoea. Higher levels of negative symptoms were associated with deceased libido in both males and females. With the exception of amenorrhoea and galactorrhoea, there was no difference in the prevalence of sexual dysfunction between the different antipsychotics studied in EUFEST.

Sexual dysfunction has been largely attributed to antipsychotic medication [28]; however, there is some evidence to suggest that it may be a consequence of the disorder. In order to disentangle this relationship, Marques et al. [29] examined the prevalence of sexual dysfunction in individuals at ultra-high risk for psychosis and compared the prevalence to the rates in FEP and in healthy controls. The study found that 50% of the ultra-high-risk group, who were not receiving antipsychotic medication, experienced at least one type of clinical sexual dysfunction, compared with 65% of the FEP group and 21% of the control group. These findings suggest that the sexual dysfunction experienced in early psychosis is partially contributed to by antipsychotic medication.

Despite the prevalence of this side effect, there are limited guidelines on how to sufficiently manage sexual dysfunction. The Australian Clinical Guidelines for Early Psychosis recommends that if sexual dysfunction occurs and is related to pharmacotherapy, then the dose should be reduced or the individual could be switched to a different antipsychotic medication [13]. A Cochrane review on the management of sexual dysfunction due to antipsychotic medication has been conducted; however, there were only four studies with a total of 138 participants [30]. The Cochrane review concluded that more interventions need to be trialed with the aim of reducing antipsychotic-induced sexual dysfunction.

Compliance/Adherence

Adherence to prescribed antipsychotic medication is a significant challenge in the treatment of early psychosis, as overall rates of non-adherence have been estimated to be less than 50% in individuals with an FEP [31, 32]. In the aforementioned EUFEST study, Czobor et al. [33] found that low levels of insight at baseline in individuals with a first episode of a schizophrenia spectrum disorder predicted non-adherence after 1 month and 1 year, and the presence of hostility predicted non-adherence in the short term. Leclerc et al. [34] conducted a review on the determinants of adherence to treatment in FEP that included 33 articles. The review found that non-adherence is multifactorial and is associated with individual level factors (lower educational level, substance use, forensic history, unemployment), environmental factors (no family involvement), medication-related factors (negative attitudes towards medication) and disorder-related factors (severe positive symptoms, longer duration of untreated psychosis). A further study by Drake et al. [35] identified five constructs that were associated with adherence: attitudes towards medication, self-esteem, accepting the need for treatment, self-rated insight and objective insight.

Despite the high prevalence of non-adherence and its clinical significance, as it is associated with higher relapse rates and hospitalization [36], knowledge is limited about how to improve adherence to antipsychotic medication. A systematic review was performed by Zygmunt et al. [37] in 2002 and an update on the intervention studies over the subsequent decade was performed by Barkhof et al. [38]. The reviews found that interventions that incorporated problem solving or motivational interviewing were more likely to be effective than more broadly based interventions, while interventions that relied on psychoeducation alone were typically ineffective. Interventions that involved supportive and rehabilitative community-based services were also more likely to be effective. Furthermore, interventions that offered more sessions during a longer period of time and focused continuously on adherence were also more likely to be effective, which demonstrates the challenges involved in non-adherence and the need to address it over the long term.

Other strategies of addressing adherence in the treatment of early psychosis include the use of long-acting injectable (LAI) antipsychotic medications [39]. While the use of LAIs have been shown to reduce relapse rates and readmission to hospital [40], it has been argued that LAIs are underutilized in early psychosis, possibly due to the stigma associated with this method of delivery and an underestimation of non-adherence in psychiatrists own patients [41].

How Long Should Antipsychotic Medication Be Continued?

The first episode represents a unique period in the management of psychosis where by definition there is no history of pattern of illness, diagnostic certainty is rare and the individual usually does not have any prior exposure to medications. Therefore, each management decision needs to be considered following a risk-benefit analysis taking into account the context of the individual [42]. There is uncertainty in the field as to how long antipsychotic medications should be continued after an FEP. On one hand, high relapse rates are observed in years following discontinuation of antipsychotic medication, with some studies reporting relapse rates of more than 80% within 5 years [43]. On the other hand, antipsychotic medications are associated with serious side effects that can interfere with the individual's quality of life. Clinical guidelines recommend the maintenance of antipsychotic medication for the first year after the onset of the disorder; however, there is no consensus in regard to longer periods of maintenance treatment [44].

A number of studies have attempted to address this important clinical question in regard to how long antipsychotic medication should be continued. Chen et al. [45] conducted a double-blind randomized controlled trial of maintenance treatment with 400 mg of quetiapine versus discontinuation (placebo) after 1 year of treatment in individuals who had achieved remission from an FEP. After 12 months, the proportion who relapse in the quetiapine group was 41% (95% CI: 29–53) compared to

79% (95% CI: 68–90) in the placebo group. A diagnosis of schizophrenia was a predictor of relapse. Two earlier studies, by Crow et al. [46] and Hogarty and Ulrich [47], found a higher rate of relapse following discharge from hospital in individuals with a first episode of schizophrenia who received placebo compared to an antipsychotic medication.

While these studies have demonstrated a higher relapse rate in individuals who discontinue their antipsychotic medication earlier, a study published by Wunderink et al. [48] has introduced another important aspect for consideration in the reduction or discontinuation of antipsychotic medications. In the initial study, Wunderink et al. [49] conducted an open trial in which 131 individuals with an FEP were randomized to maintenance treatment or discontinuation strategy. Similar to the previous studies, there was an initial higher rate of relapses in the group who attempted to discontinue their antipsychotic medication compared to the maintenance group (43 vs. 21%). However, a 7-year follow-up of this cohort found that while the initial relapse rates were higher in the discontinuation group, after approximately 3 years there was no difference in relapse rates between the groups. Furthermore, the main finding from this follow-up study was that despite symptom remission being similar across groups after 7 years, recovery rates were significantly higher in the individuals who received dose reduction/discontinuation compared to those that remained on maintenance treatment (40.4 vs. 17.6%). These findings by Wunderink et al. challenge the traditional thinking that relapse prevention is the top priority in treatment as opposed to an intermediate goal on the path to recovery [50]. Neurocognitive testing was conducted on a subgroup of this cohort and it was found that while neurocognition improved significantly in both groups, those who received dose reduction/discontinuation improved significantly more in verbal fluency and speed of processing [51]. While these findings need to replicated, the study poses an important question as to whether an initial higher rate of relapse could be a price worth paying for better longer-term functional recovery.

Controversies with Antipsychotic Medication

One of the controversies involving antipsychotic medication is the suggestion that they can significantly affect brain structure and account for progressive brain changes observed during the illness. Fusar-Poli et al. [52] undertook a meta-analysis of longitudinal MRI studies that had measures of brain volumes before and after the exposure to antipsychotic medication. The meta-analysis included 1,046 individuals with a diagnosis of schizophrenia and 780 controls, and found that there were progressive gray matter volume decreases and enlargement of the lateral ventricles in individuals with schizophrenia but not controls. The decreases in gray matter volume were inversely correlated with cumulative exposure to antipsychotic medication but not duration of illness or severity. The study concluded that some of the neuroanatomical alterations may be associated with antipsychotic medication; however, the study design could not determine causality. A similar systematic review on the MRI findings on brain structure changes associated with the use of antipsychotic medication was conducted by Navari and Dazzan [53] and found that the volumetric changes were of a greater magnitude with typical antipsychotic medications compared to the atypicals. The systematic review concluded that antipsychotic medication could potentially contribute to the brain structural changes observed in psychosis.

Another meta-analysis that included 43 studies was undertaken by Radua et al. [54] and it included all studies that reported whole-brain structural or cognitive functional imaging findings in individuals with an FEP. The meta-analysis on brain structure consisted of 965 individuals with an FEP matched with 1,040 controls and the meta-analysis on the functional imaging included 362 first episode cases and 403 controls. The meta-regression analysis indicated that gray matter volume in the anterior cingulate and left insular clusters was associated with exposure to antipsychotics and that individuals who had received antipsychotic medication were more likely to show structural abnormalities in these areas. However, as with the previous meta-analysis by Fusar-Poli, [52] the study design cannot determine causality.

Conclusion

Individuals experiencing an FEP represent a unique group in regard to treatment with antipsychotic medication. An approach of 'start low, go slow' can help ensure individuals receive the lowest effective dose, which will also help to minimize side effects. Meta-analyses have identified the antipsychotic medications which are more effective and specific early psychosis guidelines have made recommendations on second- and third-line treatment options.

Despite their established effectiveness, knowledge is still required on the optimal length of treatment with antipsychotic medications following remission of an FEP. Furthermore, strategies and interventions to reduce the adverse effects of antipsychotic medications are lacking and the development of such interventions could lead to improved adherence and quality of life for individuals with a psychotic disorder.

References

1 Howes O, McCutcheon R, Stone J: Glutamate and dopamine in schizophrenia: an update for the 21st century. J Psychopharmacol 2015;29:97–115.
2 Abi-Dargham A: Do we still believe in the dopamine hypothesis? New data bring new evidence. Int J Neuropsychopharmacol 2004;7(suppl 1):S1–S5.
3 Curran C, Byrappa N, McBride A: Stimulant psychosis: systematic review. Br J Psychiatry 2004;185:196–204.
4 Laruelle M, Abi-Dargham A, Gil R, Kegeles L, Innis R: Increased dopamine transmission in schizophrenia: relationship to illness phases. Biol Psychiatry 1999;46:56–72.
5 Abi-Dargham A, Rodenhiser J, Printz D, Zea-Ponce Y, Gil R, Kegeles LS, et al: Increased baseline occupancy of D2 receptors by dopamine in schizophrenia. Proc Natl Acad Sci U S A 2000;97:8104–8109.

6 Davis KL, Kahn RS, Ko G, Davidson M: Dopamine in schizophrenia: a review and reconceptualization. Am J Psychiatry 1991;148:1474–1486.

7 Howes OD, Kapur S: The dopamine hypothesis of schizophrenia: version III – the final common pathway. Schizophr Bull 2009;35:549–562.

8 Creese I, Burt D, Snyder S: Dopamine receptor binding predicts clinical and pharmacological potencies of antischizophrenic drugs. Science 1976;192:481–483.

9 International Early Psychosis Association Writing Group: International clinical practice guidelines for early psychosis. Br J Psychiatry 2005;187:s120–s124.

10 Buchanan RW, Kreyenbuhl J, Kelly DL, Noel JM, Boggs DL, Fischer BA, et al: The 2009 Schizophrenia PORT psychopharmacological treatment recommendations and summary statements. Schizophr Bull 2010;36:71–93.

11 National Institute for Health and Care Excellence Guidelines: Psychosis and Schizophrenia in Adults. Treatment and Management. London, NICE, 2014.

12 Taylor D, Paton C, Kapur S: The Maudsley Prescribing Guidelines in Psychiatry, ed 11. Hoboken, Wiley-Blackwell, 2012.

13 Early Psychosis Guidelines Writing Group: Australian Clinical Guidelines for Early Psychosis: A Brief Summary for Practitioners, ed 2. Melbourne, Orygen Youth Health, 2010.

14 Kahn RS, Fleischhacker WW, Boter H, Davidson M, Vergouwe Y, Keet IP, et al: Effectiveness of antipsychotic drugs in first-episode schizophrenia and schizophreniform disorder: an open randomised clinical trial. Lancet 2008;371:1085–1097.

15 National Institute for Health and Care Excellence Guidelines: Psychosis and Schizophrenia in Children and Young People: Recognition and Management. London, NICE, 2013. http://www.nice.org.uk/guidance/cg155.

16 Leucht S, Corves C, Arbter D, Engel RR, Li C, Davis JM: Second-generation versus first-generation antipsychotic drugs for schizophrenia: a meta-analysis. Lancet 2009;373:31–41.

17 Leucht S, Cipriani A, Spineli L, Mavridis D, Orey D, Richter F, et al: Comparative efficacy and tolerability of 15 antipsychotic drugs in schizophrenia: a multiple-treatments meta-analysis. Lancet 2013;382:951–962.

18 Agid O, Remington G, Kapur S, Arenovich T, Zipursky RB: Early use of clozapine for poorly responding first-episode psychosis. J Clin Psychopharmacol 2007;27:369–373.

19 Leucht S, Winter-van Rossum I, Heres S, Arango C, Fleischhacker WW, Glenthøj B, et al: The Optimization of Treatment and Management of Schizophrenia in Europe (OPTiMiSE) Trial: rationale for its methodology and a review of the effectiveness of switching antipsychotics. Schizophr Bull 2015;41:549–558.

20 Correll CU, Carlson HE: Endocrine and metabolic adverse effects of psychotropic medications in children and adolescents. J Am Acad Child Adolesc Psychiatry 2006;45:771–791.

21 Alvarez-Jimenez M, Gonzalez-Blanch C, Crespo-Facorro B, Hetrick S, Rodriguez-Sanchez JM, Perez-Iglesias R, et al: Antipsychotic-induced weight gain in chronic and first-episode psychotic disorders: a systematic critical reappraisal. CNS Drugs 2008;22:547–562.

22 Maayan L, Correll CU: Weight gain and metabolic risks associated with antipsychotic medications in children and adolescents. J Child Adolesc Psychopharmacol 2011;21:517–535.

23 Alvarez-Jimenez M, Hetrick SE, González-Blanch C, Gleeson JF, McGorry PD: Non-pharmacological management of antipsychotic-induced weight gain: systematic review and meta-analysis of randomised controlled trials. Br J Psychiatry 2008;193:101–107.

24 Curtis J, Watkins A, Rosenbaum S, Teasdale S, Kalucy M, Samaras K, et al: Evaluating an individualized lifestyle and life skills intervention to prevent antipsychotic-induced weight gain in first-episode psychosis. Early Interv Psychiatry 2015, Epub ahead of print.

25 Correll CU, Sikich L, Reeves G, Riddle M: Metformin for antipsychotic-related weight gain and metabolic abnormalities: when, for whom, and for how long? Am J Psychiatry 2013;170:947–952.

26 Macdonald S, Halliday J, MacEwan T, Sharkey V, Farrington S, Wall S, et al: Nithsdale Schizophrenia Surveys 24: sexual dysfunction. Case-control study. Br J Psychiatry 2003;182:50–56.

27 Malik P, Kemmler G, Hummer M, Riecher-Roessler A, Kahn RS, Fleischhacker WW: Sexual dysfunction in first-episode schizophrenia patients: results from European First Episode Schizophrenia Trial. J Clin Psychopharmacol 2011;31:274–280.

28 Cutler AJ: Sexual dysfunction and antipsychotic treatment. Psychoneuroendocrinology 2003;28(suppl 1):69–82.

29 Marques TR, Smith S, Bonaccorso S, Gaughran F, Kolliakou A, Dazzan P, et al: Sexual dysfunction in people with prodromal or first-episode psychosis. Br J Psychiatry 2012;201:131–136.

30 Schmidt HM, Hagen M, Kriston L, Soares-Weiser K, Maayan N, Berner MM: Management of sexual dysfunction due to antipsychotic drug therapy. Cochrane Database Syst Rev 2012;11:CD003546.

31 Coldham EL, Addington J, Addington D: Medication adherence of individuals with a first episode of psychosis. Acta Psychiatr Scand 2002;106:286–290.

32 Hill M, Crumlish N, Whitty P, Clarke M, Browne S, Kamali M, et al: Nonadherence to medication four years after a first episode of psychosis and associated risk factors. Psychiatr Serv 2010;61:189–192.

33 Czobor P, Volavka J, Derks EM, Bitter I, Libiger J, Kahn RS, et al: Insight and hostility as predictors and correlates of nonadherence in the European First Episode Schizophrenia Trial. J Clin Psychopharmacol 2013;33:258–261.

34 Leclerc E, Noto C, Bressan RA, Brietzke E: Determinants of adherence to treatment in first-episode psychosis: a comprehensive review. Rev Bras Psiquiatr 2015;37:168–176.

35 Drake RJ, Nordentoft M, Haddock G, Arango C, Fleischhacker WW, Glenthøj B, et al: Modeling determinants of medication attitudes and poor adherence in early nonaffective psychosis: implications for intervention. Schizophr Bull 2015;41:584–596.

36 Masand PS, Roca M, Turner MS, Kane JM: Partial adherence to antipsychotic medication impacts the course of illness in patients with schizophrenia: a review. Prim Care Companion J Clin Psychiatry 2009; 11:147–154.

37 Zygmunt A, Olfson M, Boyer CA, Mechanic D: Interventions to improve medication adherence in schizophrenia. Am J Psychiatry 2002;159:1653–1664.

38 Barkhof E, Meijer CJ, de Sonneville LMJ, Linszen DH, de Haan L: Interventions to improve adherence to antipsychotic medication in patients with schizophrenia – a review of the past decade. Eur Psychiatry 2012;27:9–18.

39 Kane JM: Strategies for improving compliance in treatment of schizophrenia by using a long-acting formulation of an antipsychotic: clinical studies. J Clin Psychiatry 2003;64(suppl 16):34–40.

40 Tiihonen J, Walhbeck K, Lönnqvist J, Klaukka T, Ioannidis JP, Volavka J, et al: Effectiveness of antipsychotic treatments in a nationwide cohort of patients in community care after first hospitalisation due to schizophrenia and schizoaffective disorder: observational follow-up study. BMJ 2006;333:224.

41 Patel MX, Taylor M, David AS: Antipsychotic long-acting injections: mind the gap. Br J Psychiatry Suppl 2009;52:S1–S4.

42 Malhi G, Adams D, Moss B, Walter G: To medicate or not to medicate, when diagnosis is in question: decision-making in first episode psychosis. Australas Psychiatry 2010;18:230–237.

43 Robinson D, Woerner MG, Alvir JJ, et al: Predictors of relapse following response from a first episode of schizophrenia or schizoaffective disorder. Arch Gen Psychiatry 1999;56:241–247.

44 Kane JM, Leucht S: Unanswered questions in schizophrenia clinical trials. Schizophr Bull 2008;34:302–309.

45 Chen EY, Hui CL, Lam MM, Chiu CP, Law CW, Chung DW, et al: Maintenance treatment with quetiapine versus discontinuation after one year of treatment in patients with remitted first episode psychosis: randomised controlled trial. BMJ 2010;341:c4024.

46 Crow TJ, MacMillan JF, Johnson AL, Johnstone EC: A randomised controlled trial of prophylactic neuroleptic treatment. Br J Psychiatry 1986;148:120–127.

47 Hogarty GE, Ulrich RF: The limitations of antipsychotic medication on schizophrenia relapse and adjustment and the contributions of psychosocial treatment. J Psychiatr Res 1998;32:243–250.

48 Wunderink L, Nieboer RM, Wiersma D, Sytema S, Nienhuis FJ: Recovery in remitted first-episode psychosis at 7 years of follow-up of an early dose reduction/discontinuation or maintenance treatment strategy: long-term follow-up of a 2-year randomized clinical trial. JAMA Psychiatry 2013;70:913–920.

49 Wunderink L, Nienhuis FJ, Sytema S, Slooff CJ, Knegtering R, Wiersma D: Guided discontinuation versus maintenance treatment in remitted first-episode psychosis: relapse rates and functional outcome. J Clin Psychiatry 2007;68:654–661.

50 McGorry P, Alvarez-Jimenez M, Killackey E: Antipsychotic medication during the critical period following remission from first-episode psychosis: less is more. JAMA Psychiatry 2013;70:898–900.

51 Faber G, Smid HG, Van Gool AR, Wiersma D, Van Den Bosch RJ: The effects of guided discontinuation of antipsychotics on neurocognition in first onset psychosis. Eur Psychiatry 2012;27:275–280.

52 Fusar-Poli P, Smieskova R, Kempton MJ, Ho BC, Andreasen NC, Borgwardt S: Progressive brain changes in schizophrenia related to antipsychotic treatment? A meta-analysis of longitudinal MRI studies. Neurosci Biobehav Rev 2013;37:1680–1691.

53 Navari S, Dazzan P: Do antipsychotic drugs affect brain structure? A systematic and critical review of MRI findings. Psychol Med 2009;39:1763–1777.

54 Radua J, Borgwardt S, Crescini A, Mataix-Cols D, Meyer-Lindenberg A, McGuire PK, et al: Multimodal meta-analysis of structural and functional brain changes in first episode psychosis and the effects of antipsychotic medication. Neurosci Biobehav Rev 2012;36:2325–2333.

Dr. Brian O'Donoghue
Orygen, The National Centre of Excellence in Youth Mental Health
University of Melbourne
35 Poplar Road, Parkville, VIC 3052 (Australia)
E-Mail briannoelodonoghue@gmail.com

Riecher-Rössler A, McGorry PD (eds): Early Detection and Intervention in Psychosis: State of the Art and Future Perspectives. Key Issues Ment Health. Basel, Karger, 2016, vol 181, pp 179–189 (DOI: 10.1159/000440924)

Early Detection and Intervention in Psychosis

Anita Riecher-Rössler[a] · Patrick D. McGorry[b]

[a]Center for Gender Research and Early Detection, University of Basel Psychiatric Clinics, Basel, Switzerland;
[b]Orygen, The National Centre of Excellence in Youth Mental Health, University of Melbourne, Parkville, Vic., Australia

Abstract

As this volume shows, early detection of and intervention in psychosis is a rapidly evolving and highly promising field of psychiatry. Starting with the early detection of frank psychosis and building up services for these patients, the field has in the meantime developed much further and deeper. There is now clear and accumulating evidence that early detection is also possible before transition to frank psychosis in the early prodromal and subthreshold psychotic states, i.e. in the sense of risk-assessment. Moreover, there is a large body of evidence regarding early intervention. However, it is also clear that there are still some unsolved problems and questions, and a lot has still to be done.

© 2016 S. Karger AG, Basel

Early Detection

As vigorous research during the last decades has demonstrated, early detection should be performed in a stepwise approach, using risk-enrichment strategies. Informing the public with a focus on risk groups and professionals about the early signs of psychosis and the possible steps to seek help is of utmost importance. Regular information campaigns, websites with self-screening instruments, helplines and all modern information technology should be used [1]. Psychiatrists and other medical staff should be trained using checklists and other materials.

With those seeking help or identified by primary care, specialized centers should perform further screening using established instruments such as the Comprehensive

Assessment of At-Risk Mental States (CAARMS) [2] or the Basel Screening Instrument for Psychosis (BSIP) [3]. These clinical instruments for detecting an at-risk state have a considerable diagnostic power which is even more enhanced when different instruments and assessment domains are combined.

Thus, not only so-called 'attenuated subthreshold symptoms' should be assessed, but also so-called 'basic symptoms' indicating the first subtle disturbances of information processing [see chapters by Klosterkötter, this vol., pp. 1–14, and Schultze-Lutter, this vol., pp. 29–41]. Thereby, early detection can be made more sensitive and start at an even earlier stage of the evolving disease when individuals still have full insight and do not yet suffer from functional decline. Furthermore, studies have shown that predictive accuracy could be improved by stronger weighting of selected positive and negative symptoms. Thus, high suspiciousness in the beginning seems to be a strong predictor of later transition [4–6]. The same seems to be true for high levels of anhedonia/asociality, especially withdrawal from peers [4, 7].

Assessments of psychopathology as early indicators of disease should always be accompanied by assessment of other risk factors such as genetic risk or drug abuse. For example, cannabis use is associated with a higher risk for psychosis [8] and should therefore be used for assessment of risk, just as any other known risk factors [for reviews, see 9, 10].

In a next step, neurocognitive testing, EEG and structural MRI of the brain should be performed in a research setting, followed by other domains such as functional MRI, PET, quantitative EEG, etc. These biomarkers allow for a more exact clinical staging of the risk [10].

We have established that patients with an at-risk mental state (ARMS) as compared to healthy controls show significant *cognitive disturbances* which are qualitatively similar but quantitatively not yet as severe as in first-episode psychosis patients [4, 10, 11]. Within the ARMS group, those with later progression to full psychosis already suffer from more marked deficits when they seek help at a specialized service than those without later transition. Impaired performance across a wide range of cognitive domains and especially in the areas of working memory, verbal fluency, verbal memory and speed of information processing could potentially be used for improving the accuracy of prediction [4, 11] [see chapter by Studerus et al., this vol., pp. 116–132]. When neurocognitive assessments were supplemented by measures of fine motor functioning, prediction accuracy could be improved [12]. Several studies have shown that integrative models combining neurocognitive performance with psychopathology show an added predictive value [4], although these integrative models still have some methodological limitations.

Clinical routine EEG as well as quantitative EEG can potentially further improve prediction accuracy if combined with symptomatology [13–15]. Other potential neurophysiological predictors have been described [10] [see chapter by Ruhrmann, this vol., pp. 133–141].

Table 1. Recommendations for daily clinical practice: stepwise diagnosis

Improve referrals through information campaigns, self-screening, etc.
Use instruments for clear clinical detection of ARMS or first-episode psychosis (e.g. BSIP or
  CAARMS and SPIA)
Use neurocognitive testing for
  better staging of risk within ARMS;
  planning of more specific, targeted therapy
Use EEG and MRI for
  exclusion of organic/exogenous causes;
  better staging of risk
Use further assessment domains (if available)

There is an especially large body of neuroimaging research which has taught us that there are not only structural and functional differences between ARMS and healthy controls, but also differences within the ARMS group: similar as in other domains, those with later transition to frank psychosis already at first presentation to a specialized service show more severe disturbances than those without later transition. The differences are seen in different regions of the brain and worsen with transition to psychosis [10, 16–20] [see chapter by Dwyer and McGuire, this vol., pp. 83–94].

Positron emission tomography studies indicate elevated striatal dopamine synthesis in high-risk individuals that is greater in those who later convert to psychosis [21, 22]. Several critical reviews and meta-analyses of structural, functional and neurochemical imaging findings in ARMS patients are now available [for a review, see 23]. Newer studies also show abnormal connectivity in emerging psychosis and in unaffected siblings of psychosis patients, potentially indicating enhanced vulnerability [see chapter by Schmidt and Borgwardt, this vol., pp. 103–115].

The main problem with MRI analyses has been that they can only contribute to prediction on a group level, not at the individual level. This problem may soon be solved by new methods of analysis such as the support vector machine [24] [see chapter by Koutsouleris, this vol., pp. 95–102]. Further biomarkers might emerge from psychoendocrinology, especially regarding altered stress hormones with HPA axis abnormalities [10] and HPG axis including prolactin abnormalities [25–27]. Also, inflammatory and oxidative stress markers as well as sleep and chronobiological markers and fatty acid markers might in the future contribute to refine clinical staging and sharpen prediction [10].

Based on these research findings, recommendations for clinicians regarding the stepwise diagnostic process have been issued in the meantime by the European Association of Psychiatry [28]. Apart from the aforementioned stepwise enrichment strategy and the multidomain assessments in the last steps, the process should also include a staging of the risk [10], differential diagnosis and exclusion of organic or exogenous causes of the clinical symptoms (table 1).

Table 2. Recommendations for daily clinical practice: early intervention in first-episode psychosis

Reduce stress/stimuli
Ensure sufficient sleep
Psychotherapeutic interventions to reduce anxiety, agitation and panic
Benzodiazepines until diagnosis is clear
Second-generation antipsychotics in minimal effective dosage for about 1 year
Treat comorbid disorders, esp. drug/cannabis abuse
Psychoeducation
Cognitive behavioral case management
Psychological training programs/cognitive remediation, etc.
Involvement of significant others (if patient agrees)
Treatment of physical disease
Social work
Reintegration into job/education
Assertive community treatment

Early Intervention

Regarding treatment approaches in emerging psychosis, there also is a substantial body of evidence.

Early Intervention in First-Episode Psychosis

One of the main goals of early detection services is the reduction of untreated psychosis as this has been shown to influence prognosis dramatically [see the Preface and Introduction by Riecher-Rössler and McGorry, this vol., pp. X–XIV]. Treatment and intervention services have shown how to do this (e.g. TIPS program, www.tips-info.com). As soon as a patient has made the transition to frank psychosis, there are quite clear guidelines for early intervention from different societies such as the World Psychiatric Association (WPA), World Federation of Societies of Biological Psychiatry (WFSBP), National Institute for Health and Clinical Excellence (NICE) and the Deutsche Gesellschaft für Psychiatrie und Psychotherapie (DGPPN; German Association for Psychiatry and Psychotherapy). More or less, they comprise similar recommendations such as reducing stress and stimuli, ensuring sleep, treatment with benzodiazepines until the diagnosis is clear and then second-generation antipsychotics [for reviews, see 29 and the chapter by McGorry and Goldstone, this vol., pp. 15–28, for pharmacological treatment, see chapter by O'Donoghue et al. this vol., pp. 168–178]. Table 2 lists some important interventions which might be helpful in first-episode patients.

Early Intervention in ARMS

Regarding early intervention in ARMS, we have also gathered a lot of experience. Most importantly, the setting to deliver help must be low threshold, low stigma and not a traditional psychiatric setting. The best approach is to focus on the need for care and the presenting problems which the patient is already aware of. The risk of a

Table 3. Recommendations for daily clinical practice: staged interventions in ARMS

Low risk:
  Treating the presenting symptoms and comorbidities: general symptomatic nonspecific
    supportive treatment and care [supportive therapy or cognitive behavioral case
    management, stress reduction, sleep regulation, medication as necessary for symptom
    management (no antipsychotics), social work, reduction of drug and cannabis use, etc.]
  Building a therapeutic relationship, information and education
  Monitoring the development of the disease
Greater risk:
  More specific and more intense psychotherapy (e.g. specific cognitive behavioral therapy)
  Psychological training programs, cognitive remediation according to needs
  Involvement of significant others (if patient agrees)
Transition to psychosis:
  Reduce Duration of Untreated Psychosis (DUP) and offer rapid specific treatment
  (see table 2)

---

worsening of the symptoms and transition to psychosis should be addressed, but not as the actual main issue. Initial studies examined different psychotherapeutic interventions, mainly cognitive behavioral therapy, and clarified that antipsychotic medications should not be offered as the first-line treatment. Currently, psychosocial treatments are the treatments of choice, especially cognitive behavioral therapy which might prevent transition to psychosis [30, 31] [see chapter by Müller and Bechdolf, this vol., pp. 142–158].

Treating patients without full-blown psychosis with antipsychotics is highly questionable. Newer studies have therefore explored alternative substances [see chapter by Conus, this vol., pp. 159–167]. Thus, other substances, especially omega-3 fatty acids as potential neuroprotective agents, were tested. In a preliminary study, they showed an astonishing improvement of symptoms and transition rates in young ARMS individuals [32]. A large multicenter replication study has recently been completed, data are now being analysed [33].

Based on the current state of knowledge, some recommendations for clinicians can be given. Most importantly, early interventions should be chosen according to the suspected stage of the disease respective to the degree of risk for psychosis and to the needs of the individual. This includes many unspecific supportive measures (table 3). Recently, the European Association of Psychiatry (EPA) has given evidence-based recommendations [34].

Problems to Be Solved

A lot has been achieved within a very short time [35]. Nevertheless, there are still many questions and problems to be solved.

Questions Regarding Early Detection

First of all, there are still some ethical problems to be resolved [36]. Unfortunately, there is hardly any data on the subjective experience of individuals being informed of having a potential risk status [37, 38] [see chapter by Uttinger et al., this vol., pp. 69–82]. Which effects on subjective well-being does this information have? Does it help to have an explanation for the changes being experienced or is it disturbing and leads to even more stigma and discrimination than the symptoms and impairments themselves? What about those individuals who do not transit to psychosis: can they nevertheless benefit from early intervention as their presenting symptoms and comorbidities are treated? Or do the negative consequences outweigh the benefits?

How should the diagnostic information be communicated to induce positive instead of negative consequences? How can we educate clinicians to diagnose the presenting symptoms, risk and comorbidities more exactly, to communicate results in a nontraumatic way and deliver care according to the needs and risk state of the patient? We already know quite a lot about this, but have not yet evaluated how to train clinicians and service planners.

In order to develop clearer guidelines on how to diagnose the different stages (risks), how to communicate results and to intervene accordingly, there is a clear need for more and better data. Researchers will have to further improve the accuracy of individual prediction – sensitivity as well as specificity. This is feasible by further evaluating stepwise enrichment strategies and diagnostic algorithms including different assessment domains such as neuropsychology, neurophysiology and neuroimaging in a stepwise approach. For generating more reliable data, larger sample sizes and longer follow-ups are urgently needed. Several new large multicenter studies are on their way (e.g. EU-GEI [39], NEURAPRO [33], PREVENT [40] or PRONIA, Personalized Prognostic Tools for Early Psychosis Management), but assessment methods still could be made more comparable among these large studies.

Statistical methods used so far should be reviewed more critically; for example, stricter independent external and internal validation studies should be performed [see chapter by Studerus et al., this vol., pp. 116–132]. Hopefully, multivariate prediction models for prediction in the clinic as well as algorithms for staging risk could be further improved for use in the clinic for individual patients.

More long-term data are needed on the many patients who do *not* convert to psychosis within the first years. There is only one study so far with a long-term follow-up of up to 14 years [41] which shows that these individuals are at significant risk of continued attenuated psychotic symptoms, persistent or recurrent disorders, and incident disorders. This finding has to be replicated in other settings and there is the question of how to predict long-term development of the symptoms and impairments.

Regarding those who convert to frank psychosis – what subgroups with potentially different etiologies and further courses can we define? What are the influencing factors and helpful interventions? To date, the focus has mainly been on positive symptoms. However, there is increasing evidence that negative symptoms and impaired cognitive and social functioning may be just as important for the outcome [42].

Last but not least, more research on the special features and needs of certain subgroups of patients is needed. Thus, children and young adolescents have to be diagnosed and treated especially carefully [see chapters by Simon, this vol., pp. 42–54, and Schultze-Lutter, this vol., pp. 29–41]. And finally, what about the specificities of both genders? So far, only very little is known about that particular topic [43, 44] [for review, see 45]. Women, especially the 20% with an onset after the age of 40 [46], are so far quite neglected in early detection and early intervention services and studies.

Questions Regarding Early Intervention

With regard to early intervention, it is important to note that the current preventative interventions regarding psychosis are already just as good as some established preventative interventions in internal medicine. For example, preventative cognitive behavioral therapies are associated with a 0.5 relative risk reduction and a number needed to treat of 14, which is similar to interventions for prediabetes and far superior to that of statins in cardiovascular high-risk subjects to prevent serious events (number needed to treat: 25) [47]. Incidentally, both of the latter interventions focus on asymptomatic patients in contrast to the subthreshold psychosis state where symptoms and impairment already exist and treatment of some kind is indicated. This means we can expect an additional clinical benefit of treating the presenting symptoms, the distress and impaired functioning independent of reducing the risk of transition to psychosis.

Nevertheless, better preventative intervention strategies should be developed. The ideal solution for this would be more extensive research for a better understanding of the pathogenetic mechanisms underlying the emergence of psychotic disorders, including the definition of different etiological subtypes, which would allow profiling and personalized or stratified medicine.

At the same time – based on the hypotheses we have so far – we should perform more well-controlled sequential or stepwise clinical trials with larger sample sizes assessing interventions specific for the different risk states/stages of the emerging disease [48]. For example, this includes testing of different substances including neuroprotective agents, but also of different psychotherapeutic approaches. Future trials should not only focus on transition to psychosis, but also on reduction of presenting symptoms, cognitive and functional impairments. Interventions should be developed regarding the reduction of pathogenic factors such as stress or cannabis [49, 50] as well as on enhancing resilience. For first-line treatment, simple, safe and benign interventions should be tested, and more complex treatments in those at high risk or those who fail to respond [48]. Also, the optimal duration of treatment is far from clear, including questions of tapering down treatments and optimal follow-up.

There also is an urgent need for research on service delivery, including implementation studies in various clinical settings and societal circumstances. How can we tailor our services to the specific needs of our clients – patients as well as relatives and professionals from different disciplines? How can we address potential stigma and discrimination? How can we deliver in a more sustained and comprehensive fashion?

It should always be kept in mind that services for early detection and intervention have several main goals, and service delivery should be evaluated regarding:

Early detection
- Early detection of frank psychosis
- Differential diagnosis regarding other mental disorders
- Exclusion of organic/exogenic causes
- Early reliable assessment of an ARMS with staging

Early intervention
- In first-episode psychosis according to guidelines
- In ARMS according to stage with the aim of treating the presenting symptoms and comorbidities (esp. drug/cannabis abuse), prevention/delay of transition to psychosis, and prevention of social decline

Last but not least, health economics is an important topic. How can we show that services for early detection and intervention are cost-effective for society as a whole, and how can we make sure that these services are not competing for money with services for the chronically mentally ill? That is, how can we convince politicians that extra money is needed, and that money will produce savings in many other areas such as welfare payments and the costs of incarceration? As psychiatrists we know that, in order to be convincing, one has to have good self-esteem. However, psychiatry and psychiatrists have – just as their patients – for a long time suffered from stigma, self-stigmatization and low self-esteem. Thus, the key to solving some problems might be to develop more self-esteem and confidence as psychiatrists – clinicians and researchers – based on what we have achieved and fight for our patients and the improvement of our services in a more self-confident manner. Looking at the developments outlined, we think we can be quite proud and confident about the future. We have introduced a modern predictive, preventative and personalized approach into psychiatry as is already common in general medicine. We have moved from a largely palliative approach in treating schizophrenia to an evidence-based, optimistic, recovery-oriented treatment of different stages of emerging psychotic disorders.

Some are still questioning the validity of the 'attenuated psychosis syndrome' [51] [see chapter by Rutigliano et al., this vol., pp. 55–68]. The DSM-5 working group therefore only integrated it into the appendix of the DSM-5 as a condition for further study. Nevertheless it still states, '…that secondary prevention of full psychosis may offer substantial life-course benefits. It seems likely that psychiatry will move in this direction with a number of disorders in the future' [51, p. 34]. In fact, we can see that this movement which started with psychosis is broadening into other fields and has the potential to revolutionize psychiatry.

References

1 Riecher-Rössler A, Aston J, Borgwardt S, Bugra H, Fuhr P, Gschwandtner U, Koutsouleris N, Pflueger M, Tamagni C, Radü EW, Rapp C, Smieskova R, Studerus E, Walter A, Zimmermann R: Vorhersage von Psychosen durch stufenweise Mehrebenenabklärung – Das Basel Fepsy-Projekt. [Prediction of Psychosis by Stepwise Multilevel Assessment – The Basel FePsy (Early Recognition of Psychosis)-Project]. Fortschr Neurol Psychiatr 2013;81:265–275.

2 Yung AR, Stanford C, Cosgrave E, Killackey E, Phillips L, Nelson B, McGorry PD: Testing the Ultra High Risk (prodromal) criteria for the prediction of psychosis in a clinical sample of young people. Schizophr Res 2006;84:57–66.

3 Riecher-Rössler A, Aston J, Ventura J, Merlo M, Borgwardt S, Gschwandtner U, Stieglitz RD: Das Basel Screening Instrument für Psychosen (BSIP): Entwicklung, Aufbau, Reliabilität und Validität. [The Basel Screening Instrument for Psychosis (BSIP): Development, Structure, Reliability and Validity]. Fortschr Neurol Psychiatr 2008;76:207–216.

4 Riecher-Rössler A, Pflueger MO, Aston J, Borgwardt SJ, Brewer WJ, Gschwandtner U, Stieglitz RD: Efficacy of using cognitive status in predicting psychosis: a 7-year follow-up. Biol Psychiatry 2009;66:1023–1030.

5 Haroun N, Dunn L, Haroun A, Cadenhead KS: Risk and protection in prodromal schizophrenia: ethical implications for clinical practice and future research. Schizophr Bull 2006;32:166–178.

6 Cannon TD, Cadenhead K, Cornblatt B, Woods SW, Addington J, Walker E, Seidman LJ, Perkins D, Tsuang M, McGlashan T, Heinssen R: Prediction of psychosis in youth at high clinical risk: a multisite longitudinal study in North America. Arch Gen Psychiatry 2008;65:28–37.

7 Mason O, Startup M, Halpin S, Schall U, Conrad A, Carr V: Risk factors for transition to first episode psychosis among individuals with 'at-risk mental states'. Schizophr Res 2004;71:227–237.

8 Bugra H, Rapp C, Studerus E, Aston J, Borgwardt S, Riecher-Rössler A: Kann Cannabis das Risiko für schizophrene Psychosen erhöhen? [Can Cannabis Use increase the risk for Schizophrenic Psychoses?]. Fortschr Neurol Psychiatr 2012;80:635–643.

9 Riecher-Rössler A, Gschwandtner U, Borgwardt S, Aston J, Pflüger M, Rössler W: Early detection and treatment of schizophrenia: how early? Acta Psychiatr Scand Suppl 2006;113:73–80.

10 McGorry P, Keshavan M, Goldstone S, Amminger P, Allott K, Berk M, Lavoie S, Pantelis C, Yung A, Wood S, Hickie I: Biomarkers and clinical staging in psychiatry. World Psychiatry 2014;13:211–223.

11 Fusar-Poli P, Deste G, Smieskova R, Barlati S, Yung AR, Howes O, Stieglitz RD, Vita A, McGuire P, Borgwardt S: Cognitive functioning in prodromal psychosis: a meta-analysis. Arch Gen Psychiatry 2012;69:562–571.

12 Gschwandtner U, Pflüger M, Aston J, Borgwardt S, Drewe M, Stieglitz RD, Riecher-Rössler A: Fine motor function and neuropsychological deficits in individuals at risk for schizophrenia. Eur Arch Psychiatry Clin Neurosci 2006;256:201–206.

13 Gschwandtner U, Pflüger MO, Semenin V, Gaggiotti M, Riecher-Rössler A, Fuhr P: EEG: a helpful tool in the prediction of psychosis. Eur Arch Psychiatry Clin Neurosci 2009;259:257–262.

14 Ramyead A, Kometer M, Studerus E, Koranyi S, Ittig S, Gschwandtner U, Fuhr P, Riecher-Rössler A: Aberrant current source-density and lagged phase synchronization of neural oscillations as markers for emerging psychosis. Schizophr Bull 2015;41:919–929.

15 Gschwandtner U, Zimmermann R, Pflüger MO, Riecher-Rössler A, Fuhr P: Negative symptoms in neuroleptic-naive patients with first-episode psychosis correlate with QEEG parameters. Schizophr Res 2009;115:231–236.

16 Borgwardt SJ, McGuire PK, Aston J, Berger G, Dazzan P, Gschwandtner U, Pflüger M, D'Souza M, Radü EW, Riecher-Rössler A: Structural brain abnormalities in individuals with an at-risk mental state who later develop psychosis. Br J Psychiatry Suppl 2007;51:s69–s75.

17 Mechelli A, Riecher-Rössler A, Meisenzahl EM, Tognin S, Wood SJ, Borgwardt SJ, Koutsouleris N, Yung AR, Stone JM, Phillips LJ, McGorry PD, Valli I, Velakoulis D, Woolley J, Pantelis C, McGuire P: Neuroanatomical abnormalities that predate the onset of psychosis: a multicenter study. Arch Gen Psychiatry 2011;68:489–495.

18 Borgwardt SJ, McGuire PK, Aston J, Gschwandtner U, Pflüger MO, Stieglitz RD, Radü EW, Riecher-Rössler A: Reductions in frontal, temporal and parietal volume associated with the onset of psychosis. Schizophr Res 2008;106:108–114.

19 Fusar-Poli P, Smieskova R, Serafini G, Politi P, Borgwardt S: Neuroanatomical markers of genetic liability to psychosis and first episode psychosis: a voxelwise meta-analytical comparison. World J Biol Psychiatry 2014;15:219–228.

20 Bois C, Whalley H, McIntosh A, Lawrie S: Structural magnetic resonance imaging markers of susceptibility and transition to schizophrenia: a review of familial and clinical high risk population studies. J Psychopharmacol 2015;29:144–154.

21 Howes OD, Montgomery AJ, Asselin MC, Murray RM, Valli I, Tabraham P, Bramon-Bosch E, Valmaggia L, Johns L, Broome M, McGuire PK, Grasby PM: Elevated striatal dopamine function linked to prodromal signs of schizophrenia. Arch Gen Psychiatry 2009;66:13–20.

22 Howes OD, Bose SK, Turkheimer F, Valli I, Egerton A, Valmaggia LR, Murray RM, McGuire P: Dopamine synthesis capacity before onset of psychosis: a prospective [18F]-DOPA PET imaging study. Am J Psychiatry 2011;168:1311–1317.

23 Fusar-Poli P, Borgwardt S, Bechdolf A, Addington J, Riecher-Rössler A, Schultze-Lutter F, Keshavan M, Wood S, Ruhrmann S, Seidman LJ, Valmaggia L, Cannon T, Velthorst E, De Haan L, Cornblatt B, Bonoldi I, Birchwood M, McGlashan T, Carpenter W, McGorry P, Klosterkötter J, McGuire P, Yung A: The psychosis high-risk state: a comprehensive state-of-the-art review. JAMA Psychiatry 2013;70:107–120.

24 Koutsouleris N, Borgwardt S, Meisenzahl EM, Bottlender R, Möller HJ, Riecher-Rössler A: Disease prediction in the at-risk mental state for psychosis using neuroanatomical biomarkers: results from the FePsy Study. Schizophr Bull 2011;38:1234–1246.

25 Aston J, Rechsteiner E, Bull N, Borgwardt S, Gschwandtner U, Riecher-Rössler A: Hyperprolactinaemia in early psychosis-not only due to antipsychotics. Prog Neuropsychopharmacol Biol Psychiatry 2010;34:1342–1344.

26 Riecher-Rössler A, Rybakowski JK, Pflueger MO, Beyrau R, Kahn RS, Malik P, Fleischhacker WW: Hyperprolactinemia in antipsychotic-naive patients with first-episode psychosis. Psychol Med 2013;43:2571–2582.

27 Büschlen J, Berger GE, Borgwardt SJ, Aston J, Gschwandtner U, Pflüger MO, Kuster P, Radü EW, Stieglitz RD, Riecher-Rössler A: Pituitary volume increase during emerging psychosis. Schizophr Res 2011;125:41–48.

28 Schultze-Lutter F, Michel C, Schmidt SJ, Schimmelmann BG, Maric NP, Salokangas RK, Riecher-Rössler A, van der Gaag M, Nordentoft M, Raballo A, Meneghelli A, Marshall M, Morrison A, Ruhrmann S, Klosterkötter J: EPA guidance on the early detection of clinical high risk states of psychoses. Eur Psychiatry 2015;30:405–416.

29 Nordentoft M, Jeppesen P, Petersen L, Bertelsen M, Thorup A: The rationale for early intervention in schizophrenia and related disorders. Early Interv Psychiatry 2009;3(suppl 1):S3–S7.

30 Stafford MR, Jackson H, Mayo-Wilson E, Morrison AP, Kendall T: Early interventions to prevent psychosis: systematic review and meta-analysis. BMJ 2013;346:185–198.

31 van der Gaag M, Smit F, Bechdolf A, French P, Linszen DH, Yung AR, McGorry P, Cuijpers P: Preventing a first episode of psychosis: meta-analysis of randomized controlled prevention trials of 12 month and longer-term follow-ups. Schizophr Res 2013;149:56–62.

32 Amminger GP, McGorry PD: Update on omega-3 polyunsaturated fatty acids in early-stage psychotic disorders. Neuropsychopharmacol 2012;37:309–310.

33 Markulev C, McGorry PD, Nelson B, Yuen HP, Schaefer M, Yung AR, et al: The NEURAPRO-E study protocol: A multicentre RCT of omega-3 fatty acids and cognitive-behavioural case management for patients at ultra high risk of schizophrenia and other psychotic disorders. Early Interv Psychiatry 2015, Epub ahead of print. DOI: 10.1111/eip.12260.

34 Schmidt SJ, Schultze-Lutter F, Schimmelmann BG, Maric NP, Salokangas RK, Riecher-Rössler A, van der Gaag M, Meneghelli A, Nordentoft M, Marshall M, Morrison A, Raballo A, Klosterkötter J, Ruhrmann S: EPA guidance on the early intervention in clinical high risk states of psychoses. Eur Psychiatry 2015;30:388–404.

35 Schvarcz A, Bearden CE: Early detection of psychosis: recent updates from clinical high-risk research. Curr Behav Neurosc Rep 2015;2:90–101.

36 Mittal VA, Dean DJ, Mittal J, Saks ER: Ethical, legal, and clinical considerations when disclosing a high-risk syndrome for psychosis. Bioethics 2015;29:543–556.

37 Welsh P, Tiffin PA: Observations of a small sample of adolescents experiencing an at-risk mental state (ARMS) for psychosis. Schizophr Bull 2012;38:215–218.

38 Milton AC, Mullan BA: Diagnosis telling in people with psychosis. Curr Opin Psychiatry 2014;27:302–307.

39 European Network of National Networks Studying Gene-Environment Interactions in Schizophrenia (EU-GEI), van Os J, Rutten BP, Myin-Germeys I, et al: Identifying gene-environment interactions in schizophrenia: contemporary challenges for integrated, large-scale investigations. Schizophr Bull 2014;40:729–736.

40 Bechdolf A, Müller H, Stutzer H, Wagner M, Maier W, Lautenschlager M, Heinz A, de Millas W, Janssen B, Gaebel W, Michel TM, Schneider F, Lambert M, Naber D, Brune M, Kruger-Ozgurdal S, Wobrock T, Riedel M, Klosterkötter J; PREVENT Study Group: Rationale and baseline characteristics of PREVENT: a second-generation intervention trial in subjects at-risk (prodromal) of developing first-episode psychosis evaluating cognitive behavior therapy, aripiprazole, and placebo for the prevention of psychosis. Schizophr Bull 2011;37(suppl 2):S111–S121.

41 Lin A, Wood SJ, Nelson B, Beavan A, McGorry P, Yung AR: Outcomes of nontransitioned cases in a sample at ultra-high risk for psychosis. Am J Psychiatry 2015;172:249–258.

42 Yung AR, Nelson B: The ultra-high risk concept – a review. Can J Psychiatry 2013;58:5–12.

43 González-Rodríguez A, Studerus E, Spitz A, Bugra H, Aston J, Borgwardt S, Rapp C, Riecher-Rössler A: Gender differences in the psychopathology of emerging psychosis. Isr J Psychiatry Relat Sci 2014; 51:85–93.

44 Ittig S, Studerus E, Papmeyer M, Uttinger M, Koranyi S, Ramyead A, Riecher-Rössler A: Sex differences in cognitive functioning in at-risk mental state for psychosis, first episode psychosis and healthy control subjects. Eur Psychiatry 2015;30:242–250.

45 Barajas A, Ochoa S, Obiols JE, Lalucat-Jo L: Gender differences in individuals at high-risk of psychosis: a comprehensive literature review. ScientificWorldJournal 2015;2015:430735.

46 Riecher-Rössler A: 50 Jahre nach Manfred Bleuler. Was wissen wir heute über die Spätschizophrenie(n)? [50 years after Manfred Bleuler. What do we know today about late-onset schizophrenia(s)?]. Nervenarzt 1997;68:159–170.

47 Fusar-Poli P, Carpenter W, Woods SW, McGlashan TH: Attenuated Psychosis Syndrome: Ready for DSM-5.1? Ann Rev Clin Psychiatry 2014;10:155–192.

48 McGorry P, Johannessen JO, Lewis S, Birchwood M, Malla A, Nordentoft M, Addington J, Yung A: Early intervention in psychosis: keeping faith with evidence-based health care. Psychol Med 2010;40:399–404.

49 Addington J, Case N, Saleem MM, Auther AM, Cornblatt BA, Cadenhead KS: Substance use in clinical high risk for psychosis: a review of the literature. Early Interv Psychiatry 2014;8:104–112.

50 Rapp C, Walter A, Studerus E, Bugra H, Tamagni C, Röthlisberger M, Borgwardt S, Aston J, Riecher-Rössler A: Cannabis use and brain structural alterations of the cingulate cortex in early psychosis. Psychiatry Res 2013;214:102–108.

51 Tsuang MT, Van Os J, Tandon R, Barch DM, Bustillo J, Gaebel W, Gur RE, Heckers S, Malaspina D, Owen MJ, Schultz S, Carpenter W: Attenuated psychosis syndrome in DSM-5. Schizophr Res 2013;150:31–35.

Prof. Anita Riecher-Rössler
Center for Gender Research and Early Detection, University of Basel Psychiatric Clinics
Kornhausgasse 7
CH–4051 Basel (Switzerland)
E-Mail Anita.Riecher@upkbs.ch

Author Index

Subject Index

Depersonalization, adolescent psychosis
   high-risk state 47, 48
Dopamine hypothesis, antipsychotic
   mechanism of action 169
DUP, *see* Duration of untreated psychosis
Duration of untreated psychosis (DUP) 56–58
Dysbindin, variants in psychosis 2

Early Detection and Intervention Evaluation
   (EDIE) 149
Economic impact, psychosis 2, 142
EDIE, *see* Early Detection and Intervention
   Evaluation
EEG, *see* Electroencephalography
E-EPA, *see* Ethyl-eicosapentaenoic acid
Eicosapentaenoic acid, *see*
   Ethyl-eicosapentaenoic acid
Electroencephalography (EEG), psychosis
   high-risk state prediction
   mismatch negativity 137, 138
   overview 12, 133, 134, 180
   P300 135–137
   prospects 138, 139
   quantitative parameters 134, 135
EPOS, *see* European Prediction of Psychosis
   Study
ERIraos 60
Ethyl-eicosapentaenoic acid (E-EPA), early
   intervention in ultra-high risk patients 161,
   162
EUFEST, *see* European First-Episode
   Schizophrenia Trial
European First-Episode Schizophrenia Trial
   (EUFEST) 170, 172, 173
European Prediction of Psychosis Study
   (EPOS) 10, 11, 134

Family-focused therapy (FFT), early
   intervention 150
FEP, *see* First-episode psychosis
FETZ 125
FFT, *see* Family-focused therapy
First-episode psychosis (FEP)
   basic symptoms, *see* Basic symptoms
   early detection of risk 2–4
   early interventions 182
   health service approaches to maximize
      recovery 22, 23
   interventions 19
   pharmacological interventions
      adherence 173, 174

antipsychotic mechanism of action 169
controversies 175, 176
duration of treatment 174, 175
effectiveness 170, 171
side effects and management 171–173
treatment guidelines and dosing 169,
   170
recovery and critical period 19–21
stigma in early detection, *see* Stigmatization
treatment resistance identification 21, 22
Functional magnetic resonance imaging, *see*
   Magnetic resonance imaging

GAF, *see* General Assessment of Functioning
General Assessment of Functioning
   (GAF) 124
Genetic risk and deterioration syndrome
   (GRD) 59
German Research Network Schizophrenia
   (GRNS) 34, 35
Glutathione, levels in ultra-high risk
   patients 164, 165
GRD, *see* Genetic risk and deterioration
   syndrome
GRNS, *see* German Research Network
   Schizophrenia

Hallucinations, adolescent psychosis high-risk
   state 45, 46
High-risk state, *see* Psychosis high-risk state
HRS, *see* Psychosis high-risk state
Hypochondriasis, adolescent psychosis
   high-risk state 46, 47

Intelligence quotient, *see* Cognitive function,
   psychosis prediction

Magnetic resonance imaging (MRI)
   pattern recognition, *see* Multivariate pattern
      analysis
   predictive marker rationale 83, 84
   psychosis high-risk state
      fMRI
         connectivity analysis 88, 89
         task-based studies 87, 88
      structural MRI
         manual tracing of images 84
         predictive value 85–87
         prospects 89
         whole-brain analysis 85
   research consortia 89

Metabolic syndrome, antipsychotic drug
   association 22
N-Methyl-D-aspartate receptor (NMDAR),
   agonists for early intervention in ultra-high
   risk patients 163, 164
Mismatch negativity, *see*
   Electroencephalography
Motor function, psychosis prediction
   added predictive value 123–125
   at-risk mental state patients transitioning to
      psychosis versus not transitioning 119–
      123
   limitations 126–128
   overview 116–118
   prospects 128
MRI, *see* Magnetic resonance imaging
Multivariate pattern analysis (MVPA)
   connectivity abnormalities
      fractional anisotropy studies 104–106
      functional connectivity abnormalities
         diffusion tensor imaging 104, 110,
            111
         prospects for study 109–112
         resting state studies 106, 107
         task-induced studies 107–109
      imaging techniques 104
   overview 95–97
   psychosis early recognition
      challenges 100, 101
      magnetic resonance imaging 99, 100
   techniques
      machine learning 97, 98
      prediction rule visualization 99
      support vector machine 98–100
      validation of predictive models 98, 99
MVPA, *see* Multivariate pattern analysis

NAC, *see* N-Acetyl cysteine
NAPLS, *see* North American Prodrome
   Longitudinal Study
Neuregulin-1, variants in psychosis 2
NICE guidelines 169, 170, 182
NMDAR, *see* N-Methyl-D-aspartate receptor
North American Prodrome Longitudinal Study
   (NAPLS) 124

Obesity, antipsychotic drug association 22
Obsessive-compulsive symptoms (OCS),
   adolescent psychosis high-risk state 48
Obsessive ideas, adolescent psychosis high-risk
   state 48, 49

OCS, *see* Obsessive-compulsive symptoms
Omega-3 fatty acids, early intervention in
   ultra-high risk patients 161, 162
OPTiMiSE trial 171

P300, *see* Electroencephalography
PACE, *see* Personal Assessment and Crisis
   Evaluation
PANNS, *see* Positive and Negative Syndrome
   Scale
Pattern recognition, *see* Multivariate pattern
   analysis
Personal Assessment and Crisis Evaluation
   (PACE) 58, 124
PET, *see* Positron emission tomography
Polyunsaturated fatty acids (PUFAs), early
   intervention in ultra-high risk
   patients 161–163
PORT guidelines 170
Positive and Negative Syndrome Scale
   (PANNS) 30
Positron emission tomography (PET),
   psychosis prediction 181
PQ, *see* Prodromal screening questionnaire
Prevalence, psychosis lifetime prevalence 1, 2
PREVENT study 12, 184
Prodromal screening questionnaire (PQ) 60
PRONIA 184
Psychosis high-risk state (HRS)
   adolescents
      autism spectrum disorders 49, 50
      body perceptions 46
      Bruderholtz Early Psychosis Outpatient
         Service for Adolescents and Adults
         study 44, 45
      cenesthopathy 46
      delusional ideas 48, 49
      depersonalization 47, 48
      hallucinations, isolated 45, 46
      hypochondriasis 46, 47
      obsessive-compulsive symptoms 48
      obsessive ideas 48, 49
      overview 42, 43
   clinical relevance 56–58
   duration of untreated psychosis 56–58
   electroencephalography, *see*
      Electroencephalography
   interventions 61–63
   magnetic resonance imaging findings, *see*
      Magnetic resonance imaging
   patient characteristics 143, 144